Urticaria and Angioedema

Torsten Zuberbier • Clive Grattan
Marcus Maurer
Editors

Urticaria and Angioedema

Second Edition

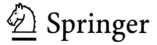

Editors
Torsten Zuberbier
Institute for Allergology
Charité – Universitätsmedizin
Berlin
Germany

Clive Grattan
St John's Institute of Dermatology
Guy's Hospital
London
UK

Marcus Maurer
Fraunhofer Institute for Translational
Medicine and Pharmacology ITMP
Allergology and Immunology
Berlin
Germany

ISBN 978-3-030-84576-6   ISBN 978-3-030-84574-2   (eBook)
https://doi.org/10.1007/978-3-030-84574-2

© Springer Nature Switzerland AG 2010, 2021
This work is subject to copyright. All rights are reserved by the Publisher, whether the whole or part of the material is concerned, specifically the rights of translation, reprinting, reuse of illustrations, recitation, broadcasting, reproduction on microfilms or in any other physical way, and transmission or information storage and retrieval, electronic adaptation, computer software, or by similar or dissimilar methodology now known or hereafter developed.
The use of general descriptive names, registered names, trademarks, service marks, etc. in this publication does not imply, even in the absence of a specific statement, that such names are exempt from the relevant protective laws and regulations and therefore free for general use.
The publisher, the authors, and the editors are safe to assume that the advice and information in this book are believed to be true and accurate at the date of publication. Neither the publisher nor the authors or the editors give a warranty, expressed or implied, with respect to the material contained herein or for any errors or omissions that may have been made. The publisher remains neutral with regard to jurisdictional claims in published maps and institutional affiliations.

This Springer imprint is published by the registered company Springer Nature Switzerland AG
The registered company address is: Gewerbestrasse 11, 6330 Cham, Switzerland

Preface to the First Edition

Urticaria is one of the most common diseases in dermatology and allergy. Unlike many other diseases, the fleeting nature of the wheals makes first diagnosis by both patients and physicians in many cases easy. However, this only refers to the ordinary wheals. The disease itself is highly complex in nature, with a variety of clinical manifestations ranging from pinpoint-sized wheals to extensive angioedema. Complexity is also seen in the diversity of possible eliciting factors, the many different clinical subtypes, and the therapeutic responsiveness. Only in recent years has a better understanding of the diversity in the different subtypes led to new classifications and new evidence-based guidelines for diagnostics and management of the disease. While mast cells are in the center of most urticaria reactions, it is now clearly understood that the responsible mediators are not only limited to histamines. This book appears in a series of books by Springer. In 1986, the first monograph was edited by Professor Henz née Chanewsky. Since then, two updates of the book have appeared in the German language with Professor Henz as the first editor and Torsten Zuberbier, J. Grabbe, and E. Monroe as the co-editors of the most recent English version, published in 1998. All these books have been written as a joint effort of Professor Henz together with her team at the Department of Dermatology at the Virchow Clinic, Humboldt University, Berlin. With the retirement of Professor Henz from her chair as head of the Department of Dermatology and novel guidelines available, the current group of editors has taken up the task of developing a completely new setup for the book. A group of internationally known authors in the field of urticaria have been asked to write different chapters, focusing on practical guidelines regarding diagnosis and therapy. This book is designed to be a useful reference for dermatologists, allergologists, pediatricians, and practitioners in general medicine, laying out clear-cut standard operating procedures on how to manage this disease efficiently.

Berlin, Germany	Torsten Zuberbier
Norwich, UK	Clive Grattan
Berlin, Germany	Marcus Maurer

Preface

In the 1998 edition, it was stated that urticaria is one of the most common dermatological and allergological cutaneous conditions and, compared to other dermatoses, it is usually recognized easily by patients and physicians alike. Nevertheless, urticaria is highly complex regarding its eliciting causes, its clinical manifestations, and therapy.

All of this remains true 23 years later. Urticaria continues to be a highly complex disease and is heavily researched. We still do not understand the underlying pathomechanisms and eliciting factors as much as we would like to, but unlike in the 1990s, when few people were interested in this disease, we are now in the good position that urticaria has come into the focus of many clinicians, researchers, and the pharmaceutical industry. We are also in the good position that we have global guidelines, and many advances have been made in the management of chronic urticaria. Today, we have reliable tools to measure patient-related outcomes to better monitor disease activity, and impact and treatment options have improved considerably. We now have a licensed biological, omalizumab, available for the treatment of chronic spontaneous urticaria, and many new trials are ongoing for further treatment options. When in the 1980s, a famous New York dermatologist stated that he would rather have a lion than a patient with chronic urticaria walk into his office; this is surely no longer any physician's wish.

Urticaria by definition is a disease characterized by the sudden appearance of wheals, angioedema, or both, and the unpredictable occurrence of symptoms is a factor, which has a high impact on the quality of life of our patients. The best support for them is a knowledgeable physician.

This book summarizes in a comprehensive and easy-to-follow approach the current knowledge on urticaria as well as tips and tricks for better treating our patients.

Berlin, Germany	Torsten Zuberbier
Norwich, UK	Clive Grattan
Berlin, Germany	Marcus Maurer

Contents

1. **History of Urticaria** 1
   M. Greaves and Torsten Zuberbier

2. **Aetiopathogenesis of Urticaria** 9
   Clive Grattan and Martin K. Church

3. **Classification and Diagnosis of Urticaria** 25
   Torsten Zuberbier

4. **Impact of Chronic Urticaria and How to Measure It** 39
   Karsten Weller

5. **Acute Urticaria** 57
   Torsten Zuberbier and Zuotao Zhao

6. **Chronic Spontaneous Urticaria** 65
   Dorothea Terhorst-Molawi and Marcus Maurer

7. **Chronic Spontaneous Urticaria and Comorbidities** 77
   Pavel Kolkhir and Marcus Maurer

8. **Inducible Urticarias** 109
   Sabine Altrichter, Markus Magerl, and Martin Metz

9. **Angioedema** 133
   L. Bouillet

10. **Management Principles in Urticaria** 149
    Torsten Zuberbier, Marcus Maurer, and Clive Grattan

11. **Antihistamines** 153
    Martin K. Church

12. **Omalizumab in the Treatment of Urticaria** 167
    Torsten Zuberbier, Tamara Dörr, Clive Grattan,
    and Marcus Maurer

13	**Other Interventions for Chronic Urticaria**............................ 177
	Clive Grattan, Torsten Zuberbier, and Marcus Maurer
14	**Urticaria in Pediatrics and During Pregnancy and Lactation: Highlights on Epidemiology, Diagnosis, and Management**.......... 207
	Moshe Ben-Shoshan and Petra Staubach
15	**Urticaria Therapy and Management. Looking Forward**........... 227
	Emek Kocatürk, Zuotao Zhao, and Ana M. Giménez-Arnau

Index 247

Contributors

Sabine Altrichter Institute for Allergology, Charité – Universitätsmedizin, Berlin, Germany

Department of Dermatology and Venerology, Kepler University Hospital, Linz, Austria

Moshe Ben-Shoshan Division of Allergy Immunology and Dermatology, Montreal Children's Hospital, Montreal, QC, Canada

L. Bouillet French National Reference Center for Angioedema (CREAK), Internal Medicine/Clinical Immunology Department, Grenoble University Hospital, Grenoble, France

Martin K. Church Institute for Allergology, Charité – Universitätsmedizin, Berlin, Germany

Tamara Dörr Institute for Allergology, Charité – Universitätsmedizin, Berlin, Germany

Ana M. Giménez-Arnau Department of Dermatology, Hospital del Mar, IMIM, Universitat Autònoma, Barcelona, Spain

Clive Grattan St John's Institute of Dermatology, Guy's Hospital, London, UK

M. Greaves Cutaneous Allergy Clinic, St. Johns Institute of Dermatology, St. Thomas Hospital, London, UK

Emek Kocatürk Department of Dermatology, Koç University School of Medicine, Istanbul, Turkey

Pavel Kolkhir Institute for Allergology, Charité – Universitätsmedizin, Berlin, Germany

Fraunhofer Institute for Translational Medicine and Pharmacology ITMP, Allergology and Immunology, Berlin, Germany

Division of Immune-mediated Skin Diseases, I.M. Sechenov First Moscow State Medical University (Sechenov University), Moscow, Russian Federation

Markus Magerl Institute for Allergology, Charité – Universitätsmedizin, Berlin, Germany

Marcus Maurer Institute for Allergology, Charité – Universitätsmedizin, Berlin, Germany

Fraunhofer Institute for Translational Medicine and Pharmacology ITMP, Allergology and Immunology, Berlin, Germany

Martin Metz Institute for Allergology, Charité – Universitätsmedizin, Berlin, Germany

Petra Staubach Department of Dermatology, University Medical Center, Mainz, Germany

Dorothea Terhorst-Molawi Institute for Allergology, Charité – Universitätsmedizin, Berlin, Germany

Fraunhofer Institute for Translational Medicine and Pharmacology ITMP, Allergology and Immunology, Berlin, Germany

Karsten Weller Institute for Allergology, Charité – Universitätsmedizin, Berlin, Germany

Zuotao Zhao Department of Dermatology and Venereology, Peking University First Hospital, Beijing, China

Torsten Zuberbier Institute for Allergology, Charité – Universitätsmedizin, Berlin, Germany

Fraunhofer Institute for Translational Medicine and Pharmacology ITMP, Allergology and Immunology, Berlin, Germany

History of Urticaria

M. Greaves and Torsten Zuberbier

Core Messages
- The beginning of the twentieth century ushered in the era of molecular medicine, eventually leading to unravelling of the molecular and immunological basis of urticaria.
- The mast cell and its histamine content remain central to the pathophysiology of the pruritic wheal in most forms of urticaria, and the synthesis, storage, regulation of release of histamine as well as molecular characterisation of its receptors, are becoming well understood.
- The challenge of the past 50 years has been to understand the causation of the promiscuous activation of dermal and mucosal mast cells in urticaria forming both wheals in a highly diverse clinical appearance as well as angioedema.
- The discovery in the 1980s of autoreactivity in the serum of some patients with chronic urticaria (the autologous serum skin test) was a major step forward and prompted attempts to identify and characterise this activity.
- The subsequent finding in chronic urticaria of specific complement-dependent autoantibodies, which release histamine and other mediators from mast cells and basophils via dimerisation of their high affinity IgE receptors, has stimulated intense interest in the multifactorial modes of activation of mast cells and basophils in this disorder.
- Antihistamines, discovered in the 1940s, remain the cornerstone of treatment of most types of urticaria. Although recent derivative ("second-generation") com-

M. Greaves
Cutaneous Allergy Clinic, St. Johns Institute of Dermatology, St. Thomas Hospital,
London, UK
e-mail: malcolmgreaves@clinidermsolutions.co.uk

T. Zuberbier (✉)
Institute for Allergology, Charité – Universitätsmedizin, Berlin, Germany

Fraunhofer Institute for Translational Medicine and Pharmacology ITMP,
Allergology and Immunology, Berlin, Germany
e-mail: Torsten.Zuberbier@charite.de

© Springer Nature Switzerland AG 2021
T. Zuberbier et al. (eds.), *Urticaria and Angioedema*,
https://doi.org/10.1007/978-3-030-84574-2_1

pounds manifest greatly refined properties, they are often only moderately effective and need updosing.
- Licensing of omalizumab as the first biological for CSU, now nearly worldwide, has been a major breakthrough, giving hope for antihistamine refractory patients. New therapeutic approaches "round the corner" are already in clinical trials and are discussed in this book.

1.1 Introduction

The history of urticaria divides itself conveniently into the early, clinically descriptive, and later pathophysiological eras. Much has been written on the early history of urticaria as a clinical entity, from Hippocrates in the fourth century BC to Heberden and Willan at the end of the eighteenth century AD. For useful accounts of urticaria in early Western writings, the reader is referred to publications by Czarnetzki [1] and Humphreys [2] and the ESHDV Special Annual Lecture entitled "The History of Urticaria and Angioedema" delivered by the late Lennart Juhlin in 2000, a transcript of which is available online. However, in the last hundred years, a dramatic increase in the understanding of the cellular and molecular basis of some common forms of urticaria took place, the foundations for which were laid down by pioneers in the latter years of the nineteenth century and in the early and later twentieth century. This period is the focus of the present account, which attempts to reveal to the reader a historical perspective on "how we got to where we are" today in urticaria.

1.2 The Cellular and Molecular Basis of Urticaria: First Steps

Although the mast cell ("mastzellen") was discovered by Paul Ehrlich in 1877 [3], it is the principal source and repository of tissue histamine (including the skin) was not appreciated until the seminal work of Riley and West was published in a series of papers in the 1950s. The correlation between histamine levels and mast cell content of skin of several species is well described in several publications summarised by Riley [4]. Histamine was discovered in 1906 by Dale in extracts of ergot [5] and he described all the important actions of histamine except for stimulation of gastric acid secretion. Dale also established the famous "Dale criteria", which should be fulfilled by a mediator deemed to be responsible for a given inflammatory response. Indeed, these criteria are only completely satisfied by histamine in the pruritic wheals of urticaria—hence we have previously designated histamine as the "quintessential mediator" [6].

It was Lewis who first delineated the potency of histamine as a mediator of whealing in human skin [7]. Lewis showed that, in low dosage, histamine could produce central whealing (vasopermeability) redness (vasodilation) and a surrounding bright red axon reflex flare (Lewis's triple response) characteristic of the urticarial wheal. Curiously, in all his intensive studies of actions of histamine in skin, he never once mentions itching! We now know that, in addition to itching (and pain), intracutaneous injection of histamine can also cause alloknesis (perception of itching in response to local nonpruritic stimuli such as fine touch or even temperature change) [8]. These vascular effects are receptor-mediated and involve two subclasses of histamine receptors, H1 and H2, both of which were cloned and sequenced in the early 1990s [9, 10]. Histamine-induced itching is served by H1 receptors. First evidence of the effectiveness of H1 antagonists in the treatment of urticaria emerged in the late 1940s [11, 12]. Recently described and characterised H4 receptors and their antagonists [13] are currently under scrutiny regarding possible relevance to urticaria and its management. That histamine released in lesional skin of chronic urticaria has been demonstrated repeatedly in skin tissue fluid, and more recently by skin microdialysis technology [14, 15]. However, histamine, although playing a significant role, is clearly not the only mediator, especially in chronic urticaria and this supposition is supported by kinetic studies [16].

1.3 The Enigma of Chronic "Idiopathic" Urticaria

The problem of how, in urticaria, the dermal mast cell is prompted to relieve itself of its burden of histamine and other mediators have puzzled investigators in the post Second World War era. The discovery and characterisation of the "reaginic" IgE immunoglobulin by Ishizaka [17] enabled elucidation of the relatively uncomplicated acute allergic urticaria, which could be explained by a straightforward immediate Gell and Coombs type I reaction [18] between dermal mast cell-bound IgE and specific allergen, leading to release of histamine and other mast cell-derived mediators. However, the aetiology and pathogenesis of chronic "idiopathic" urticaria (CIU) remained obscure. Even in the twenty-first century there remain numerous unanswered questions. Why do the dermal mast cells degranulate explosively in a seemingly random way with no evident triggering factor?

In the 1960s and 1970s, attempts were made, mainly in Europe, to popularise the role of common food additives, colouring agents, and preservatives such as tartrazine, sodium benzoate, and antioxidants as aetiological agents in CIU. Protagonists of this theory included Juhlin, Doeglas, and Warner [19–21]. Complex exclusion diets were devised and successes were claimed. Some of these regimes did include challenge tests, but were not adequately controlled and the reproducibility of apparent positive reactions was not investigated. Latterly, this approach has been revived and refined, food additives now being described as "pseudoallergens" [22], further successes being claimed following use of pseudoallergen-free diets in CIU, but this issue, which was reviewed in more detail recently [23], remains controversial.

Foci of infections are always liable to be invoked to explain otherwise inexplicable relapses in any chronic diseases, and chronic urticaria is no exception. The literature contains numerous usually anecdotal accounts of patients with severe chronic and recalcitrant urticaria who made a dramatic recovery following removal of an infected gallbladder/tooth, or treatment of an infected sinus or urinary tract. The 1980s saw the emergence of a new putative microbial culprit—Helicobacter pylori. Because of its ubiquity, especially in European populations, it was frequently found in patients with CIU. When patients with Helicobacter were treated, some got better both from the infection and from the urticaria. Although carefully controlled studies have not substantiated an aetiological relationship between H. pylori and urticaria despite its frequency in these patients [24], a more indirect role in the pathogenesis has been proposed [25].

The notion that antibodies may be causative in CIU is an old one. As long ago as 1962, Rorsman, a Swedish dermatologist, reported the striking basopenia in chronic urticaria and remarked on its absence in physical urticarias. He also pointed out that "In cases where the basopenia is marked it appears probable that antigen–antibody reactions … bring about degranulation of basophil leukocytes" [26]. Over 20 years later [27], we noted the impaired histamine release evoked by anti-IgE in basophils from patients with CIU. In 1988, Gruber et al. found that more than 50% of patients with cold urticaria, CIU and urticarial vasculitis had IgG autoantibodies directed against IgE [28]. There was also indirect evidence arising from the strong association between autoimmune thyroid disease and CIU [29]. The HLA class 11 DRB1*04 alleles were increased in frequency in CIU, consistent with a possible role for autoimmunity in CIU [30]. However, at this juncture there was no convincing evidence that any autoantibodies found in CIU were anything more than passive bystanders in the pathogenesis of this disorder.

Against this background, an important observation was made in 1986 by Grattan [31]. He demonstrated that the serum of some but not all patients with CIU would cause whealing when reinjected intracutaneously in an autologous fashion into the same patient's clinically uninvolved skin. This finding greatly encouraged attempts to identify circulating vasoactive factors in the blood of CIU patients [32, 33]. As had previously been suspected by earlier writers [26, 28], the culprit turned out to be a functional, histamine-releasing autoantibody—at least in some patients. Hide et al. in 1993 and subsequently Fiebiger et al. and Tong et al. found that in 30–50% of patients with CIU, a circulating histamine-releasing factor with the characteristics of an IgG anti-FcεR1 autoantibody was demonstrable in serum [34–37]. Indirect evidence as well as successful passive transfer [38] supported the view that these autoantibodies are the cause of the whealing in those patients that have them. Although "autoimmune urticaria" has yet to justify, in a strict sense, its designation as an autoimmune disease (there is no animal model), these advances have for the first time put the investigation and treatment of chronic urticaria on a sound scientific basis. Lack of a convenient specific and sensitive screening test for autoimmune urticaria remains the main drawback to further progress.

However in the recent years also new discoveries identifying autologous proteins as targets of autoimmune responses were made such as IgE antibodies against IL-24 [39].

1.4 Treatment of Urticaria: Antihistamines

Fortunately, most patients with chronic urticaria, whatever the cause, can be effectively managed by H1 antihistamines. These were first characterised by Bovet and Staub [40], a discovery which was, in part, responsible for conferment of the Nobel Prize on Bovet in 1957. Their use in treatment of chronic urticaria was explored intensively after the end of World War II [11, 12]. O'Leary and Farber, referring in 1947 to diphenhydramine [11] stated that it is effective in chronic urticaria and also pointed out that it "is not a potent antipruritic drug"—a view that present-day clinicians will echo in respect of its present-day successors. These early "first-generation" antihistamines, though carrying a baggage of annoying rather than serious side effects, are still very much in use today by urticaria sufferers. Although initially believed to be competitive antagonists of histamine at the H1 receptor, all currently available H1 antihistamines are now considered to behave as inverse agonists—that is, they downregulate and stabilise the constitutively activated state of the H1 receptor [41]. H2 histamine receptors are also expressed by human skin blood vessels [42] and the possibility was entertained that combination of H2 receptor antagonists (e.g. cimetidine) with first-generation H1 antihistamines would have a "sparing" effect on the latter, thus mitigating the unwanted effects of H1 antihistamines. Although some benefits were established for use of this combination [43], they were small and in any case their use was largely superseded by the advent of second-generation antihistamines.

Second-generation H1 antihistamines, as defined by Simons [44], are essentially H1 antihistamines with low or non-sedating properties at therapeutic dosages. Many of these are active metabolites or enantiomers of first-generation compounds. Their usage over the past 15 years in chronic urticaria, especially as daytime treatment, has greatly improved the quality of life of otherwise severely handicapped sufferers [45–48]. However, they are less effective in relieving whealing than itching in urticaria and sedative first-generation antihistamines still have a place in the management of nocturnal pruritus in urticaria sufferers. Combination of montelukast, a leucotriene inhibitor, with an H1 antihistamine has been advocated in the past, but results have been variable, new studies are missing [49] and they are no longer recommended in the treatment algorithm. The cloning and sequencing of the H1 receptor in 1991 [9, 50] have laid the foundation for emergence of a truly new "third generation" of antihistamines for clinicians and patients alike to look forward to.

Future developments in the diagnosis and management of urticaria have also been greatly encouraged by the recent establishment of European Guidelines for urticaria now published in the fifth update with the collaboration of more than 40 international societies becoming a truly global guideline [51]. These should also give much needed help to clinicians faced with investigation and treatment of urticaria.

Take Home Pearls

- The autologous serum skin test established that in patients with chronic "idiopathic" urticaria, the causation was endogenous rather than due to external factors such as food allergy or pseudoallergy, and "focal infection".
- In some patients, this endogenous activity turned out to be attributable to specific autoantibodies (autoimmune urticaria), which promiscuously activate dermal mast cells and basophils and this has led to advent of immunotherapy (e.g. cyclosporine) in selected patients.
- The "cause" of chronic urticaria is, however, multifactorial and other factors such as dysregulation of intracellular signal transduction in dermal mast cells and basophils are likely to be important in other patients.
- With the current algorithm of using modern H1 antihistamines, updosing these and in the third step adding omalizumab, a big step forward has been taken in the last two decades but still some patients remain refractory and more research is needed.
- As knowledge of the pathomechanisms of urticaria advances, novel treatments are appearing, including the anti-IgE monoclonal ligelizumab, IgE trap molecules, and small molecules. Thus history of urticaria is currently being rewritten.

References

1. Czarnetzki BM. The history of urticaria. Int J Dermatol. 1989;28(1):52–7.
2. Humphreys F. Major landmarks in the history of urticarial disorders. Int J Dermatol. 1997;36(10):793–6.
3. Ehrlich P. Beiträge zur Kenntnis der Anilinfärbungen und ihrere in der Verwendung mikroskopischen Technik. Arch Mikro Anat. 1877;13:263–77.
4. Riley JF. Mast cells and histamine in the skin. The mast cells. Edinburgh: E&S Livingstone; 1959. p. 144–59.
5. Dale HH. On some physiological actions of ergot. J Physiol. 1906;34(3):163–206.
6. Greaves MW, Sabroe RA. Histamine: the quintessential mediator. J Dermatol. 1996;23:735–40.
7. Lewis T. The blood vessels of the human skin and their responses. London: Shaw; 1927.
8. Simone DA, Alreja M, LaMotte RH. Psychophysical studies of the itch sensation and itchy skin ("alloknesis") produced by intracutaneous injection of histamine. Somatosens Mot Res. 1991;8(3):271–9.
9. Le Coniat M, Traiffort E, Ruat M, Arrang JM, Berger R. Chromosomal localisation of the human histamine H1 receptor gene. Hum Genet. 1994;94:186–8.
10. Gantz I, Schaffer M, DelValle J, Logsdon C, Campbell V, Uhler M, Yamada T. Molecular cloning of a gene encoding the histamine H2 receptor. Proc Natl Acad Sci U S A. 1991;88(2):429–33.
11. O'Leary PA, Farber EM. Benadryl in the treatment of certain diseases of the skin. J Am Med Assoc. 1947;134(12):1010–3.
12. Bain WA, Hellier FF, Warin RP. Some aspects of the action of histamine antagonists. Lancet. 1948;2(6538):964–9.
13. Fung-Leung WP, Thurmond RL, Ling P, Karlsson L. Histamine H4 receptor antagonists: the new antihistamines? Curr Opin Investig Drugs. 2004;5(11):1174–83.
14. Kaplan AP, Horakova Z, Katz SI. Assessment of tissue fluid histamine levels in patients with urticaria. J Allergy Clin Immunol. 1978;61(6):350–4.
15. Okahara K, Murakami T, Yamamoto S, Yata N. Skin microdialysis: detection of in vivo histamine release in cutaneous allergic reactions. Skin Pharmacol. 1995;8(3):113–8.

16. Cook J, Shuster S. Histamine weal formation and absorption in man. Br J Pharmacol. 1980;69(4):579–85.
17. Ishizaka K, Ishizaka T, Hornbrook MM. Physicochemical properties of reaginic antibody. V. Correlation of reaginic activity with gamma-E-globulin antibody. J Immunol. 1966;97(6):840–53.
18. Gell PGH, Coombs RR. Clinical aspects of immunology. Oxford: Blackwell; 1963. p. 317–20.
19. Michaelsson G, Juhlin L. Urticaria induced by preservatives and dye additives in food and drugs. Br J Dermatol. 1973;88:525–32.
20. Doeglas HM. Reactions to aspirin and food additives in patients with chronic urticaria, including the physical urticarias. Br J Dermatol. 1975;93(2):135–44.
21. Supramaniam G, Warner JO. Artificial food additive intolerance in patients with angio-oedema and urticaria. Lancet. 1986;2(8512):907–9.
22. Zuberbier T, Chantraine-Hess S, Hartmann K, Czarnetzki BM. Pseudoallergen-free diet in the treatment of chronic urticaria. A prospective study. Acta Derm Venereol. 1995;75(6):484–7.
23. Greaves MW. Food intolerance in urticaria and angioedema and urticarial vasculitis. In: Brostoff J, Challacombe S, editors. Food allergy and intolerance. 2nd ed. Philadelphia: WB Saunders; 2002. p. 623–69.
24. Burova GP, Mallet AI, Greaves MW. Is Helicobacter pylori a cause of chronic urticaria. Br J Dermatol. 1998;139(Suppl 51):42.
25. Greaves MW. Chronic idiopathic urticaria and Helicobacter pylori: not directly related—but could there be a link? ACI Int. 2001;13:23–6.
26. Rorsman H. Basophilic leucopenia in different forms of urticaria. Acta Allergol. 1962;17:168–84.
27. Greaves MW, Plummer VM, McLaughlan P, Stanworth DR. Serum and cell bound IgE in chronic urticaria. Clin Allergy. 1974;4(3):265–71.
28. Gruber BL, Baeza ML, Marchese MJ, Agnello V, Kaplan AP. Prevalence and functional role of anti-IgE autoantibodies in urticarial syndromes. J Invest Dermatol. 1988;90(2):213–7.
29. Leznoff A, Sussman GL. Syndrome of idiopathic chronic urticaria and angioedema with thyroid autoimmunity: a study of 90 patients. J Allergy Clin Immunol. 1989;84(1):66–71.
30. O'Donnell BF, O'Neill CM, Francis DM, Niimi N, Barr RM, Barlow RJ, Kobza Black A, Welsh KI, Greaves MW. Human leucocyte antigen class II associations in chronic idiopathic urticaria. Br J Dermatol. 1999;140(5):853–8.
31. Grattan CE, Wallington TB, Warin RP, Kennedy CT, Bradfield JW. A serological mediator in chronic idiopathic urticaria a clinical, immunological and histological evaluation. Br J Dermatol. 1986;114(5):583–90.
32. Claveau J, Lavoie A, Brunet C, Bedard PM, Hebert J. Chronic idiopathic urticaria: possible contribution of histamine-releasing factor to pathogenesis. J Allergy Clin Immunol. 1993;92(1 Pt 1):132–7.
33. MacDonald SM, Rafnar T, Langdon J, Lichtenstein LM. Molecular identification of an IgE-dependent histamine-releasing factor. Science. 1995;269(5224):688–90.
34. Hide M, Francis DM, Grattan CE, Hakimi J, Kochan JP, Greaves MW. Autoantibodies against the high-affinity IgE receptor as a cause of histamine release in chronic urticaria. N Engl J Med. 1993;328(22):1599–604.
35. Niimi N, Francis DM, Kermani F, O'Donnell BF, Hide M, Kobza-Black A, Winkelmann RK, Greaves MW, Barr RM. Dermal mast cell activation by autoantibodies against the high affinity IgE receptor in chronic urticaria. J Invest Dermatol. 1996;106(5):1001–6.
36. Fiebiger E, Maurer D, Holub H, Reininger B, Hartmann G, Woisetschlager M, Kinet JP, Stingl G. Serum IgG autoantibodies directed against the alpha chain of Fc epsilon RI: a selective marker and pathogenetic factor for a distinct subset of chronic urticaria patients? J Clin Invest. 1995;96(6):2606–12.
37. Tong LJ, Balakrishnan G, Kochan JP, Kinet JP, Kaplan AP. Assessment of autoimmunity in patients with chronic urticaria. J Allergy Clin Immunol. 1997;99(4):461–5.
38. Grattan CEH, Francis DM. Autoimmune urticaria. Adv Dermatol. 1999;15:311–40.

39. Schmetzer O, Lakin E, Topal FA, Preusse P, Freier D, Church MK, Maurer M. IL-24 is a common and specific autoantigen of IgE in patients with chronic spontaneous urticaria. J Allergy Clin Immunol. 2018;142(3):876–82.
40. Staub A, Bovet D. Actions de la thymoethyl-diethylamine (929F) et des ethersphenoliques sur le choc anaphylactique du cobaye. CR Soc Biol. 1937;128:818–25.
41. Leurs R, Church MK, Taglialatela M. H1-antihistamines: inverse agonism, anti-inflammatory actions and cardiac effects. Clin Exp Allergy. 2002;32(4):489–98.
42. Marks R, Greaves MW. Vascular reactions to histamine and compound 48/80 in human skin: suppression by a histamine H2-receptor blocking agent. Br J Clin Pharmacol. 1977;4(3):367–9.
43. Bleehen SS, Thomas SE, Greaves MW, Newton J, Kennedy CT, Hindley F, Marks R, Hazell M, Rowell NR, Fairiss GM, et al. Cimetidine and chlorpheniramine in the treatment of chronic idiopathic urticaria: a multi-centre randomized double-blind study. Br J Dermatol. 1987;117(1):81–8.
44. Simons FER, Simons KJ. The pharmacology and use of H1 receptor antagonist drugs. N Eng J Med. 1994;330:1663–70.
45. Breneman DL. Cetirizine versus hydroxyzine and placebo in chronic idiopathic urticaria. Ann Pharmacother. 1996;30(10):1075–9.
46. Finn AF Jr, Kaplan AP, Fretwell R, Qu R, Long J. A double-blind, placebo-controlled trial of fexofenadine HCl in the treatment of chronic idiopathic urticaria. J Allergy Clin Immunol. 1999;104(5):1071–8.
47. Paul E, Berth-Jones J, Ortonne J-P, Stern M, Paul E, Berth-Jones J, Ortonne J-P, Stern M. Fexofenadine hydrochloride in the treatment of chronic idiopathic urticaria: a placebo—controlled parallel group, dose ranging study. J Dermatol Treat. 1998;9:143–9.
48. Zuberbier T, Munzberger C, Haustein U, Trippas E, Burtin B, Mariz SD, Henz BM. Double-blind crossover study of high-dose cetirizine in cholinergic urticaria. Dermatology. 1996;193(4):324–7.
49. Di Lorenzo G, Pacor ML, Mansueto P, Esposito Pellitteri M, Lo Bianco C, Ditta V, Martinelli N, Rini GB. Randomized placebo-controlled trial comparing desloratadine and montelukast in monotherapy and desloratadine plus montelukast in combined therapy for chronic idiopathic urticaria. J Allergy Clin Immunol. 2004;114(3):619–25.
50. Yamashita M, Fukui H, Sugama K, Horio Y, Ito S, Mizuguchi H, Wada H. Expression cloning of a cDNA encoding the bovine histamine H1 receptor. Proc Natl Acad Sci U S A. 1991;88(24):11515–9.
51. Zuberbier T, Aberer W, Asero R, Abdul Latiff AH, Baker D, Ballmer-Weber B, Bernstein JA, Bindslev-Jensen C, Brzoza Z, Buense Bedrikow R, Canonica GW, Church MK, Craig T, Danilycheva IV, Dressler C, Ensina LF, Gimenez-Arnau A, Godse K, Goncalo M, Grattan C, Hebert J, Hide M, Kaplan A, Kapp A, Katelaris CH, Kocaturk E, Kulthanan K, Larenas-Linnemann D, Leslie TA, Magerl M, Mathelier-Fusade P, Meshkova RY, Metz M, Nast A, Nettis E, Oude-Elberink H, Rosumeck S, Saini SS, Sanchez-Borges M, Schmid-Grendelmeier P, Staubach P, Sussman G, Toubi E, Vena GA, Vestergaard C, Wedi B, Werner RN, Zhao Z, Maurer M, Endorsed by the following societies: AAAAI AADAAAAABADBCDACCDD, WAO. The EAACI/GA(2)LEN/EDF/WAO guideline for the definition, classification, diagnosis and management of urticaria. Allergy. 2018;73(7):1393–414.

Aetiopathogenesis of Urticaria

Clive Grattan and Martin K. Church

Core Messages
- Urticaria is a disease with a diversity of clinical presentations and aetiologies.
- The cutaneous mast cell is the primary effector cell.
- As well as inflammatory events happening in lesional skin of spontaneous urticaria patients, non-lesional skin appears primed for whealing.
- Histamine released from mast cells during degranulation is the primary mediator of itch and swelling.
- Leukotrienes and platelet activating factor may also be important.
- Bradykinin is the primary mediator of angioedema in patients with C1 inhibitor deficiency and those with angiotensin converting enzyme inhibitor (ACEI)-induced angioedema.
- Mast cell degranulation from immunological activation of the high affinity IgE receptor (FcεRI) by functional autoantibodies may involve co-factor augmentation, including C5a.
- Type I hypersensitivity reactions due to binding of allergen to specific IgE on mast cells is one cause of acute urticaria but is not a cause of chronic urticaria in adults.
- Type I hypersensitivity reactions to autoallergens may be important in the aetiopathogenesis of chronic spontaneous urticaria (autoallergic urticaria). Type I hypersensitivity reactions to neoantigens may also be relevant to inducible urticarias.

C. Grattan (✉)
St John's Institute of Dermatology, Guy's Hospital, London, UK
e-mail: Clive.E.Grattan@gstt.nhs.uk

M. K. Church
Institute for Allergology, Charité – Universitätsmedizin, Berlin, Germany
e-mail: M.K.Church@soton.ac.uk

- Type IIb (non-cytotoxic) hypersensitivity reactions due to binding of functional IgG autoantibodies to IgE or the FcεRI on mast cells and basophils occur in 30–50% of patients with chronic spontaneous urticaria (autoimmune urticaria).
- External aggravating factors, including local heat and pressure, stress and viral infections, acting independently or together, may account for the variable and unpredictable course of this multifactorial illness.

Urticaria is defined clinically by the sudden appearance of wheals, angioedema or both. Wheals are superficial and resolve completely within hours. Deeper swellings, angioedema can last up to 3 days. Superficial wheals usually start as sharply defined elevations of variable size with a surrounding red flare. They nearly always itch intensely before changing from a pale colour to pink, spreading outwards and becoming flatter and more diffuse before fading. The deeper swellings of angioedema are predominantly located in the loose connective tissue below the skin and mucosa of the mouth and genitalia but not the bowel or bladder. Involvement of the respiratory tract is very rare with the exception of occasional acute allergic urticaria presenting with throat swelling, wheeze or both. This is in contrast to hereditary angioedema where upper respiratory tract and bowel swellings are common. Angioedema swellings tend to be pale and painful and last longer than wheals. Urticaria has many presentations that can usually be grouped into patterns on the strength of clinical features. These patterns may help clinicians to investigate and manage individual patients appropriately but, in themselves, do not define aetiology or pathogenesis, which often remains poorly understood and difficult to demonstrate. The aim of this chapter is to step backwards from the patient and explore the pathways that mediate urticaria, illustrating the diversity and overlap that may occur.

Acute urticaria, arbitrarily defined by up to 6 weeks duration, is more common than chronic urticaria and mainly affects children or young adults (Chap. 14). Both children and adults may develop chronic urticaria but it is more common in adults. It is now accepted that patients with continuous chronic urticaria have an endogenous illness that can be exacerbated by external factors but is hardly ever a type I allergy. The reason why chronic urticaria begins for the first time is often unclear but there may be a history of a preceding minor viral infection, for instance, leading to an altered immunological state in the skin resulting in persistent enhanced 'releasability' of cutaneous mast cells.

Clinical experience indicates that external aggravating factors influence the day-to-day variability of the illness. These include localised heat, cold, pressure, skin friction, hormone fluctuations in women, some medicines (especially nonsteroidal anti-inflammatory drugs, NSAIDs), dietary pseudoallergens, alcohol, stress and infections. In acute urticaria, by contrast, an identifiable exogenous cause (infectious, allergic or pseudoallergic) may be found in about 50% of patients [1] but many cases remain unexplained after evaluation and some will evolve into chronic disease. Although the causes of spontaneous urticaria may vary, it is likely that the mediators involved in wheal pathogenesis are similar.

In acute and chronic spontaneous urticaria (CSU) the eruption of wheals and angioedema is unpredictable, unlike the inducible urticarias in which lesions are elicited by a reproducible trigger or triggers. Overlaps between spontaneous and inducible urticarias may occur. The clinician should try to identify this trigger since the activity of inducible urticaria can, in theory, be reduced by avoiding its stimulus. Despite defining inducible urticarias clinically by their eliciting event, their cause remains unknown. Passive transfer research over four decades ago implicating immunoglobulin E in cold, cholinergic, solar and dermographic urticaria has not been explored further to date. It is likely that differences will emerge between the mediators of inducible and spontaneous urticaria to account for the different clinical behaviours as more becomes known about the local mediator and cytokine profiles in lesional and non-lesional skin.

Although urticarial vasculitis has been included historically in classifications of urticaria because of the similarity in the appearance of the skin lesions with spontaneous wheals, it really should be considered as a pattern of small vessel vasculitis. Hereditary angioedema, due to mutations in the gene for C1-inhibitor on chromosome 11q11 resulting in complement consumption and kinin formation, and the urticarial autoinflammatory syndromes, defined by mutations of *NLRP3* on chromosome 1q44 resulting in activation of the *NALP3* inflammasome complex [2] with generation of interleukin 1β and -18, illustrate the fundamental differences in aetiopathogenesis that exist between different clinical patterns of urticaria, and the implications for investigation and management that flow from this.

2.1 Lessons Learned from Histopathology

The histology of urticaria may seem bland and non-specific but the pathological features complement and extend what can be deduced from the clinical features. The intensity and depth of dermal oedema depend on the timing and depth of the swelling, favouring the papillary dermis in wheals and the deep dermis and subcutis in angioedema.

The development of an urticarial wheal resembles the triple response to skin stroking/histamine described by Thomas Lewis in 1924 [3]. Initially there is a very early red spot due to local capillary dilatation. Around this, redness in the surrounding area develops due to arteriolar dilatation mediated by a local axon reflex. This is the so-called flare. Finally, exudation of fluid from capillaries and post-capillary venules causes the development of a pale coloured wheal. Within plasma, high molecular weight proteins, including immunoglobulins, are then able to pass temporarily from the lumina to the interstitium until the leak repairs. Fluid is removed via lymphatic vessels that become dilated early during wheal formation. Although small blood vessels are functionally impaired by these events, they are not damaged, unlike the changes that are seen in small vessel vasculitis where the post-capillary venules are disrupted to the point of necrosis with fibrinoid change, leading to passive extravasation of red cells in addition to plasma proteins and recruitment of inflammatory cells. Morphology of the endothelial changes can be best appreciated on semi-thin sections or ultrastructural examination. Inflammatory infiltrates are initially perivascular as leucocytes are recruited actively from the circulation by upregulation of adhesion molecules under the influence of chemokines and then become more diffusely distributed.

Biopsies taken from patients diagnosed with CSU have shown a spectrum of changes ranging from mild mononuclear perivascular infiltrates to full-blown changes of small vessel vasculitis with numerous neutrophils and eosinophils in a minority [4–6]. This diversity probably reflects a lack of definition of clinical patterns and the severity of urticaria at the time of biopsy but may also depend on the timing of biopsy in relation to the onset of the lesion. Accurate timing of spontaneous wheals is always problematical, but it does appear that acute inflammatory cells predominate in the early stages of wheal formation and that mononuclear cells follow later. More neutrophils and eosinophils were present in lesions over 12 h than below 4 h in biopsies of spontaneous wheals of CSU patients [7]. A 'neutrophilic' pattern of urticaria may be seen in patients with wide-ranging clinical patterns from cold urticaria to acute spontaneous urticaria [8]. Neutrophilic urticaria is distinct from the diffuse intense neutrophilic infiltrates with leukocytoclasia described in neutrophilic urticarial dermatosis (NUD) biopsies of autoinflammatory syndromes and systemic lupus erythematosus.

Lesional biopsies of patients with CSU show a Th0 cytokine profile [9]. Increased expression of Th2-initiating cytokines (IL-33, IL-25 and thymic stromal lymphopoetin) in lesional skin in CSU suggested that innate pathways might play a role in the mechanism of whealing [6] alongside cutaneous mast cell degranulation. Lesional skin in CSU contained significantly more CD31+ endothelial cells; CD31+ blood vessels, neutrophils, eosinophils, basophils and macrophages; and CD3+ T cells than non-lesional skin. Uninvolved skin from CSU also contained significantly more CD31+ endothelial cells, CD31+ blood vessels and eosinophils compared with the control subjects, suggesting that clinically uninvolved skin is primed for whealing, [5] probably after mast cell degranulation. Increased CGRP and VEGF expression was detected in lesional, but not uninvolved, skin co-localised to UEA-1+ blood vessels indicating that these potent vasoactive agents may play a role in whealing and tissue oedema [10].

The qualitative and quantitative features of inflammatory infiltrates do not help to define a specific pathogenesis or aetiology for an individual patient with urticaria, in general. Exceptions are urticaria patients with functional autoantibodies which show an increased number of activated eosinophils in biopsies of 12 h old wheals [7], delayed pressure urticaria with deep mixed infiltrates and urticarial vasculitis which is defined by leukocytoclasia with red cell extravasation.

2.2 A Central Role for the Mast Cell

The role of mast cells in urticaria has recently been the subject of a comprehensive review [11]. In urticaria patients, as in healthy individuals, mast cells are located in the upper and lower dermis with a prevalent perivascular and periadnexal pattern [12]. Highest numbers are found in superficial dermal skin lesions and the lowest numbers in lower reticular dermis [13, 14]. Mast cell density was found to be highest in peripheral sites of healthy skin, especially the chin and nose, but independent of age or gender in one study [15] and highest on distal limb sites in another [16].

2 Aetiopathogenesis of Urticaria

Although the disposition of mast cells in the skin of urticaria patients is normal, do their numbers change in chronic urticaria? Reports about this are conflicting. The earliest study in CSU reported an increase in the percentage of dermal mast cells from 11 to 14% [17]. Increased mast cell numbers in both lesional and non-lesional skin have been reported [10, 18] whealing or recent whealing [19–23] or in both lesional and uninvolved skin of patients with prolonged (>10 weeks) disease [14]. One study, which compared mast cell subtypes in lesional skin of CSU patients and healthy skin, is particularly noteworthy [24]. This study showed that there were no differences between the numbers of MC_{TC}, known as the connective tissue mast cell, between the two groups. However, the increased number of MC_T in CSU lesional skin was highly significant ($P < 0.001$). As it is the MC_T subtype of mast cells that is particularly associated with allergic disease [25], this would support an allergic mechanism for CSU. By contrast, other studies found no difference between mast cell numbers in the skin of chronic urticaria patients and healthy individuals [26–29].

2.3 Mast Cell Mediators of Urticaria

2.3.1 Histamine

It is now more than 50 years since the first demonstration of histamine in the plasma of a patient with cold urticaria [30, 31]. This observation has been repeated for CSU [24, 32, 33] and many types of inducible urticaria including cold urticaria [34–40], heat-induced urticaria [34, 41–43], solar urticaria [44] symptomatic dermographism [45], cholinergic urticaria [35], delayed pressure urticaria [46] and aspirin-induced urticaria [47]. Increased levels of histamine in the tissues have also been demonstrated. More recently, histamine liberated into the tissues in cold-induced urticaria in response to cold provocation was demonstrated by dermal microdialysis [48].

Binding of histamine H_1 receptors on small cutaneous blood vessels mediates vasopermeability and vasodilatation. It also mediates itch through stimulation of cutaneous nociceptors and the surrounding flare by antidromic stimulation of local C-fibre networks. The flare response is mediated by calcitonin gene related peptide (CGRP) release from cutaneous nerve endings rather than histamine [49, 50]. Stimulation of H_2 receptors on cutaneous blood vessels may also be responsible for vasodilatation and vasopermeability within the wheal but not itch or flare. Effects of histamine on the cellular immune system [51] and some proinflammatory cytokines [48] have been demonstrated but their relevance to urticaria is yet to be determined.

2.3.2 Cysteinyl Leukotrienes and Platelet Activating Factor

The cysteinyl leukotrienes (LT) may contribute to vasopermeability and vasodilatation in urticaria but are secondary in importance to histamine. Synthesis of LTC_4, D_4, E_4 by mast cells at the time of degranulation and subsequently by infiltrating basophils and eosinophils may be a factor in the prolongation of urticaria wheals in some types of urticaria, particularly aspirin-sensitive urticaria, autoimmune urticaria and delayed

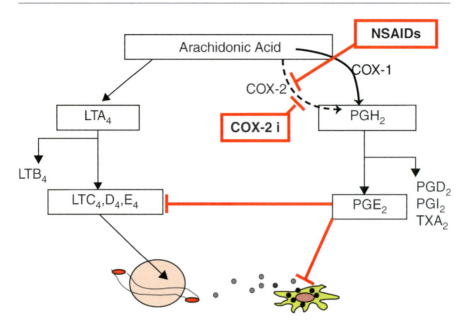

Fig. 2.1 Inhibition of the cyclo-oxygenase (COX) pathway by non-selective NSAIDS results in diversion of arachidonic acid metabolism from prostaglandins to leukotrienes. PGE_2 normally has an inhibitory action on immunological mast cell degranulation and cysteinyl leukotriene production. Reduced PGE_2 formation has a permissive effect on immunological mast cell degranulation that is not seen with selective COX-2 inhibitors

pressure urticaria. It is thought that aspirin and other non-selective NSAIDs may activate mast cells indirectly by inhibiting formation of prostaglandin E_2 (PGE_2) via the cyclo-oxygenase (COX) for which there is some evidence of an inhibitory effect on immunological mast cell activation [52] (Fig. 2.1). Selective inhibitors of inducible COX-2 are less likely to exacerbate aspirin-sensitive urticaria than non-selective COX-1 and -2 inhibitors since PGE_2 production by the constitutively expressed COX-1 isoform is not affected. Evidence of thrombin generation in citrated plasma of CSU patients was related to CSU severity [53] suggesting that coagulation factors may enhance vascular permeability or induce mast cell degranulation.

Platelet activating factor (PAF) may also contribute to vasopermeability and vasodilatation in urticaria. A recent study showed that patients with CSU, particularly those with H1-antihistamine refractoriness, showed significantly increased serum PAF levels, as compared to healthy controls [54].

2.4 Involvement of Other Inflammatory Cells in Urticaria

Although the cutaneous mast cell is the primary effector cell of the early phase of urticaria, eosinophils, basophils and lymphocytes almost certainly play a significant role afterwards in the evolution of wheals and angioedema. Eosinophils contain toxic granules including major basic protein (MBP) and eosinophil cationic protein (ECP) that are released on activation. MPB can degranulate mast cells non-immunologically thereby enhancing the level of histamine in the lesion. Basophils are thought to migrate from peripheral blood into wheals of CSU at the time of their formation [55–58] and probably perpetuate the inflammatory oedema by releasing histamine and leukotrienes. No specific role for polymorphonuclear neutrophils has been identified, but it is possible that they are involved with oxygen free radical formation. There is some evidence for oxidative stress being important in the lesional skin of patients with CSU but the antioxidant activity in plasma and erythrocytes was similar to that of healthy controls [59]. The contribution of lesional skin lymphocytes to urticaria pathogenesis is uncertain but upregulation of immunoreactivity for interleukin-3 (IL-3) and tumour necrosis factor alpha (TNF-α) was seen in perivascular cells in the upper dermis of patients with acute urticaria and delayed pressure urticaria, but not CSU [60]. CD40L expression was higher on activated circulating T cells in CSU than healthy controls implying that co-stimulatory signals for B-cell activation are upregulated and Bcl-2 protein expression on blood B and T cells was enhanced in severe CSU, consistent with their prolonged survival and proliferation [61]. Aberrant signalling through the p21Ras pathway in lymphocytes of patients with CSU supports the autoimmune basis of this disease [62]. Peripheral blood lymphocyte numbers were consistently lower in untreated active CSU patients than controls on automated differential counts [55] although any significance of this has yet to be determined.

2.5 The Role of Bradykinin in Angioedema

There is currently no evidence that bradykinin is a mediator of urticaria. By contrast, bradykinin generated by the action of kallikrein on kininogen is the primary mediator of hereditary angioedema [63] (Fig. 2.2). Here, C1 inhibitor prevents initiation of the intrinsic coagulation pathway by activated Hagemann Factor (XIIa), plasmin formation, the classical pathway of complement activation and the kallikrein–kininogen–kinin system. Kininase II (also known as angiotensin converting enzyme, ACE) inhibition by angiotensin converting enzyme inhibitors (ACEI) may result in accumulation of kinins leading to angioedema *without* wheals but is not a cause of angioedema *with* wheals (Fig. 2.3).

2.6 What Causes Mast Cell Mediator Release in the First Place?

Understanding the stimulus for mast cell mediator secretion is the key to diagnosis and appropriately directed management in clinical practice. The stimulus may be immunological, non-immunological or, perhaps, a combination of both in some situations. Certainly, the effectiveness of omalizumab (anti-IgE) in the majority of

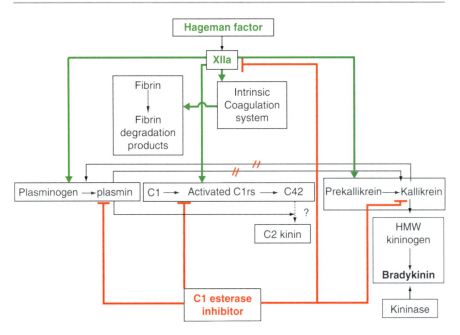

Fig. 2.2 Stimulation of Hageman Factor XII activates the intrinsic coagulation system, generation of plasmin and production of bradykinin by the action of kallikrein on high molecular weight kininogen. There is a complex interconnecting system of feedback loops involving C 1 esterase inhibitor, which has a controlling inhibitory influence on the complement, kallikrein, coagulation and fibrinolytic systems

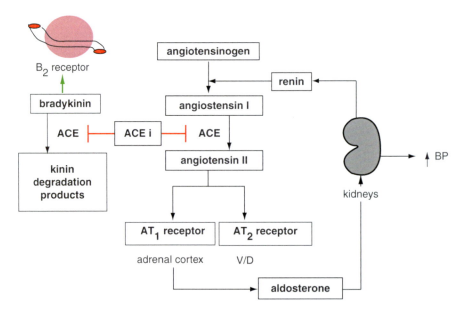

Fig. 2.3 Inhibitors of angiotensin converting enzyme (ACE) block the angiotensin-renin system that controls blood pressure and the breakdown of bradykinin, which may lead to angio-oedema through stimulation of B_2 receptors on blood vessels

CSU patients in whom H_1-antihistamines are poorly effective [64] would support an immunological basis of the condition.

The first evidence that CSU may have an immunological basis started with the report that, in some patients, autologous sera with CSU re-injected intradermally produced a wheal at the site of injection [65]. This is known as the autologous serum skin test (ASST). Subsequent studies showed that IgG antibodies to the patient's own IgE or its high affinity receptor (FcεRI) were instrumental in causing basophil [66, 67] and mast cell degranulation [68] with subsequent wheal development. The evidence in support of this mechanism of CSU has been reviewed recently [69, 70]. Removal of IgE and subsequent loss of cutaneous mast cell FcεRI would explain the slow onset of action of omalizumab seen in up to 30% of patients responding to omalizumab [71, 72]. This IgG-mediated CSU is called autoimmune CSU (aiCSU). Characteristically aiCSU patients have low total IgE levels and high IgG-anti-TPO levels [73].

Of biomarkers, positive basophil activation tests (BAT) and basophil activation tests (BHRA) tests were 69% and 88% predictive of aiCSU, respectively.

Some 60% of responders to omalizumab become symptom free quite rapidly, usually within a week [64, 74]. In these individuals, a Type-1 allergic mechanism appears likely even though there is no obvious external allergen as in classical allergy (Fig. 2.4). Thus, an autoallergic CSU (aaCSU) has been proposed in which IgE is directed to an element of self [7], i.e. an autoantigen. This is supported by studies that have shown that patients with CSU have high levels of IgE autoantibodies such as IgE-anti-TPO [74] and IgE-anti-dsDNA in their blood [75]. More recently, using array analyses, over 200 IgE-autoantigens were found in CSU patients that were not present in controls. Of these, IgE-anti-IL-24 was found in all

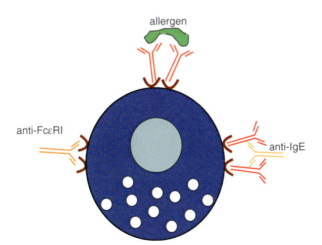

Fig. 2.4 Type I autoallergic urticaria (aaCSU) is thought to be due to specific IgE on mast cells and basophils binding to autoantigens. Type IIb autoimmune urticaria (aiCSU) involves IgG directed against the high affinity IgE receptor on mast cells and basophils or IgE bound to its receptor

CSU patients indicating IL-24 to be a dermal autoantigen in CSU [76]. While this study focussed on CSU, the effectiveness of omalizumab in a wide range of chronic inducible urticarias [64, 77, 78] raises the possibility that similar autoantigens and IgE-dependent mechanisms may also underlie these forms of urticaria [79] although other mechanisms, such as neuropeptide-induced degranulation are possible, and this might account for the very rapid onset and resolution of most inducible urticarias.

In addition to the two mechanisms described above, IgG autoantibodies have been described against the low affinity IgE receptor (FcεRII) on eosinophils that cause release of major basic protein (MBP), which, in turn, may lead to non-immunological degranulation of mast cells [80]. Urticaria mediated by this mechanism would be unresponsive to omalizumab. The main receptor responsible for mast activation by MBP appears to be Mas-related G protein-coupled receptor X2 (MRGPRX2) [81, 82]. Human skin mast cells also express CD88/C5aR allowing them to be activated by complement peptide C5a [83, 84].

2.7 Tests for Autoimmune and Autoallergic Urticaria

2.7.1 Autologous Serum Skin Test (ASST)

The autologous serum skin test originally described by Grattan and colleagues in 1996 [65] was widely used to screen for histamine releasing factors in blood but it has been criticised for having only moderate specificity and sensitivity for *in vitro* basophil histamine release in CSU [85] and is no longer so popular. It was not abolished by IgG depletion and heat decomplementation [86]. Skin testing with low molecular weight fractions of autologous CSU sera between 30 and 1 KD elicited a positive response indicating that the serum response is probably due to low molecular weight vasoactive substances in addition to functional autoantibodies [87] and this could account for the subsequent findings of Fagiolo [86]. Intradermal skin testing with autologous citrated plasma gave a higher proportion of positive results than autologous plasma and some ASST-negative patients gave a positive APST result [54] but this was not confirmed subsequently [88]. Patients with CSU and thyroid autoimmunity were more likely to have a positive ASST than those without; the ASST remained positive in the majority of patients with thyroid autoantibodies after clinical remission of their urticaria [89]. Reversion of a positive to a negative response one year after clinical remission was reported in the original description of the ASST [65]. The autologous serum skin test remains, nevertheless, a relatively safe and simple test to perform, provides a convincing demonstration for patients that their urticaria has an endogenous cause if positive and may be a useful predictive test for the detection of functional autoantibodies, provided the results are interpreted with caution [90]. Combining information from ASSTs and thyroid antibodies in patients with CSU for clinicians without access to basophil activation assays may increase its predictive value for functional autoantibodies.

2.7.2 Basophil Activation Assays

Basophil activation assays are now widely used as functional assays of histamine release factors in serum, including IgG autoantibodies against FcεRI and IgE. Two assays are available. The first is the basophil histamine release assay (BHRA) [66, 67, 72, 91]. The second is the basophil activation test (BAT), which was developed following the development of flow cytometry, discovery of activation markers such as CD63 and unique markers identifying basophil granulocytes [92, 93]. In a study of IgG-mediated autoimmune CSU, positive BAT and BHRA tests were 69% and 88% predictive, respectively [73].

2.7.3 Immunoassays for Autoantibodies in Autoimmune CSU

Assays of IgG-anti-FcεRIα IgG-anti-IgE and auto-IgE antibodies are being developed in order to distinguish between IgG-mediated autoimmune CSU (aiCSU) and IgE-mediated autoallergic CSU (aaCSU) [73, 74, 76, 94, 95]. However, these assays are undergoing development and are currently not available in the clinic; their utility is unknown since they detect both functional and non-functional autoantibodies and the latter may not be directly relevant in disease pathogenesis. There is currently no diagnostic test for aaCSU although many patients will have an increased total IgE.

2.8 Conclusions

Urticaria is a common illness with a common pathway centred on the cutaneous mast cell with histamine as a primary mediator. However, the clinical presentation and the events leading to activation of the mast cell are diverse, requiring further detailed research.

References

1. Zuberbier T, Ifflander J, Semmler C, Henz BM. Acute urticaria: clinical aspects and therapeutic responsiveness. Acta Derm Venereol. 1996;76(4):295–7.
2. Shinkai K, McCalmont TH, Leslie KS. Cryopyrin-associated periodic syndromes and autoinflammation. Clin Exp Dermatol. 2008;33(1):1–9.
3. Lewis T, Grant RT. Vascular reactions of the skin to injury. The liberation of a histamine-like substance in injured skin; the underlying cause of factitious urticaria and of wheals produced by burning: and observations upon the nervous control of certain skin reactions. Heart. 1924;11:209–65.
4. Jones RR, Bhogal B, Dash A, Schifferli J. Urticaria and vasculitis: a continuum of histological and immunopathological changes. Br J Dermatol. 1983;108(6):695–703.
5. Kay AB, Ying S, Ardelean E, Mlynek A, Kita H, Clark P, Maurer M. Elevations in vascular markers and eosinophils in chronic spontaneous urticarial weals with low-level persistence in uninvolved skin. Br J Dermatol. 2014;171(3):505–11.

6. Kay AB, Clark P, Maurer M, Ying S. Elevations in T-helper-2-initiating cytokines (interleukin-33, interleukin-25 and thymic stromal lymphopoietin) in lesional skin from chronic spontaneous ('idiopathic') urticaria. Br J Dermatol. 2015;172(5):1294–302.
7. Sabroe RA, Poon E, Orchard GE, Lane D, Francis DM, Barr RM, Black MM, Black AK, Greaves MW. Cutaneous inflammatory cell infiltrate in chronic idiopathic urticaria: comparison of patients with and without anti-FcepsilonRI or anti-IgE autoantibodies. J Allergy Clin Immunol. 1999;103(3 Pt 1):484–93.
8. Toppe E, Haas N, Henz BM. Neutrophilic urticaria: clinical features, histological changes and possible mechanisms. Br J Dermatol. 1998;138(2):248–53.
9. Ying S, Kikuchi Y, Meng Q, Kay AB, Kaplan AP. TH1/TH2 cytokines and inflammatory cells in skin biopsy specimens from patients with chronic idiopathic urticaria: comparison with the allergen-induced late-phase cutaneous reaction. J Allergy Clin Immunol. 2002;109(4):694–700.
10. Kay AB, Ying S, Ardelean E, Mlynek A, Kita H, Clark P, Maurer M. Calcitonin gene-related peptide and vascular endothelial growth factor are expressed in lesional but not uninvolved skin in chronic spontaneous urticaria. Clin Exp Allergy. 2014;44(8):1053–60.
11. Church MK, Kolkhir P, Metz M, Maurer M. The role and relevance of mast cells in urticaria. Immunol Rev. 2018;282(1):232–47.
12. Caproni M, Giomi B, Melani L, Volpi W, Antiga E, Torchia D, Fabbri P. Cellular infiltrate and related cytokines, chemokines, chemokine receptors and adhesion molecules in chronic autoimmune urticaria: comparison between spontaneous and autologous serum skin test induced wheal. Int J Immunopathol Pharmacol. 2006;19(3):507–15.
13. Haas N, Toppe E, Henz BM. Microscopic morphology of different types of urticaria. Arch Dermatol. 1998;134(1):41–6.
14. Terhorst D, Koti I, Krause K, Metz M, Maurer M. In chronic spontaneous urticaria, high numbers of dermal endothelial cells, but not mast cells, are linked to recurrent angio-oedema. Clin Exp Dermatol. 2018;43(2):131–6.
15. Weber A, Knop J, Maurer M. Pattern analysis of human cutaneous mast cell populations by total body surface mapping. Br J Dermatol. 2003;148(2):224–8.
16. Janssens AS, Heide R, den Hollander JC, Mulder PG, Tank B, Oranje AP. Mast cell distribution in normal adult skin. J Clin Pathol. 2005;58(3):285–9.
17. Elias J, Boss E, Kaplan AP. Studies of the cellular infiltrate of chronic idiopathic urticaria: prominence of T-lymphocytes, monocytes, and mast cells. J Allergy Clin Immunol. 1986;78(5 Pt 1):914–8.
18. Czarnetzki BM, Zwadlo-Klarwasser GZ, Brocker EB, Sorg C. Macrophage subsets in different types of urticaria. Arch Dermatol Res. 1990;282(2):93–7.
19. Czarnetzki BM, Meentken J, Kolde G, Brocker EB. Morphology of the cellular infiltrate in delayed pressure urticaria. J Am Acad Dermatol. 1985;12(2 Pt 1):253–9.
20. Kobza Black A, Dover J, Greaves M. The histological features of induced delayed pressure urticaria. Br J Dermatol. 1987;(116):427–428.
21. Barlow RJ, Ross EL, MacDonald DM, Kobza Black A, Greaves MW. Mast cells and T lymphocytes in chronic urticaria. Clin Exp Allergy. 1995;25(4):317–22.
22. Toyoda M, Maruyama T, Morohashi M, Bhawan J. Free eosinophil granules in urticaria: a correlation with the duration of wheals. Am J Dermatopathol. 1996;18(1):49–57.
23. Hong GU, Ro JY, Bae Y, Kwon IH, Park GH, Choi YH, Choi JH. Association of TG2 from mast cells and chronic spontaneous urticaria pathogenesis. Ann Allergy Asthma Immunol. 2016;117(3):290–7.
24. Nettis E, Dambra P, Loria MP, Cenci L, Vena GA, Ferrannini A, Tursi A. Mast-cell phenotype in urticaria. Allergy. 2001;56(9):915.
25. Bradding P, Okayama Y, Howarth PH, Church MK, Holgate ST. Heterogeneity of human mast cells based on cytokine content. J Immunol. 1995;155(1):297–307.
26. English JS, Murphy GM, Winkelmann RK, Bhogal B. A sequential histopathological study of dermographism. Clin Exp Dermatol. 1988;13(5):314–7.
27. Smith CH, Kepley C, Schwartz LB, Lee TH. Mast cell number and phenotype in chronic idiopathic urticaria. J Allergy Clin Immunol. 1995;96(3):360–4.

28. Caproni M, Volpi W, Macchia D, Giomi B, Manfredi M, Campi P, Cardinali C, D'Agata A, Fabbri P. Infiltrating cells and related cytokines in lesional skin of patients with chronic idiopathic urticaria and positive autologous serum skin test. Exp Dermatol. 2003;12(5):621–8.
29. Moy AP, Murali M, Nazarian RM. Identification of a Th2- and Th17-skewed immune phenotype in chronic urticaria with Th22 reduction dependent on autoimmunity and thyroid disease markers. J Cutan Pathol. 2016;43(4):372–8.
30. Henderson LL, Code CF, Roth GM. Increased blood histamine in thermal intolerance. J Allergy. 1958;29(2):122–9.
31. Spuzic I, Ivkovic L. Histamine in plasma in the induced urticaria due to cold. Acta Allergol. 1961;16:228–31.
32. Phanuphak P, Schocket AL, Arroyave CM, Kohler PF. Skin histamine in chronic urticaria. J Allergy Clin Immunol. 1980;65(5):371–5.
33. Guida B, De Martino CD, De Martino SD, Tritto G, Patella V, Trio R, D'Agostino C, Pecoraro P, D'Agostino L. Histamine plasma levels and elimination diet in chronic idiopathic urticaria. Eur J Clin Nutr. 2000;54(2):155–8.
34. Beall GN. Plasma histamine concentrations in allergic diseases. J Allergy. 1963;34:8–15.
35. Kaplan AP, Gray L, Shaff RE, Horakova Z, Beaven MA. In vivo studies of mediator release in cold urticaria and cholinergic urticaria. J Allergy Clin Immunol. 1975;55(6):394–402.
36. Bentley-Phillips CB, Black AK, Greaves MW. Induced tolerance in cold urticaria caused by cold-evoked histamine release. Lancet. 1976;2(7976):63–6.
37. Soter NA, Wasserman SI, Austen KF. Cold urticaria: release into the circulation of histamine and eosinophil chemotactic factor of anaphylaxis during cold challenge. N Engl J Med. 1976;294(13):687–90.
38. Wasserman SI, Austen KF, Soter NA. The functional and physicochemical characterization of three eosinophilotactic activities released into the circulation by cold challenge of patients with cold urticaria. Clin Exp Immunol. 1982;47(3):570–8.
39. Grandel KE, Farr RS, Wanderer AA, Eisenstadt TC, Wasserman SI. Association of platelet-activating factor with primary acquired cold urticaria. N Engl J Med. 1985;313(7):405–9.
40. Ormerod AD, Kobza Black A, Dawes J, Murdoch RD, Koro O, Barr RM, Greaves MW. Prostaglandin D2 and histamine release in cold urticaria unaccompanied by evidence of platelet activation. J Allergy Clin Immunol. 1988;82(4):586–9.
41. Atkins PC, Zweiman B. Mediator release in local heat urticaria. J Allergy Clin Immunol. 1981;68(4):286–9.
42. Grant JA, Findlay SR, Thueson DO, Fine DP, Krueger GG. Local heat urticaria/angioedema: evidence for histamine release without complement activation. J Allergy Clin Immunol. 1981;67(1):75–7.
43. Irwin RB, Lieberman P, Friedman MM, Kaliner M, Kaplan R, Bale G, Treadwell G, Yoo TJ. Mediator release in local heat urticaria: protection with combined H1 and H2 antagonists. J Allergy Clin Immunol. 1985;76(1):35–9.
44. Hawk JL, Eady RA, Challoner AV, Kobza-Black A, Keahey TM, Greaves MW. Elevated blood histamine levels and mast cell degranulation in solar urticaria. Br J Clin Pharmacol. 1980;9(2):183–6.
45. Garafalo J, Kaplan AP. Histamine release and therapy of severe dermatographism. J Allergy Clin Immunol. 1981;68(2):103–5.
46. Czarnetzki BM, Meentken J, Rosenbach T, Pokropp A. Clinical, pharmacological and immunological aspects of delayed pressure urticaria. Br J Dermatol. 1984;111(3):315–23.
47. Asad SI, Murdoch R, Youlten LJ, Lessof MH. Plasma level of histamine in aspirin-sensitive urticaria. Ann Allergy. 1987;59(3):219–22.
48. Krause K, Spohr A, Zuberbier T, Church MK, Maurer M. Up-dosing with bilastine results in improved effectiveness in cold contact urticaria. Allergy. 2013;68(7):921–8.
49. Petersen LJ, Church MK, Skov PS. Histamine is released in the wheal but not the flare following challenge of human skin in vivo: a microdialysis study. Clin Exp Allergy. 1997;27(3):284–95.
50. Schmelz M, Luz O, Averbeck B, Bickel A. Plasma extravasation and neuropeptide release in human skin as measured by intradermal microdialysis. Neurosci Lett. 1997;230(2):117–20.

51. Jutel M, Akdis CA. Histamine as an immune modulator in chronic inflammatory responses. Clin Exp Allergy. 2007;37(3):308–10.
52. Chan CL, Jones RL, Lau HY. Characterization of prostanoid receptors mediating inhibition of histamine release from anti-IgE-activated rat peritoneal mast cells. Br J Pharmacol. 2000;129(3):589–97.
53. Asero R, Tedeschi A, Riboldi P, Cugno M. Plasma of patients with chronic urticaria shows signs of thrombin generation, and its intradermal injection causes wheal-and-flare reactions much more frequently than autologous serum. J Allergy Clin Immunol. 2006;117(5):1113–7.
54. Ulambayar B, Yang EM, Cha HY, Shin YS, Park HS, Ye YM. Increased platelet activating factor levels in chronic spontaneous urticaria predicts refractoriness to antihistamine treatment: an observational study. Clin Transl Allergy. 2019;9:33.
55. Grattan CE, Dawn G, Gibbs S, Francis DM. Blood basophil numbers in chronic ordinary urticaria and healthy controls: diurnal variation, influence of loratadine and prednisolone and relationship to disease activity. Clin Exp Allergy. 2003;33(3):337–41.
56. Vasagar K, Vonakis BM, Gober LM, Viksman A, Gibbons SP Jr, Saini SS. Evidence of in vivo basophil activation in chronic idiopathic urticaria. Clin Exp Allergy. 2006;36(6):770–6.
57. Vonakis BM, Vasagar K, Gibbons SP Jr, Gober L, Sterba PM, Chang H, Saini SS. Basophil FcepsilonRI histamine release parallels expression of Src-homology 2-containing inositol phosphatases in chronic idiopathic urticaria. J Allergy Clin Immunol. 2007;119(2):441–8.
58. Saini SS. Chronic spontaneous urticaria: etiology and pathogenesis. Immunol Allergy Clin North Am. 2014;34(1):33–52.
59. Kasperska-Zajac A, Brzoza Z, Polaniak R, Rogala B, Birkner E. Markers of antioxidant defence system and lipid peroxidation in peripheral blood of female patients with chronic idiopathic urticaria. Arch Dermatol Res. 2007;298(10):499–503.
60. Hermes B, Prochazka AK, Haas N, Jurgovsky K, Sticherling M, Henz BM. Upregulation of TNF-alpha and IL-3 expression in lesional and uninvolved skin in different types of urticaria. J Allergy Clin Immunol. 1999;103(2 Pt 1):307–14.
61. Toubi E, Adir-Shani A, Kessel A, Shmuel Z, Sabo E, Hacham H. Immune aberrations in B and T lymphocytes derived from chronic urticaria patients. J Clin Immunol. 2000;20(5):371–8.
62. Confino-Cohen R, Aharoni D, Goldberg A, Gurevitch I, Buchs A, Weiss M, Weissgarten J, Rapoport MJ. Evidence for aberrant regulation of the p21Ras pathway in PBMCs of patients with chronic idiopathic urticaria. J Allergy Clin Immunol. 2002;109(2):349–56.
63. Cicardi M, Johnston DT. Hereditary and acquired complement component 1 esterase inhibitor deficiency: a review for the hematologist. Acta Haematol. 2012;127(4):208–20.
64. Metz M, Ohanyan T, Church MK, Maurer M. Omalizumab is an effective and rapidly acting therapy in difficult-to-treat chronic urticaria: a retrospective clinical analysis. J Dermatol Sci. 2014;73(1):57–62.
65. Grattan CE, Wallington TB, Warin RP, Kennedy CT, Bradfield JW. A serological mediator in chronic idiopathic urticaria—a clinical, immunological and histological evaluation. Br J Dermatol. 1986;114(5):583–90.
66. Grattan CE, Francis DM, Hide M, Greaves MW. Detection of circulating histamine releasing autoantibodies with functional properties of anti-IgE in chronic urticaria. Clin Exp Allergy. 1991;21(6):695–704.
67. Hide M, Francis DM, Grattan CE, Hakimi J, Kochan JP, Greaves MW. Autoantibodies against the high-affinity IgE receptor as a cause of histamine release in chronic urticaria. N Engl J Med. 1993;328(22):1599–604.
68. Niimi N, Francis DM, Kermani F, et al. Dermal mast cell activation by autoantibodies against the high affinity IgE receptor in chronic urticaria. J Invest Dermatol. 1996;106(5):1001–6.
69. Kolkhir P, Church MK, Weller K, Metz M, Schmetzer O, Maurer M. Autoimmune chronic spontaneous urticaria: what we know and what we do not know. J Allergy Clin Immunol. 2017;139(6):1772–178.
70. Kolkhir P, Metz M, Altrichter S, Maurer M. Comorbidity of chronic spontaneous urticaria and autoimmune thyroid diseases: a systematic review. Allergy. 2017;72(10):1440–60.

71. Chang TW, Chen C, Lin CJ, Metz M, Church MK, Maurer M. The potential pharmacologic mechanisms of omalizumab in patients with chronic spontaneous urticaria. J Allergy Clin Immunol. 2015;135(2):337–42.
72. Gericke J, Metz M, Ohanyan T, Weller K, Altrichter S, Skov PS, Falkencrone S, Brand J, Kromminga A, Hawro T, Church MK, Maurer M. Serum autoreactivity predicts time to response to omalizumab therapy in chronic spontaneous urticaria. J Allergy Clin Immunol. 2017;139(3):1059–61.
73. Schoepke N, Asero R, Ellrich A, Ferrer M, Gimenez-Arnau A, Grattan CE, Jakob T, Konstantinou GN, Raap U, Skov PS, Staubach P, Kromminga A, Zhang K, Bindslev-Jensen C, Daschner A, Kinaciyan T, Knol EF, Makris M, Marrouche N, Schmid-Grendelmeir P, Sussman G, Toubi E, Church MK, Maurer M. Biomarkers and clinical characteristics of autoimmune chronic spontaneous urticaria: results of the PURIST Study. Allergy. 2019;74(12):2427–36.
74. Altrichter S, Peter HJ, Pisarevskaja D, Metz M, Martus P, Maurer M. IgE mediated autoallergy against thyroid peroxidase—a novel pathomechanism of chronic spontaneous urticaria? PLoS One. 2011;6(4):e14794.
75. Hatada Y, Kashiwakura J, Hayama K, Fujisawa D, Sasaki-Sakamoto T, Terui T, Ra C, Okayama Y. Significantly high levels of anti-dsDNA immunoglobulin E in sera and the ability of dsDNA to induce the degranulation of basophils from chronic urticaria patients. Int Arch Allergy Immunol. 2013;161(Suppl 2):154–8.
76. Schmetzer O, Lakin E, Topal FA, et al. IL-24 is a common and specific autoantigen of IgE in patients with chronic spontaneous urticaria. J Allergy Clin Immunol. 2018;142(3):876–82.
77. Maurer M, Church MK, Goncalo M, Sussman G, Sanchez-Borges M. Management and treatment of chronic urticaria (CU). J Eur Acad Dermatol Venereol. 2015;29(Suppl 3):16–32.
78. Maurer M, Metz M, Brehler R, Hillen U, Jakob T, Mahler V, Pfohler C, Staubach P, Treudler R, Wedi B, Magerl M. Omalizumab treatment in patients with chronic inducible urticaria: a systematic review of published evidence. J Allergy Clin Immunol. 2018;141(2):638–49.
79. Hiragun M, Hiragun T, Ishii K, Suzuki H, Tanaka A, Yanase Y, Mihara S, Haruta Y, Kohno N, Hide M. Elevated serum IgE against MGL_1304 in patients with atopic dermatitis and cholinergic urticaria. Allergol Int. 2014;63(1):83–93.
80. Puccetti A, Bason C, Simeoni S, et al. In chronic idiopathic urticaria autoantibodies against Fc epsilonRII/CD23 induce histamine release via eosinophil activation. Clin Exp Allergy. 2005;35(12):1599–607.
81. Tatemoto K, Nozaki Y, Tsuda R, Konno S, Tomura K, Furuno M, Ogasawara H, Edamura K, Takagi H, Iwamura H, Noguchi M, Naito T. Immunoglobulin E-independent activation of mast cell is mediated by Mrg receptors. Biochem Biophys Res Commun. 2006,349(4):1322 8.
82. Fujisawa D, Kashiwakura J, Kita H, Kikukawa Y, Fujitani Y, Sasaki-Sakamoto T, Kuroda K, Nunomura S, Hayama K, Terui T, Ra C, Okayama Y. Expression of Mas-related gene X2 on mast cells is upregulated in the skin of patients with severe chronic urticaria. J Allergy Clin Immunol. 2014;134(3):622–33. e629
83. el-Lati SG, Dahinden CA, Church MK. Complement peptides C3a- and C5a-induced mediator release from dissociated human skin mast cells. J Invest Dermatol. 1994;102(5):803–6.
84. Fureder W, Agis H, Willheim M, Bankl HC, Maier U, Kishi K, Muller MR, Czerwenka K, Radaszkiewicz T, Butterfield JH, Klappacher GW, Sperr WR, Oppermann M, Lechner K, Valent P. Differential expression of complement receptors on human basophils and mast cells. Evidence for mast cell heterogeneity and CD88/C5aR expression on skin mast cells. J Immunol. 1995;155(6):3152–60.
85. Sabroe RA, Grattan CE, Francis DM, Barr RM, Kobza Black A, Greaves MW. The autologous serum skin test: a screening test for autoantibodies in chronic idiopathic urticaria. Br J Dermatol. 1999;140(3):446–52.
86. Fagiolo U, Kricek F, Ruf C, Peserico A, Amadori A, Cancian M. Effects of complement inactivation and IgG depletion on skin reactivity to autologous serum in chronic idiopathic urticaria. J Allergy Clin Immunol. 2000;106(3):567–72.

87. Grattan CE, Hamon CG, Cowan MA, Leeming RJ. Preliminary identification of a low molecular weight serological mediator in chronic idiopathic urticaria. Br J Dermatol. 1988;119(2):179–83.
88. Metz M, Giménez-Arnau A, Borzova E, Grattan CE, Magerl M, Maurer M. Frequency and clinical implications of skin autoreactivity to serum versus plasma in patients with chronic urticaria. J Allergy Clin Immunol. 2009;123(3):705–6.
89. Fusari A, Colangelo C, Bonifazi F, Antonicelli L. The autologous serum skin test in the follow-up of patients with chronic urticaria. Allergy. 2005;60(2):256–8.
90. Konstantinou GN, Asero R, Maurer M, Sabroe RA, Schmid-Grendelmeier P, Grattan CE. EAACI/GA(2)LEN task force consensus report: the autologous serum skin test in urticaria. Allergy. 2009;64(9):1256–68.
91. Altrich ML, Halsey JF, Altman LC. Comparison of the in vivo autologous skin test with in vitro diagnostic tests for diagnosis of chronic autoimmune urticaria. Allergy Asthma Proc. 2009;30(1):28–34.
92. Hoffmann HJ, Santos AF, Mayorga C, Nopp A, Eberlein B, Ferrer M, Rouzaire P, Ebo DG, Sabato V, Sanz ML, Pecaric-Petkovic T, Patil SU, Hausmann OV, Shreffler WG, Korosec P, Knol EF. The clinical utility of basophil activation testing in diagnosis and monitoring of allergic disease. Allergy. 2015;70(11):1393–405.
93. Hoffmann HJ, Knol EF, Ferrer M, Mayorga L, Sabato V, Santos AF, Eberlein B, Nopp A, MacGlashan D. Pros and cons of clinical basophil testing (BAT). Curr Allergy Asthma Rep. 2016;16(8):56.
94. Kolkhir P, Andre F, Church MK, Maurer M, Metz M. Potential blood biomarkers in chronic spontaneous urticaria. Clin Exp Allergy. 2017;47(1):19–36.
95. Lakin E, Church MK, Maurer M, Schmetzer O. On the lipophilic nature of the autoreactive IgE in chronic spontaneous urticaria. Theranostics. 2019;9:829–36.

Classification and Diagnosis of Urticaria

Torsten Zuberbier

Core Messages
- Urticaria is primarily mast-cell-induced.
- Depending on the level in the skin where mast cells degranulate, the clinical signs are superficial (hives) or deep swellings (angioedema).
- Urticaria is a disease entity with many subtypes and from various causes.
- The main classification method of urticaria is based on its symptoms, duration, frequency, and causes. The disease severity is patient-reported according to a 7-day urticaria activity score (UAS7).

3.1 Definition

Urticaria is defined by the rapid appearance of wheals, angioedema, or both (Figs. 3.1, 3.2, 3.3, 3.4, 3.5, and 3.6). Urticaria is a disease entity that encompasses several distinct subtypes. These subtypes need to be clearly differentiated, as diagnosis and treatment differ greatly. Furthermore, it must be emphasized that urticaria is a disease. Wheals and angioedema, the clinical symptoms, can also occur independently, e.g., in anaphylaxis. It is important to note that approximately 10–20% of urticaria patients present with angioedema only, yet if other sources of angioedema are ruled out, the mast cell driven histaminergic pathogenesis is the same as in wheals and angioedema.

T. Zuberbier (✉)
Institute for Allergology, Charité – Universitätsmedizin, Berlin, Germany

Fraunhofer Institute for Translational Medicine and Pharmacology ITMP, Allergology and Immunology, Berlin, Germany
e-mail: Torsten.Zuberbier@charite.de

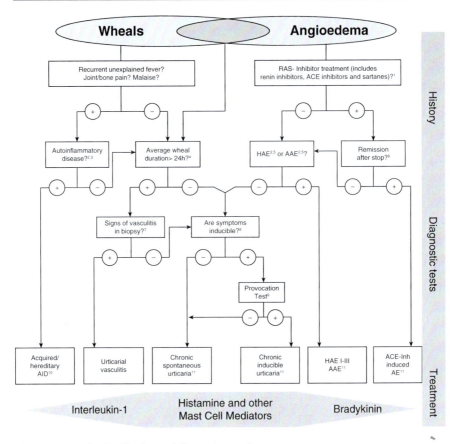

Fig. 3.1 Urticaria classification and diagnosis overview

Fig. 3.2 Spontaneous, single wheal in acute urticaria. ©ECARF

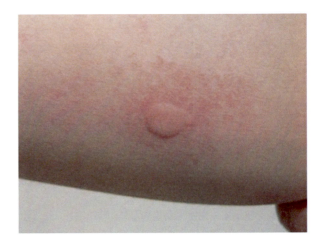

3 Classification and Diagnosis of Urticaria

Fig. 3.3 Annular wheals in chronic urticaria. ©ECARF

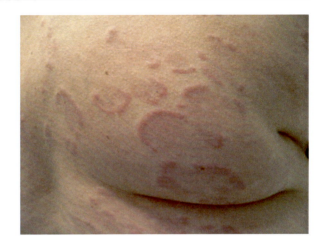

Fig. 3.4 Spontaneous angioedema. ©ECARF

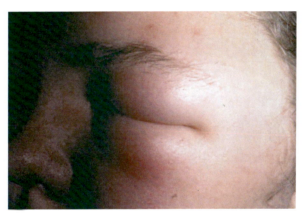

Fig. 3.5 Superficial wheals in chronic spontaneous urticaria. ©ECARF

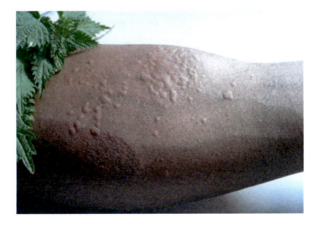

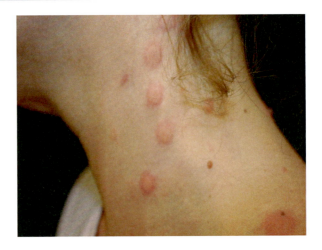

Fig. 3.6 Spontaneous wheals in chronic spontaneous urticaria resembling an ictus reaction. ©ECARF

Wheals are characterized by

- a central swelling of variable size, almost invariably surrounded by reflex erythema,
- an itching or sometimes burning sensation,
- a fleeting nature, with the skin returning to its normal appearance, usually within 30 min–24 h.

Angioedema is characterized by

- a sudden, pronounced erythematous or skin colored swelling of the lower dermis and subcutis or mucous membranes,
- sometimes pain, rather than itch.
- a resolution slower than that of wheals (can take up to 72 h).

3.2 Histology

The classic fleeting wheal displays edema of the upper- and mid-dermis, with dilatation of the post-capillary venules and lymphatic vessels of the upper dermis. Similar changes occur in angioedema, primarily in the lower dermis and the subcutis. Wheal-affected skin almost always exhibits upregulation of endothelial adhesion molecules and a mixed inflammatory perivascular infiltrate of variable intensity, consisting of neutrophils and/or eosinophils, macrophages, and T-helper lymphocytes [3]. A mild to moderate increase in mast cell numbers has also been observed. In delayed pressure urticaria, the infiltrate is typically located in the mid to lower dermis [4]. In some subtypes of urticaria, upregulation of adhesion molecules [5] and altered cytokine expression can also be seen in uninvolved skin [6].

These findings highlight the complex nature of the pathogenesis of urticaria, which has many features, in addition to the release of histamine from dermal mast cells. These changes are also seen in a wide variety of inflammatory reactions and are thus not specific or of diagnostic value.

3.3 Classification of Urticaria on the Basis of Its Symptoms, Duration, Frequency, and Causes

In the last three decades, many advances have been made in identifying the causes of the different types and subtypes of urticaria [7, 8], and the causes that are at the root of the disease's heterogeneity. Among others, chronic infections (such as Helicobacter pylori), non-allergic intolerance reactions to foods, and autoreactivity functional auto-antibodies directed against the IgE receptor have been described [9–13]. However, these different studies show considerable variation in the frequency of the eliciting factor, and in case of *Helicobacter* it could be shown that it is not the germ itself but the gastritis and reflux caused by it [14]. This may reflect differences in patient selection, underlining the need for a better classification of patients that will enable the comparison of results from different centers.

In the past, a number of attempts have been made to classify urticaria subtypes on the basis of underlying mechanisms, or in frustration of not knowing the cause using the term chronic idiopathic urticaria. The current guidelines [1] recommend a simple classification based on clinical symptoms, their duration, and if they are inducible.

However, the clinical manifestations of different urticaria subtypes also cover a very wide spectrum. Furthermore, two or more different subtypes of urticaria can coexist in any given patient. The current classification for clinical use according to the guidelines [1] is given in Table 3.1.

Urticaria pigmentosa (cutaneous mastocytosis), urticarial vasculitis, familial cold urticaria, and non-histaminergic angioedema (e.g., hereditary or acquired angioedema) are no longer considered subtypes of urticaria, but are listed in Table 3.2 for reference. Chronic urticaria or other subtypes of urticaria is observable in several eponymous syndromes (Table 3.2).

Disease activity and level of symptoms must also be considered when assessing the severity of urticaria. When symptoms arise due to physical triggers, an exact measurement of the intensity of the eliciting factor can be made, e.g., the temperature and duration of application in cold urticaria or pressure, and the duration of application until the appearance of lesions in delayed pressure urticaria. Assessing disease activity is more complex for non-physical acute and chronic urticaria. Several scoring systems have been proposed using scales from 0 to 3 or up to 10 points. The guidelines propose the use of unified scoring systems which are discussed in Chap. 4 that would facilitate comparison of study results from different centers. This simple scoring system (Table 3.3) is based on the assessment of key urticaria symptoms (wheals and pruritus). It can be used by urticaria patients and

Table 3.1 Classification of urticaria subtypes (presenting with wheals and/or angioedema)

Chronic urticaria subtypes	
Chronic spontaneous urticaria (CSU)	Inducible urticaria
Spontaneous appearance of wheals, angioedema, or both for >6 weeks due to known[a] or unknown causes	Symptomatic dermographism[b] Cold urticaria[c] Delayed pressure urticaria[d] Solar urticaria Heat urticaria[e] Vibratory angioedema Cholinergic urticaria Contact urticaria Aquagenic urticaria

[a]For example, autoreactivity, that is the presence of mast cell-activating auto-antibodies
[b]Also called urticaria factitia or dermographic urticaria
[c]Also called cold contact urticarial
[d]Also called pressure urticaria
[e]Also called heat contact urticaria

Table 3.2 Diseases related to urticaria for historical reasons and syndromes that include urticaria/angioedema [1]

- Maculopapular cutaneous mastocytosis (urticaria pigmentosa)
- Urticarial vasculitis
- Bradykinin-mediated angioedema (e.g., HAE)
- Exercise-induced anaphylaxis
- Cryopyrin-associated periodic syndromes (CAPS; urticarial rash, recurrent fever attacks, arthralgia or arthritis, eye inflammation, fatigue and headaches), that is familial cold auto-inflammatory syndrome (FCAS), Muckle–Wells syndrome (MWS) or neonatal-onset multisystem inflammatory disease (NOMID)
- Schnitzler's syndrome (recurrent urticarial rash and monoclonal gammopathy, recurrent fever attacks, bone and muscle pain, arthralgia or arthritis, and lymphadenopathy)
- Gleich's syndrome (episodic angioedema with eosinophilia)
- Well's syndrome (granulomatous dermatitis with eosinophilia/eosinophilic cellulitis)
- Bullous pemphigoid (prebullous stage)

Table 3.3 Assessment of disease activity in urticaria patients [1]

Score	Wheals	Pruritus
0	None	None
1	Mild (<20 wheals/24 h)	Mild (present but not annoying or troublesome)
2	Moderate (20–50 wheals/24 h)	Moderate (troublesome but does not interfere with normal daily activity or sleep)
3	Intense (>50 wheals/24 h or large confluent areas of wheals)	Intense (severe pruritus, which is sufficiently troublesome to interfere with normal daily activity or sleep)

Sum of score: 0–6

their treating physicians to evaluate disease activity. The UAS7 is then simply calculated by adding the results of seven consecutive days.

As urticaria symptoms frequently change in intensity during the day, overall disease activity can most effectively be monitored by having patients record 24-h self-evaluation scores over a period of several days. Additionally, a single time point evaluation and/or sequential physical examinations by the treating physician can help to make the patient's score more objective.

Other issues that have not received sufficient attention in the current guidelines and which are an urgent and unmet need in research are inter-patient and within-patient differences in the appearance of wheals before and after treatment. In general, larger and longer standing wheals indicate that the disease is more severe and more difficult to treat. However, the appearance of angioedema, often frightening patients, is not a sign of severity itself, and angioedema responds equally well to the same treatment as wheals. Regarding wheals, the color may provide a useful clue to the nature of the disease. Histamine-induced wheals are of a light color and surrounded by a pink erythema, which is caused by the dilatation of cutaneous vessels. Wheals of a dark red or violaceous color may reflect intense vascular damage and leakage in association with wheal formation, as found in urticarial vasculitis.

3.4 Diagnosis of Urticaria

3.4.1 Diagnostic Work Up in Acute Urticaria

As acute urticarial is normally self-limiting, no standard diagnostic workup is required. The only exception is the suspicion of a determinable eliciting factor such as type I food allergy in sensitized patients or nonsteroidal anti-inflammatory drugs (NSAIDs), where targeted diagnostics should be performed.

3.4.2 The Diagnostic Work Up in CU

In CSU the diagnostic work up aims at (1) exclusion of differential diagnoses, (2) assessment of disease activity, impact, and control, and (3) identification of exacerbating and underlying factors.

For the first aim it is necessary to rule out urticarial vasculitis and auto-inflammatory disorders such as Schnitzler syndrome or cryopyrin-associated periodic syndromes (CAPS) in patients with wheals (but no angioedema). In those with recurrent angioedema only (but no wheals) bradykinin-mediated angioedema-like angiotensin-converting enzyme (ACE) inhibitor-induced angioedema or other non-mast cell-related angioedema, that is HAE type 1–3, should be considered.

For (2) a baseline assessment should be made including disease activity (UAS, AAS), quality of life (CU-Q2oL, AE-QoL), and disease control (UCT). Aside from facilitating documentation work, those are necessary for guiding treatment decisions by providing insight into the patients' burden of disease.

For the identification of factors relevant for the course of the disease it is important to take a detailed history. Further diagnostic procedures based on the patient's history should be chosen carefully. Although progress has been made in the identification of causes of different types and subtypes of chronic urticarial in recent years (for example, in autoimmunity mediated by functional auto-antibodies directed against the high-affinity IgE receptor or IgE-auto-antibodies to auto-antigens, non-allergic hypersensitivity reactions to foods or drugs, and acute or chronic infections, e.g., Helicobacter pylori or Anisakis simplex) there are considerable variations in frequency and accountable triggers in the available research. This may also reflect regional differences, possibly attributable to dietary habits and prevalence of relevant infections. Therefore, the first step is a thorough history considering the following aspects:

1. Time of onset of disease
2. Shape, size, frequency/duration, and distribution of wheals
3. Associated angioedema
4. Associated symptoms, for example, bone/joint pain, fever, abdominal cramps
5. Family and personal history regarding wheals and angioedema
6. Induction by physical agents or exercise
7. Occurrence in relation to daytime, weekends, menstrual cycle, holidays, and foreign travel
8. Occurrence in relation to foods or drugs (e.g., NSAIDs, ACE inhibitors)
9. Occurrence in relation to infections, stress
10. Previous or current allergies, infections, internal/autoimmune diseases, gastric/intestinal problems or other disorders
11. Social and occupational history, leisure activities
12. Previous therapy and response to therapy including dosage and duration
13. Previous diagnostic procedures/results

The second step of the diagnosis is the physical examination of the patient. Where it is indicated by history and/or physical examination, further appropriate diagnostic tests should be performed. The selection of these diagnostic measures largely depends on the nature of the urticaria subtype, as summarized in Fig. 3.1 and Table 3.4.

It is not advised to perform general screening programmes for causes of CU which are intensive and costly. Also, the diagnostic programme should be individualized, based on patient history only. CU is extremely rarely, attributable to type I allergy, pseudo-allergic (non-allergic hypersensitivity reactions) to NSAIDs or food, however, may be more relevant for CSU. In those cases, diagnosis should be based on history of NSAID intake or a pseudo-allergic elimination diet protocol. Regarding infections, several bacterial, viral, parasitic, or fungal infections have been implicated as underlying causes of urticarial, among these *H. pylori*, streptococci, staphylococci, *Yersinia, Giardia lamblia, Mycoplasma pneumoniae*, hepatitis viruses, *norovirus, parvovirus B19, Anisakis simplex, Entamoeba* spp, and *Blastocystis* spp. [15–17]. Frequency and relevance of those, however, vary between

3 Classification and Diagnosis of Urticaria

Table 3.4 Recommended diagnostic tests in frequent urticaria subtypes [1]

Types	Subtypes	Routine diagnostic tests (recommended)	Extended diagnostic programme[a] (based on history) for identification of underlying causes or eliciting factors and for ruling out possible differential diagnoses if indicated
Spontaneous urticaria	Acute spontaneous urticaria	None	None[b]
	Chronic spontaneous urticaria	Differential blood count. ESR and/or CRP	Avoidance of suspected triggers (e.g., drugs); Conduction of diagnostic tests for (in no preferred order): (1) infectious diseases (e.g., Helicobacter pylori); (2) functional auto-antibodies (e.g., autologous skin serum test); (3) thyroid gland disorders (thyroid hormones and auto-antibodies); (4) allergy (skin tests and/or allergen avoidance test, e.g., avoidance diet); (5) concomitant CIndU, see below [35]; (6) severe systemic diseases (e.g., tryptase); (7) other (e.g., lesional skin biopsy)
Inducible urticaria	Cold urticaria	Cold provocation test and threshold test[c,d]	Differential blood count and ESR or CRP, rule out other diseases, especially infections [36]
	Delayed pressure urticaria	Pressure test and threshold test[c,d]	None
	Heat urticaria	Heat provocation and threshold test[c,d]	None
	Solar urticaria	UV and visible light of different wavelengths and threshold test[c]	Rule out other light-induced dermatoses
	Symptomatic dermographism	Elicit dermographism and threshold test[c,d]	Differential blood count, ESR or CRP
	Vibratory angioedema	Test with vibration, for example, Vortex or mixer[d]	None
	Aquagenic urticaria	Provocation testing[d]	None
	Cholinergic urticaria	Provocation and threshold testing[d]	None
	Contact urticaria	Provocation testing[d]	None

ESR erythrocyte sedimentation rate, *CRP* C-reactive protein
[a]Depending on suspected cause
[b]Unless strongly suggested by patient history, for example, allergy
[c]All tests are carried out with different levels of the potential trigger to determine the threshold
[d]For details on provocation and threshold testing see [35]

different patient groups and different geographical regions. The sea fish nematode, Anisakis simplex, for example, has only been discussed as having potential for eliciting recurrent acute spontaneous urticaria in areas of the world where raw fish is eaten frequently [18]. Also, the relevance of other infections like *H. pylori*, dental or ear, nose, and throat infections also appears to vary between patient groups [17, 19–21] and more research is needed to make definitive recommendations.

Although a slightly increased prevalence of neoplastic diseases in CU patients has been reported in Taiwan, it is also not advised to perform routine screening for malignancies since there is no sufficient evidence for a causal correlation. Of course, it should be ruled out if a patient's history suggests the possibility of a malignant disease. The only tests available for screening of auto-antibodies against either IgE or FceR1 (the high-affinity IgE receptor) are the autologous serum skin test (ASST) and basophil activation tests (BATs). The ASST evaluates the presence of serum histamine-releasing factors of any type and not only auto-antibodies. It should be performed with utmost care as the transmission of infections is possible if the patient's serums are confounded. This is also subject of a separate EAACI/GA2LEN position paper [22, 23]. In the BAT, histamine release or upregulation of activation markers of donor basophils in response to stimulation with the serum of CSU patients is assessed. BATs may be helpful to co-assess disease activity in urticarial patients [24, 25], in the diagnosis of autoimmune urticaria [26] and as marker for responsiveness to ciclosporin A or omalizumab [27, 28].

Multiple research groups noted blood basopenia and suppressed IgE receptor-mediated histamine release to anti-IgE by blood basophils in some patients with active CSU. An association of CSU remission with an increase in blood basophil numbers and IgE receptor-triggered histamine response could be seen [29, 30] as well as blood basophils in the skin lesions of CSU patients [31]. When anti-IgE-treatment is done, a rise in basophil numbers can be observed [32]. Since these findings need to be investigated further, there is currently no diagnostic recommendation, and it should be noted that a low basophil blood count should not result in further diagnostic procedures. Another known parameter is significantly elevated D-dimers in patients with active CSU and a decline of D-dimer levels correlating with the clinical response of the disease to omalizumab. As the relevance of this finding is not clear there is currently no recommendation for measuring D-dimers in CSU patients [33, 34].

3.4.2.1 Assessment of Disease Activity Impact and Control

The UAS7 is a unified and simple scoring system that has been validated for the assessment of disease activity in CSU and should be used in both clinical care and trials of CSU. It has been proposed in the last version of the urticarial guidelines and assesses the key signs and symptoms of urticaria. Since the patient is in charge of documenting the symptoms this score is especially valuable and its standardized collection of patient data facilitates the comparison of study resulting from different care and research centers. Disease activity in CSU may change frequently, therefore the overall disease activity is best monitored if the patients use 24-h self-evaluation scores once daily for several days. The UAS7 is a sum score of 7 consecutive days that should be used in routine clinical practice to assess disease activity and treatment response. For patients with angioedema, the angioedema activity score (AAS) may be used, which is validated for the assessment of angioedema. Other important factors that should be regularly assessed are the patient's quality of life and disease control, both in clinical care and research trials. The urticaria control test (UCT) has only recently proved to be a valuable tool to assess and monitor the status of the patient's disease [37, 38]. It may be used in all forms of CU (CSU and CIndU), has only 4 items with a clearly defined cut-off for patients with "well controlled" vs "poorly controlled" disease, and it is thus suited for the management of patients in routine clinical practice and in the guidance of treatment decisions. The cut-off value for a well-controlled disease is 12 of 16 possible points.

The assessment of disease activity, impact, and control should be done at the first and every follow-up visit. Some tools, like the UAS develop their informative value over time and can only be used prospectively. Others, like the UCT, allow for retrospective assessment. Validated instruments such as the UAS7, AAS, CU-Q2oL, AE-QoL, and UCT should be used in CU for this purpose.

Take Home Pearls
- Urticaria is the name of the disease independent if wheals, angioedema, or both occur.
- More than one subtype of urticaria can coexist in one patient.
- A robust score for assessing disease activity is the UAS based on 24 h self-observation of patient's grading symptoms from 0 to 3 for wheals and pruritus, for a duration of 7 days.

References

1. Zuberbier T, Aberer W, Asero R, Abdul Latiff AH, Baker D, Ballmer-Weber B, Bernstein JA, Bindslev-Jensen C, Brzoza Z, Buense Bedrikow R, Canonica GW, Church MK, Craig T, Danilycheva IV, Dressler C, Ensina LF, Gimenez-Arnau A, Godse K, Goncalo M, Grattan C, Hebert J, Hide M, Kaplan A, Kapp A, Katelaris CH, Kocaturk E, Kulthanan K, Larenas-Linnemann D, Leslie TA, Magerl M, Mathelier-Fusade P, Meshkova RY, Metz M, Nast A, Nettis E, Oude-Elberink H, Rosumeck S, Saini SS, Sanchez-Borges M, Schmid-Grendelmeier P, Staubach P, Sussman G, Toubi E, Vena GA, Vestergaard C, Wedi B, Werner RN, Zhao Z, Maurer M, Endorsed by the following societies: AAAAI AADAAAAAABADBCDACCDD, WAO. The EAACI/GA(2)LEN/EDF/WAO guideline for the definition, classification, diagnosis and management of urticaria. Allergy. 2018;73(7):1393–414.
2. Magerl M, Borzova E, Gimenez-Arnau A, Grattan CE, Lawlor F, Mathelier-Fusade P, Metz M, Mlynek A, Maurer M, EAACI/Ga2Len/EDF/UNEV. The definition and diagnostic testing of physical and cholinergic urticarias—EAACI/GA2LEN/EDF/UNEV consensus panel recommendations. Allergy. 2009;64(12):1715–21.
3. Haas N, Schadendorf D, Henz BM. Endothelial adhesion molecules in immediate and delayed urticarial whealing reactions. Int Arch Allergy Immunol. 1998;115:210–4.
4. Barlow RJ, Ross EL, MacDonald D, Black AK, Greaves MW. Adhesion molecule expression and the inflammatory cell infiltrate in delayed pressure urticaria. Br J Dermatol. 1994;131(3):341–7.

5. Zuberbier T, Schadendorf D, Haas N, Hartmann K, Henz BM. Enhanced P-selectin expression in chronic and dermographic urticaria. Int Arch Allergy Immunol. 1997;114(1):86–9.
6. Hermes B, Prochazka AK, Haas N, Jurgovsky K, Sticherling M, Henz BM. Upregulation of TNF-alpha and IL-3 expression in lesional and uninvolved skin in different types of urticaria. J Allergy Clin Immunol. 1999;103(2 Pt 1):307–14.
7. Zuberbier T. Urticaria. Allergy. 2003;58(12):1224–34.
8. Juhlin L. Recurrent urticaria: clinical investigation of 330 patients. Br J Dermatol. 1981;104(4):369–81.
9. Zuberbier T, Chantraine-Hess S, Hartmann K, Czarnetzki BM. Pseudoallergen-free diet in the treatment of chronic urticaria. A prospective study. Acta Derm Venereol. 1995;75(6):484–7.
10. Hide M, Francis DM, Grattan CE, Hakimi J, Kochan JP, Greaves MW. Autoantibodies against the high-affinity IgE receptor as a cause of histamine release in chronic urticaria. N Engl J Med. 1993;328(22):1599–604.
11. Buhner S, Reese I, Kuehl F, Lochs H, Zuberbier T. Pseudoallergic reactions in chronic urticaria are associated with altered gastroduodenal permeability. Allergy. 2004;59(10):1118–23.
12. Kolkhir P, Balakirski G, Merk HF, Olisova O, Maurer M. Chronic spontaneous urticaria and internal parasites—a systematic review. Allergy. 2016;71(3):308–22.
13. Fiebiger E, Hammerschmid F, Stingl G, Maurer D. Anti-FcepsilonRIalpha autoantibodies in autoimmune-mediated disorders. Identification of a structure-function relationship. J Clin Invest. 1998;101(1):243–51.
14. Zheleznov S, Urzhumtseva G, Petrova N, Sarsaniia Z, Didkovskii N, Dorr T, Zuberbier T. Gastritis can cause and trigger chronic spontaneous urticaria independent of the presence of Helicobacter pylori. Int Arch Allergy Immunol. 2018;175(4):246–51.
15. Imbalzano E, Casciaro M, Quartuccio S, Minciullo PL, Cascio A, Calapai G, Gangemi S. Association between urticaria and virus infections: a systematic review. Allergy Asthma Proc. 2016;37(1):18–22.
16. Minciullo PL, Cascio A, Barberi G, Gangemi S. Urticaria and bacterial infections. Allergy Asthma Proc. 2014;35(4):295–302.
17. Foti C, Nettis E, Cassano N, Di Mundo I, Vena GA. Acute allergic reactions to Anisakis simplex after ingestion of anchovies. Acta Derm Venereol. 2002;82(2):121–3.
18. Dionigi PC, Menezes MC, Forte WC. A prospective ten-year follow-up of patients with chronic urticaria. Allergol Immunopathol (Madr). 2016;44(4):286–91.
19. Shabrawy RM, Gharib K. Helicobacter pylori Infection as a risk factor in patients suffering from food allergy and urticaria. Egypt J Immunol. 2016;23(1):67–75.
20. Curth HM, Dinter J, Nigemeier K, Kutting F, Hunzelmann N, Steffen HM. Effects of Helicobacter pylori eradication in chronic spontaneous urticaria: results from a retrospective cohort study. Am J Clin Dermatol. 2015;16(6):553–8.
21. Rasooly MM, Moye NA, Kirshenbaum AS. Helicobacter pylori: a significant and treatable cause of chronic urticaria and angioedema. Nurse Pract. 2015;40(10):1–6.
22. Konstantinou GN, Asero R, Maurer M, Sabroe RA, Schmid-Grendelmeier P, Grattan CE. EAACI/GA(2)LEN task force consensus report: the autologous serum skin test in urticaria. Allergy. 2009;64(9):1256–68.
23. Konstantinou GN, Asero R, Ferrer M, Knol EF, Maurer M, Raap U, Schmid-Grendelmeier P, Skov PS, Grattan CE. EAACI taskforce position paper: evidence for autoimmune urticaria and proposal for defining diagnostic criteria. Allergy. 2013;68(1):27–36.
24. Curto-Barredo L, Yelamos J, Gimeno R, Mojal S, Pujol RM, Gimenez-Arnau A. Basophil activation test identifies the patients with chronic spontaneous urticaria suffering the most active disease. Immun Inflamm Dis. 2016;4(4):441–5.
25. Netchiporouk E, Moreau L, Rahme E, Maurer M, Lejtenyi D, Ben-Shoshan M. Positive CD63 basophil activation tests are common in children with chronic spontaneous urticaria and linked to high disease activity. Int Arch Allergy Immunol. 2016;171(2):81–8.
26. Kim Z, Choi BS, Kim JK, Won DI. Basophil markers for identification and activation in the indirect basophil activation test by flow cytometry for diagnosis of autoimmune urticaria. Ann Lab Med. 2016;36(1):28–35.

27. Iqbal K, Bhargava K, Skov PS, Falkencrone S, Grattan CE. A positive serum basophil histamine release assay is a marker for ciclosporin-responsiveness in patients with chronic spontaneous urticaria. Clin Transl Allergy. 2012;2(1):19.
28. Gericke J, Metz M, Ohanyan T, Weller K, Altrichter S, Skov PS, Falkencrone S, Brand J, Kromminga A, Hawro T, Church MK, Maurer M. Serum autoreactivity predicts time to response to omalizumab therapy in chronic spontaneous urticaria. J Allergy Clin Immunol. 2017;139(3):1059–61.e1.
29. Eckman JA, Hamilton RG, Gober LM, Sterba PM, Saini SS. Basophil phenotypes in chronic idiopathic urticaria in relation to disease activity and autoantibodies. J Invest Dermatol. 2008;128(8):1956–63.
30. Grattan CE, Dawn G, Gibbs S, Francis DM. Blood basophil numbers in chronic ordinary urticaria and healthy controls: diurnal variation, influence of loratadine and prednisolone and relationship to disease activity. Clin Exp Allergy. 2003;33(3):337–41.
31. Kay AB, Ying S, Ardelean E, Mlynek A, Kita H, Clark P, Maurer M. Elevations in vascular markers and eosinophils in chronic spontaneous urticarial weals with low-level persistence in uninvolved skin. Br J Dermatol. 2014;171(3):505–11.
32. Saini SS, Omachi TA, Trzaskoma B, Hulter HN, Rosen K, Sterba PM, Courneya JP, Lackey A, Chen H. Effect of omalizumab on blood basophil counts in patients with chronic idiopathic/spontaneous urticaria. J Invest Dermatol. 2017;137(4):958–61.
33. Kolkhir P, Andre F, Church MK, Maurer M, Metz M. Potential blood biomarkers in chronic spontaneous urticaria. Clin Exp Allergy. 2017;47(1):19–36.
34. Asero R, Marzano AV, Ferrucci S, Cugno M. D-dimer plasma levels parallel the clinical response to omalizumab in patients with severe chronic spontaneous urticaria. Int Arch Allergy Immunol. 2017;172(1):40–4.
35. Magerl M, Altrichter S, Borzova E, Gimenez-Arnau A, Grattan CE, Lawlor F, Mathelier-Fusade P, Meshkova RY, Zuberbier T, Metz M, Maurer M. The definition, diagnostic testing, and management of chronic inducible urticarias—The EAACI/GA(2) LEN/EDF/UNEV consensus recommendations 2016 update and revision. Allergy. 2016;71(6):780–802.
36. Maurer M. Cold urticaria: Wolters Kluwer Health; 2014 [updated 10 May 2019. Topic 8102 Version 21.0].
37. Ohanyan T, Schoepke N, Bolukbasi B, Metz M, Hawro T, Zuberbier T, Peveling-Oberhag A, Staubach P, Maurer M, Weller K. Responsiveness and minimal important difference of the urticaria control test. J Allergy Clin Immunol. 2017;140(6):1710–3.e11.
38. Weller K, Groffik A, Church MK, Hawro T, Krause K, Metz M, Martus P, Casale TB, Staubach P, Maurer M. Development and validation of the urticaria control test: a patient-reported outcome instrument for assessing urticaria control. J Allergy Clin Immunol. 2014;133(5):1365–72, 1372 e1–6.

Impact of Chronic Urticaria and How to Measure It

4

Karsten Weller

Core Messages
- Most CSU patients suffer from daily or almost daily occurring itchy wheals, angioedema, or both. A key characteristic of the disorder is its unpredictability, i.e., patients never know when, where, and how strong their symptoms will occur.
- CSU has a major physical, emotional, and social impact on the patients' lives and is frequently associated with an impairment of daily life activities, sleep deprivation, and psychiatric comorbidities.
- In addition to its humanistic burden, CSU often goes long with a significant economic burden, including missed school or work days, and reduced performance at work.
- Due to the fluctuating nature of CSU and since objective and specific biomarkers are not yet established, validated patient-reported outcome measures (PROMs) should be used to assess and monitor the patient's disease status and disease impact.
- Disease activity, i.e., the frequency and severity of CSU signs and symptoms, can be measured prospectively with the Urticaria Activity Score (UAS) and/or Angioedema Activity Score (AAS) in a diary-type manner.
- HRQoL can be assessed with the Chronic Urticaria Quality of Life Questionnaire (CU-Q2oL) and/or with the Angioedema Quality of Life Questionnaire (AE-QoL), which provide important insights on the disease burden from the patient perspective.
- Disease control can be determined with the Urticaria Control Test (UCT) and/or the Angioedema Control Test (AECT) to distinguish well-controlled from poorly controlled disease and to determine the need for treatment adjustments.

K. Weller (✉)
Institute for Allergology, Charité – Universitätsmedizin, Berlin, Germany
e-mail: karsten.weller@charite.de

- The clinical pattern of chronic inducible urticaria (CIndU) is different from CSU and so is its impact. In addition to troublesome signs and symptoms, disease burden is strongly determined by the required avoidance of triggers.
- First PROMs specifically designed to assess the disease status of patients with CIndU have been published recently, i.e., the Cholinergic Urticaria Activity Score (CholUAS) and the Cholinergic Urticaria Quality of Life Questionnaire (CholU-QoL). Additional tools for the most common forms of CIndU are currently under development.

The skin is the most visible organ of the human body, and the face and hands are critical for communication and social interactions [1]. Skin that appears healthy is essential for positive self-perception and social life [1]. Moreover, it is particularly abundant of sensory nerves, and any disturbance can have a great impact on physical and mental well-being [1]. Accordingly, skin diseases, even those with a benign course, can have a major impact on patients' lives [1].

Chronic urticaria (CU) belongs to the skin disorders with a particularly high disease burden, and CU frequently and substantially affects the patients' quality of life [2]. To provide a better insight into this important topic, this chapter addresses three important questions: (1) what makes urticaria such a burdensome condition, (2) what is known about the extent, pattern, and drivers of disease burden, and (3) how to best assess and monitor disease burden in real life as well as in clinical studies.

4.1　What Makes Chronic Urticaria a Burdensome Condition

Chronic spontaneous urticaria (CSU) comes with strongly fluctuating disease activity and is characterized by the recurrent and spontaneous occurrence of itchy wheals, angioedema, or both [3]. In contrast, chronic inducible urticarias (CIndUs) are characterized by specific triggers, which are required for urticarial signs and symptoms to occur and reproducibly induce them [4]. Accordingly, the characteristics and, as a consequence, also the impact of disease are different in CSU and CIndUs.

4.1.1　Physical, Social, and Emotional Burden in Chronic Spontaneous Urticaria

In CSU, various factors are responsible for its considerable disease burden (Fig. 4.1). Many patients suffer from daily or almost daily itchy wheals and/or angioedema, but the timing of their occurrence, their severity, and duration can change considerably from day to day [4]. Moreover, they often occur during the evening, night time, or early morning [5]. This makes the disorder highly unpredictable and many patients have a constant expectation or even fear of suddenly appearing new wheals and/or angioedema [6], including the fear of suffocation [7]. CSU patients never know when, where, for how long, and how strong their urticaria signs and

4 Impact of Chronic Urticaria and How to Measure It

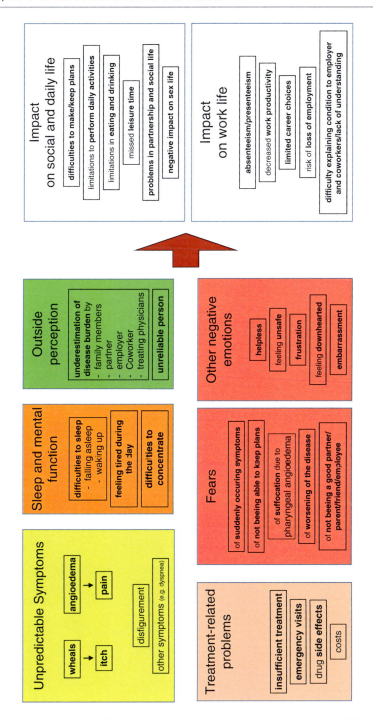

Fig. 4.1 Important factors making chronic spontaneous urticaria a burdensome condition

symptoms will occur. This causes high levels of uncertainty and many patients have the feeling of loosing control over their lives [6].

CSU has an important impact on social interactions. Affected patients are at an increased risk to be regarded as unreliable in private and work life. The unpredictability of the signs and symptoms of CSU makes it difficult to make and keep plans or require patients to unexpectedly cancel plans [6] and/or to stay at home with the consequence of missed social activities [6] and an increased risk for social isolation. Furthermore, CSU frequently has a negative impact on partnership and sex life [6, 8].

The emotional impact of CSU is high [9]. Many patients experience negative emotions related to their disease, such as self-consciousness and embarassement [6], frustration [6], feeling downhearted [10, 11], helpless, anxious [6, 9, 11, 12], or unsafe. These negative emotions may be additionally fueled by an underestimation of their disease burden by others, such as partners, family members, coworkers, employers, and even by treating physicians [13]. Notably, the perception of disease severity was found to be clearly discordant between physicians and patients in independent studies [12, 13].

4.1.2 Itch, Sleep Impairment, and Psychiatric Comorbidities in Chronic Spontaneous Urticaria

CSU has a considerable impact on sleep and cognitive functions [5, 6, 9, 11, 12, 14]. Affected patients frequently suffer from difficulties falling asleep and wake up during the night [10, 15]. As a consequence, they feel tired during the day and experience difficulties to concentrate [10]. The latter may be caused by the impaired night time sleep but also by itch during the daytime. It is well-established that chronic itch, a hallmark feature of CSU, often leads to sleep deprivation [16], and sleep deprivation in turn modulates itch perception [17]. Notably, CSU patients frequently suffer from one or more psychiatric comorbidities, such as anxiety, depression, and somatoform disorders [18]. Anxiety and depression also go along with sleep deprivation [19] and, in turn, sleep disturbance and short sleep are known risk factors for depression [20]. Finally, chronic itch may facilitate psychiatric disorders [21, 22], and these are, in turn, able to increase itch perception [15, 23]. This unfavorable triangle of interactions between chronic itch, sleep deprivation, and psychiatric disorders (Fig. 4.2) is an important aspect of CSU and relevant for its impact.

With regard to psychiatric comorbidities, it is still a subject of discussions whether CSU increases the risk of psychiatric disorders or vice versa. Notably, the results of a recent study examining the efficacy of omalizumab or placebo in CSU with angioedema indicated that at least depressive mood seems to be rather a reaction to CSU [7]. While the mean score of the WHO-5, a screening tool for depression, was <13 for both treatment groups at baseline (indicative for depression), approximately 80% of patients showed no signs of depression (≥13 points in the WHO-5) following treatment with omalizumab compared with approximately 40% in the placebo group [7]. Thus, omalizumab treatment did not only lead to an improvement of CSU signs and symptoms but also to an improvement of

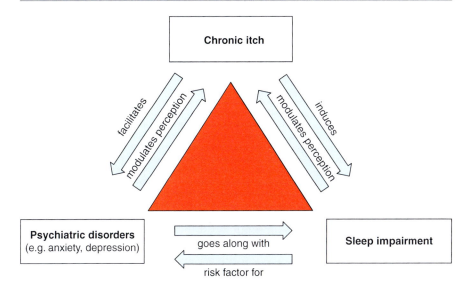

Fig. 4.2 The unfavorable triangle of chronic itch, sleep impairment, and psychiatric comorbidity in chronic spontaneous urticaria

psychological symptoms [7]. Interestingly, omalizumab has also been proven to improve sleep problems in CSU patients [24].

4.1.3 Impairment of Daily Activities and Work Productivity in Chronic Spontaneous Urticaria

CSU has a major impact on daily life activities [9, 11] and work productivity [9, 11] and causes a considerable economic burden. It frequently leads to missed working days (absenteeism) and a reduced performance at work (presenteeism) or school [6, 9, 25]. Itch and angioedema are the main drivers in this context [9] and presenteeism is the major factor [9]. For individual patients, this means to have limited career choices or even to encounter severe problems with their employer. From an overarching perspective, this implies that CSU not only goes along with considerable direct health care costs [9, 11, 26, 27], but is also a costly condition for the society [9].

4.1.4 Disease Burden in Chronic Inducible Urticaria

The impact of CIndU is different from the impact of CSU, due to its distinct clinical pattern. Apart from the physical impact caused by the signs and symptoms, disease burden in CIndUs is strongly determined by the required avoidance of triggers and the associated impairment of daily life activities and social interactions as well as their emotional impact. Even when patients seem to have relatively few signs and symptoms this might just be the result of their effective avoidance behavior and does not provide relevant information on their actual disease status and individual disease burden. This clinical pattern puts CIndU patients at a particular risk for underestimation of their disease burden.

4.2 Extent, Pattern, and Drivers of Disease Burden

The World Health Organization (WHO) defines health as a state of complete physical, mental, and social well-being. As described above, CSU has a major impact on all three of these health dimensions. It is obvious that just assessing the frequency and severity of CSU signs and symptoms is not a suitable way to gain a comprehensive picture of its overall disease burden [2]. A more holistic and comprehensive way to measure the burden of CU is the assessment of health-related quality of life (HRQoL) [2]. HRQoL assesses the patient perspective and can be defined as the way patients perceive and react to their health status [28]. With regard to its dimensions, HRQoL can be defined as a concept that measures a persons perceived well-being in physical, mental, and social domains of health as well as how well a person functions in his or her life [29].

4.2.1 HRQoL Impairment in Chronic Spontaneous Urticaria

The pioneer work examining HRQoL impairment in CSU was published almost 25 years ago by O'Donnel and coworkers [6]. They applied a self-designed disease-specific questionnaire for urticaria as well as the Nottingham health profile (NHP) [30]. With their own questionnaire, they found that CSU patients frequently have problems attributable to their skin condition in many facets of everyday life including home management, personal care, recreation and social interaction, mobility, emotional factors, sleep, rest, and work [6]. With the NHP they were able to show that CSU goes along with restrictions in the areas of mobility, sleep, energy, and demonstrated pain, social isolation, and altered emotional reactions [6]. In addition, they revealed that CSU patients and patients with severe coronary artery disease waiting for bypass grafting suffer in many aspects a comparable HRQoL impairment, i.e., energy, social isolation, and emotional reaction [6]. Asked for the worst aspects of their disease, CSU patients stressed the unpredictability of their disease, angioedema, itch, feelings of being tired, irritable, weak, or a feeling of loss of control over their lives [6]. Other problems were social restrictions, feeling embarrassed, time off work, restriction of food or clothing, side-effects of drugs, and being unable to relax or sit [6]. In summary, their results made absolutely clear that patients with CSU exhibit severe restrictions in all areas of health.

Since the work of O'Donnel and colleagues, several other studies have confirmed and extended their results [10, 31–33]. Grob and coworkers compared HRQoL impairment in CSU with that in atopic dermatitis and psoriasis with the VQ-Dermato, a multidimensional instrument in French validated for chronic skin diseases [32].

As expected, they found completely different HRQoL profiles in the three disorders, influenced by their clinical characteristics and usual treatment options, but the overall HRQoL impairment was comparable in CSU and psoriasis patients, which was later confirmed independently [11]. With their work Grob et al. corrected a common perspective, particularly of physicians, that psoriasis and atopic dermatitis but not CSU may severely affect HRQoL.

Baiardini and colleagues compared HRQoL of CU-patients to a reference sample as well as to patients with respiratory allergy employing two generic tools, the SF-36 (a health status questionnaire) and the SAT-P (a satisfaction profile) [31]. They found CSU patients to have an impairment in all examined HRQoL dimensions, and a higher impairment than respiratory allergy patients. CSU patients had low satisfaction levels with regard to sleep (quantity and quality), physical well-being, resistance to stress and mood. Compared with patients with respiratory allergy, patients with CSU reported lower satisfaction levels in many aspects of daily life related to sleep, eating behavior, psychological functioning, and work. In summary, they confirmed that the symptomatology of CU affects many daily life activities, limits and impairs physical and emotional functioning, and acts as an indirect burden on life satisfaction [31].

Lewis and Finlay published an overview of results obtained with the Dermatology Life Quality Index (DLQI), the most widely applied HRQoL measure in the field of dermatology [33]. Their results made clear that CSU belongs to a group of skin disorders with a particularly strong HRQoL impairment. In addition, they showed that (1) skin disorders with chronic itch as a major component, such as atopic dermatitis, chronic pruritus, chronic prurigo as well as (2) skin disorders with high visibility, such as acne, hirsutism, and melasma have the lowest levels of HRQoL. Both aspects are key factors of CSU.

In 2005, Baiardini et al. published the first disease-specific HRQoL questionnaire for CSU, the Chronic Urticaria Quality of Life Questionnaire (CU-Q$_2$oL) [10]. The development and selection of its questions were carefully done by including input from clinical and research experts as well as from affected patients to make sure that only those topics were included that really matter to patients [10]. The CU-Q$_2$oL results impressively confirmed the major impact of CSU on daily activities, physical and emotional well-being, and social interactions. In addition, the CU-Q$_2$oL development process highlighted sleep deprivation as a major problem in CSU patients with 3 of the 23 final items addressing sleep impairment or sleep related problems.

Further studies in different countries and different health care settings have examined and confirmed the considerable burden of CSU [34–39].

4.2.2 Drivers of HRQoL in chronic spontaneous urticaria

HRQoL impairment increases with disease activity [9, 40, 41], i.e., the frequency and severity of signs and symptoms. However, the correlation of disease activity and HRQoL is not high [40–42], indicating that there are additional drivers of

HRQoL in CSU. Certainly, the unpredictability of the disease is another important factor. In addition, age and gender seem to have an impact on some dimensions of HRQoL [43, 44], Another very important aspect are psychiatric comorbidities, such as anxiety and depression. HRQoL was found to be stronger impaired in CSU patients with a psychiatric comorbidity as compared to patients without [45–49]. Finally, also the presence or absence of effective coping strategies and social supporting systems may have an impact on the extent of HRQoL impairment.

4.2.3 HRQoL Impairment in Chronic Inducible Urticaria

As compared to CSU, HRQoL impairment in CIndUs is poorly studied. Major reasons are (1) that the clear distinction between CSU and CIndUs as it is consensus today [3] was far from clear a few years ago, which hindered research specifically aimed to better understand CIndUs, and (2) that there was, until recently, no specific tool available to determine HRQoL in any CIndU. However, some data were published: O'Donnel already showed in her pioneer work that CSU patients with comorbid CIndU have a significantly lower HRQoL as compared to patients with CSU alone [6], suggesting that CIndUs considerably affect HRQoL. These results were confirmed by Poon and coworkers, who demonstrated that subjects with delayed pressure urticaria and cholinergic urticaria had a strong HRQoL impairment, comparable to that of patients with severe atopic dermatitis and higher than that of patients with psoriasis, at least in the setting of a tertiary referral center [50].

CSU and CIndUs are distinct with regard to the triggering and appearance of signs and symptoms. Accordingly, a major difference in the extent and pattern of HRQoL impairment is to be expected. Further research is required to better understand HRQoL impairment in the different CIndUs as well as its major drivers. A first step to allow for this was recently made by Ruft and colleagues, who published the first disease-specific HRQoL questionnaire in the field of CIndUs, the Cholinergic Urticaria Quality of Life Questionnaire (CholU-QoL) [51].

4.3 How to Assess Disease Burden in CSU

4.3.1 The Use of PROMs Improves Chronic Urticaria Management

Due to the fluctuating nature of CSU, many patients do not exhibit any signs and symptoms at the time of appointments with their treating physicians, or they present with wheals or angioedema that are not typical for what they usually suffer from. Accordingly, urticaria treating physicians only rarely see a representative picture of CSU during regular patient consultations and have to fully rely on what patients report [52]. Since objective and specific biomarkers are also not available, validated patient-reported outcome measures (PROMs) should be used to assess the patients' disease activity, i.e., symptom burden, disease impact, i.e., HRQoL impairment, and disease control, i.e., the level of control over urticaria signs and symptoms as well as its impact that is achieved by the current treatment strategy. The assessment of all three concepts is essential for providing optimal care, e.g., to adjust the treatment approach as best as possible to the patient needs [4, 53], but also becomes increasingly important in clinical trials. In fact, regulatory authorities strongly encourage researchers and companies to capture the patient perspective by using PROMs, i.e., to use patient relevant outcome measures [54]. In turn, the lack of suitable and disease-specific PROMs severely hinders the conductance of clinical research.

4.3.2 What PROMs Should Be Used in Chronic Spontaneous Urticaria

In the past 15 years, several disease-specific PROMs have been developed for CSU to assess disease activity, impact, and control (Table 4.1). The symptom pattern, i.e., wheals, angioedema, or both, in individual patients is key for the selection of the most suitable PROMs. In patients who predominantly or only develop wheals, the Urticaria Activity Score (UAS) [3, 57], the Chronic Urticaria Quality of Life Questionnaire (CU-Q2oL) [10], and the Urticaria Control Test (UCT) [58] should be administered. In patients who predominantly or only have angioedema, the Angioedema Activity Score (AAS) [59], the Angioedema Quality of Life Questionnaire (AE-QoL) [60], and the Angioedema Control Test (AECT) [61] are the preferred PROMs.

The UAS is the current gold standard to assess disease activity in CSU patients who develop wheals [3] and has proven its high value as an outcome measure in numerous randomized controlled clinical trials [62–64]. It is a diary-type tool that records wheal numbers and itch intensity over 7 consecutive days (UAS7) [3]. Two versions are available and differ in their frequency of documentation (once daily vs twice daily) and in their categories for wheal numbers [65–67]. Since both versions yield comparable results [65, 66], the once daily UAS is preferred, because it is less burdensome in administration and scoring [65]. The once daily UAS is valid and reliable, and score changes of 11 points or higher can be considered as a meaningful change [57], i.e., its minimal clinically important difference (MCID). Important limitations of the UAS include (1) that the prospective assessment makes results not instantly available, (2) that a validated version for children is missing (although a modified version has already been used in a clinical trial in children) [68], (3) that it does not include angioedema, although this is a frequent and highly relevant clinical manifestation of CSU, and (4) that it is not suitable to adequately capture the disease activity in CIndU patients.

HRQoL impairment in CSU and its changes over time, e.g., before and after treatment adjustment, can be best captured with the disease-specific and guideline-recommended CU-Q2oL [3]. The CU-Q2oL has been proven to have high levels of validity and reliability [10], has been translated to many different languages [44, 55, 69–76], and was applied successfully in several clinical studies [77–79]. It is sensitive to change, and its MCID was found to be 3 and 15 in independent studies and

Table 4.1 Available patient-reported outcome measures in chronic spontaneous urticaria

	UAS	CU-Q₂oL	UCT	AAS	AE-QoL	AECT
Concept measured	Disease activity	HRQoL	Disease control	Disease activity	HRQoL	Disease control
Suitable for patients with						
– Wheals/No angioedema	+	+	+	–	–	–
– Wheals & Angioedema	+	+	+	+	+	+
– No wheals/ angioedema	–	–	+	+	+	+
Number of items	2	23	4	5	17	4
Retrospective assessment (Recall period)	–	2 weeks	4 weeks	–	4 weeks	4 weeks 3 months
Prospective assessment (frequency)	1×/day or 2×/day for 7 days	–	–	1×/day for usually 28 days	–	–
MCID	11	3–15[c]	3	8	6	not yet established
Cost-free for						
Routine patient care	+	+	+	+	+	+
Academic research	+	+	+	+	+	+
Industry studies	+	–	–	–	–	–
Language/country versions available	+[a]	Italian, German, Greek, Hebrew, Korean, Persian, Polish, Portuguese, Spanish, Thai, Turkish	>20 language versions available[b]	>70 language versions available[b]	>25 language versions available[b]	German, American-English

AAS Angioedema Activity Score, *AECT* Angioedema Control Test, *AE-QoL* Angioedema Quality of Life Questionnaire, *CU-Q₂oL* Chronic Urticaria Quality of Life Questionnaire, *HRQoL* Health-related quality of life, *MCID* Minimal Clinically Important Difference, *UAS* Urticaria Activity Score, *UCT* Urticaria Control Test

[a]The UAS is available in several languages. The original source is the EAACI/GA2LEN/EDF/WAO urticaria guideline. Due to its easy structure the UAS is usually translated but not formally linguistically validated

[b]For more details with regard to available language versions of the AAS, AE-QoL, UCT and AECT go to www.moxie-gmbh.de/additional language/country versions may be or are in preparation, for more information please contact MOXIE at info@moxie-gmbh.de

[c]The MCID of the CU-Q₂oL was determined in 2 independent studies, in different patient collectives (one study found an MCID of 3 points, the MCID identified in the other study was higher with 15 points) [55, 56]

patient collectives [55, 56]. Recently, also a short form of the CU-Q$_2$oL has been validated, the Chronic Urticaria Patient Perspective (CUPP), to facilitate assessment of HRQoL impairment in clinical practice [80]. Limitations of the CU-Q$_2$oL include (1) that it was not specifically developed to measure HRQoL impairment in CSU patients predominantly suffering from angioedema, (2) that a modified version for children is missing, and (3) that it is not a suitable PROM for the use in CIndUs.

In patient groups or countries where the CU-Q2oL is not available, it is possible to apply generic HRQoL measures designed to capture skin disorder-related HRQoL impairment, e.g., the Dermatology Life Quality Index (DLQI) [81], which has also been tested successfully in CSU [82], or other tools such as the Skindex [48, 83] and the Children's DQLI (CDLQI) [84]. However, it is important to recognize that the items of these tools are not specific for CSU, which makes them less sensitive for the CSU-related extent and pattern of HRQoL impairment, but also less sensitive to capture its changes over time, e.g., in response to treatment adjustment. The primary focus of the use of these tools should be comparisons of HRQoL between CSU patients and patients with other skin disorders, which is not possible with the CU-Q$_2$oL.

The achievement of disease control is an important aim in the treatment of CSU patients. The UCT has been specifically designed to assess the level of disease control as well as to distinguish patients with poorly-controlled and well-controlled disease in routine care and clinical trials [58]. The UCT is currently the easiest to use PROM in the field of CSU [4], has been translated and tested in different languages [85–90], and was successfully applied in several clinical studies [91–93]. It consists of 4 questions and has a minimum and maximum score of 0 and 16 points, respectively. Higher scores indicate higher levels of disease control [58], and a UCT score of 12 points is the cut-off to identify poorly-controlled vs. well-controlled CSU [58]. The concept of disease control is linked to disease activity and HRQoL, i.e., UCT scores strongly correlate with the UAS [58, 91, 92, 94, 95] and the CUQ$_2$oL total score [58, 92, 94]. The UCT has high levels of validity and reliability [58, 88], and is responsive to change, with an MCID of 3 points [88, 94]. While the UCT is suitable for all forms of CU (CSU and CIndU), a limitation includes that a children version is not available yet.

In CSU patients who predominantly develop angioedema and CSU patients who suffer from isolated recurrent angioedema without wheals, disease activity can be assessed with the AAS. Similar to the UAS, the AAS works as a prospective, diary type PROM [4]. Patients are asked to document, once daily, whether angioedema is present. If this is the case, they are requested to answer the five actual AAS questions on the duration, severity, and impact of the current angioedema episode [59]. As the UAS, the AAS also has high levels of validity and reliability [59]. The MCID is 8 points for the 7-day AAS (AAS7) [59]. Since its publication, the AAS has been applied in several randomized controlled trials, in the field of CSU [62, 79] but also in the field of hereditary angioedema [96]. Its limitations are comparable to those of the UAS, i.e., (1) that the prospective assessment makes results not instantly available and (2) that a validated version for children is missing.

The AE-QoL is the first questionnaire to evaluate angioedema-specific HRQoL impairment in patients with recurrent angioedema [60]. It has 17 questions with 5 answer options each [4]. Its results can be computed as a total score or as four different domain scores ("functioning," "fatigue/mood," "fears/shame," "food") that are each displayed on a 0–100 scale, with higher scores indicative of a higher HRQoL impairment [60]. The AE-QoL has good levels of validity and reliability [60], and is responsive to change, with an MCID of 6 points [97, 98]. As the AAS it has been a helpful outcome measure in recent clinical studies in the fields of CSU [7] and hereditary angioedema [96, 99–101]. Unfortunately, no AE-QoL pediatric version has been developed yet.

The Angioedema Control Test (AECT) is a new PROM that has been developed to assess disease control in adult patients with recurrent angioedema, such as in CSU [61]. The AECT is easy-to-administer, easy-to-complete, and easy-to-score [61]. It works in a similar way as the UCT, i.e., it captures the current level of disease control retrospectively by asking the patients 4 questions with 5 answer options each (scored from 0 to 4). Accordingly, the minimum and maximum score are 0 and 16 points, respectively, with higher scores indicating higher levels of disease control. The cut-off value to distinguish poorly-controlled from well-controlled disease is 10 points [102]. Two versions have been tested in the validation study, one with a recall period of 4 weeks and one with a recall period of three month. The results of both versions correlate strongly [102].

4.3.3 What PROMs Should Be Used in Chronic Inducible Urticaria

In patients with CIndUs, disease activity is usually determined by testing patients for their trigger thresholds. This may be complemented by the administration of CIndU-specific activity scores, which take into account the frequency and intensity of symptoms but also the trigger exposure during the assessment period. As a first of such tools, the Cholinergic Urticaria Activity Score (CholUAS) has been published recently [103], and its further validation is currently ongoing. In addition, the development of specific activity scores for cold urticaria and symptomatic dermographism, the most common forms of CIndUs next to cholinergic urticaria, is underway.

For the assessment of HRQoL impairment of CIndU patients, the first validated questionnaire has been published recently for cholinergic urticaria, the CholU-QoL [51]. It consists of 28 questions that can be grouped together to a total score as well as to 5 dimension scores ("symptoms," "functional life," "social interactions," "therapy," and "emotions") [51]. Its responsiveness to change needs to be determined yet. The development process of a specific HRQoL questionnaire for symptomatic dermographism (SD-QoL) is finished and the tool will be published shortly. A specific HRQoL questionnaire for cold urticaria is currently tested in a validation study and will also be available in the near future.

The determination of disease control of CIndU patients can be assessed with the UCT, since this PROM has been developed for all subforms of CU.

References

1. Grob JJ, Gaudy-Marqueste C. Urticaria and quality of life. Clin Rev Allergy Immunol. 2006;30:47–51.
2. Maurer M, Weller K, Bindslev-Jensen C, Gimenez-Arnau A, Bousquet PJ, Bousquet J, et al. Unmet clinical needs in chronic spontaneous urticaria. A GA(2)LEN task force report. Allergy. 2011;66:317–30.
3. Zuberbier T, Aberer W, Asero R, Abdul Latiff AH, Baker D, Ballmer-Weber B, et al. The EAACI/GA(2)LEN/EDF/WAO guideline for the definition, classification, diagnosis and management of urticaria. Allergy. 2018;73:1393–414.
4. Weller K, Siebenhaar F, Hawro T, Altrichter S, Schoepke N, Maurer M. Clinical measures of chronic urticaria. Immunol Allergy Clin North Am. 2017;37:35–49.
5. Maurer M, Ortonne JP, Zuberbier T. Chronic urticaria: an internet survey of health behaviours, symptom patterns and treatment needs in European adult patients. Br J Dermatol. 2009;160:633–41.
6. O'Donnell BF, Lawlor F, Simpson J, Morgan M, Greaves MW. The impact of chronic urticaria on the quality of life. Br J Dermatol. 1997;136:197–201.
7. Staubach P, Metz M, Chapman-Rothe N, Sieder C, Brautigam M, Maurer M, et al. Omalizumab rapidly improves angioedema-related quality of life in adult patients with chronic spontaneous urticaria: X-ACT study data. Allergy. 2018;73:576–84.
8. Ertas R, Erol K, Hawro T, Yilmaz H, Maurer M. Sexual functioning is frequently and markedly impaired in female patients with chronic spontaneous urticaria. J Allergy Clin Immunol Pract. 2020;8(3):1074–82.
9. Maurer M, Abuzakouk M, Berard F, Canonica W, Oude Elberink H, Gimenez-Arnau A, et al. The burden of chronic spontaneous urticaria is substantial: real-world evidence from ASSURE-CSU. Allergy. 2017;72:2005–16.
10. Baiardini I, Pasquali M, Braido F, Fumagalli F, Guerra L, Compalati E, et al. A new tool to evaluate the impact of chronic urticaria on quality of life: chronic urticaria quality of life questionnaire (CU-QoL). Allergy. 2005;60:1073–8.
11. Balp MM, Khalil S, Tian H, Gabriel S, Vietri J, Zuberbier T. Burden of chronic urticaria relative to psoriasis in five European countries. J Eur Acad Dermatol Venereol. 2018;32:282–90.
12. Hoskin B, Ortiz B, Paknis B, Kavati A. Exploring the real-world profile of refractory and non-refractory chronic idiopathic urticaria in the USA: clinical burden and healthcare resource use. Curr Med Res Opin. 2019;35:1387–95.
13. Sussman G, Abuzakouk M, Berard F, Canonica W, Oude Elberink H, Gimenez-Arnau A, et al. Angioedema in chronic spontaneous urticaria is underdiagnosed and has a substantial impact: analyses from ASSURE-CSU. Allergy. 2018;73:1724–34.
14. Mann C, Dreher M, Weess HG, Staubach P. Sleep disturbance in patients with urticaria and atopic dermatitis: an underestimated burden. Acta Derm Venereol. 2020;100(6):adv00073.
15. Yosipovitch G, Ansari N, Goon A, Chan YH, Goh CL. Clinical characteristics of pruritus in chronic idiopathic urticaria. Br J Dermatol. 2002;147:32–6.
16. Gupta MA, Gupta AK. Sleep-wake disorders and dermatology. Clin Dermatol. 2013;31:118–26.
17. Gupta MA, Gupta AK, Schork NJ, Ellis CN. Depression modulates pruritus perception: a study of pruritus in psoriasis, atopic dermatitis, and chronic idiopathic urticaria. Psychosom Med. 1994;56:36–40.
18. Konstantinou GN, Konstantinou GN. Psychiatric comorbidity in chronic urticaria patients: a systematic review and meta-analysis. Clin Transl Allergy. 2019;9:42.

19. Chapman DP, Presley-Cantrell LR, Liu Y, Perry GS, Wheaton AG, Croft JB. Frequent insufficient sleep and anxiety and depressive disorders among U.S. community dwellers in 20 states, 2010. Psychiatr Serv. 2013;64:385–7.
20. Kalmbach DA, Arnedt JT, Song PX, Guille C, Sen S. Sleep disturbance and short sleep as risk factors for depression and perceived medical errors in first-year residents. Sleep. 2017;40:zsw073.
21. Dalgard FJ, Svensson A, Halvorsen JA, Gieler U, Schut C, Tomas-Aragones L, et al. Itch and mental health in dermatological patients across Europe: a cross-sectional study in 13 countries. J Invest Dermatol. 2020;140(3):568–73.
22. Schut C, Mollanazar NK, Kupfer J, Gieler U, Yosipovitch G. Psychological interventions in the treatment of chronic itch. Acta Derm Venereol. 2016;96:157–61.
23. Verhoeven EW, de Klerk S, Kraaimaat FW, van de Kerkhof PC, de Jong EM, Evers AW. Biopsychosocial mechanisms of chronic itch in patients with skin diseases: a review. Acta Derm Venereol. 2008;88:211–8.
24. Gimenez-Arnau AM, Spector S, Antonova E, Trzaskoma B, Rosen K, Omachi TA, et al. Improvement of sleep in patients with chronic idiopathic/spontaneous urticaria treated with omalizumab: results of three randomized, double-blind, placebo-controlled studies. Clin Transl Allergy. 2016;6:32.
25. Vietri J, Turner SJ, Tian H, Isherwood G, Balp MM, Gabriel S. Effect of chronic urticaria on US patients: analysis of the National Health and Wellness Survey. Ann Allergy Asthma Immunol. 2015;115:306–11.
26. Broder MS, Raimundo K, Antonova E, Chang E. Resource use and costs in an insured population of patients with chronic idiopathic/spontaneous urticaria. Am J Clin Dermatol. 2015;16:313–21.
27. Delong LK, Culler SD, Saini SS, Beck LA, Chen SC. Annual direct and indirect health care costs of chronic idiopathic urticaria: a cost analysis of 50 nonimmunosuppressed patients. Arch Dermatol. 2008;144:35–9.
28. Gill TM, Feinstein AR. A critical appraisal of the quality of quality-of-life measurements. JAMA. 1994;272:619–26.
29. Karimi M, Brazier J. Health, health-related quality of life, and quality of life: what is the difference? Pharmacoeconomics. 2016;34:645–9.
30. Hunt SM, McEwen J. The development of a subjective health indicator. Sociol Health Illn. 1980;2:231–46.
31. Baiardini I, Giardini A, Pasquali M, Dignetti P, Guerra L, Specchia C, et al. Quality of life and patients' satisfaction in chronic urticaria and respiratory allergy. Allergy. 2003;58:621–3.
32. Grob JJ, Revuz J, Ortonne JP, Auquier P, Lorette G. Comparative study of the impact of chronic urticaria, psoriasis and atopic dermatitis on the quality of life. Br J Dermatol. 2005;152:289–95.
33. Lewis V, Finlay AY. 10 years experience of the Dermatology Life Quality Index (DLQI). J Investig Dermatol Symp Proc. 2004;9:169–80.
34. Dias GA, Pires GV, Valle SO, Dortas SDJ, Levy S, Franca AT, et al. Impact of chronic urticaria on the quality of life of patients followed up at a university hospital. An Bras Dermatol. 2016;91:754–9.
35. Itakura A, Tani Y, Kaneko N, Hide M. Impact of chronic urticaria on quality of life and work in Japan: results of a real-world study. J Dermatol. 2018;45:963–70.
36. Kang MJ, Kim HS, Kim HO, Park YM. The impact of chronic idiopathic urticaria on quality of life in Korean patients. Ann Dermatol. 2009;21:226–9.
37. Liu JB, Yao MZ, Si AL, Xiong LK, Zhou H. Life quality of Chinese patients with chronic urticaria as assessed by the dermatology life quality index. J Eur Acad Dermatol Venereol. 2012;26:1252–7.
38. Pherwani AV, Bansode G, Gadhia S. The impact of chronic urticaria on the quality of life in Indian patients. Indian J Dermatol. 2012;57:110–3.
39. Yun J, Katelaris CH, Weerasinghe A, Adikari DB, Ratnayake C. Impact of chronic urticaria on the quality of life in Australian and Sri Lankan populations. Asia Pac Allergy. 2011;1:25–9.

40. Koti I, Weller K, Makris M, Tiligada E, Psaltopoulou T, Papageorgiou C, et al. Disease activity only moderately correlates with quality of life impairment in patients with chronic spontaneous urticaria. Dermatology. 2013;226:371–9.
41. Weller K, Church MK, Kalogeromitros D, Krause K, Magerl M, Metz M, et al. Chronic spontaneous urticaria: how to assess quality of life in patients receiving treatment. Arch Dermatol. 2011;147:1221–3.
42. Mlynek A, Zalewska-Janowska A, Martus P, Staubach P, Zuberbier T, Maurer M. How to assess disease activity in patients with chronic urticaria? Allergy. 2008;63:777–80.
43. Maurer M, Ortonne JP, Zuberbier T. Chronic urticaria: a patient survey on quality-of-life, treatment usage and doctor-patient relation. Allergy. 2009;64:581–8.
44. Mlynek A, Magerl M, Hanna M, Lhachimi S, Baiardini I, Canonica GW, et al. The German version of the chronic urticaria quality-of-life questionnaire: factor analysis, validation, and initial clinical findings. Allergy. 2009;64:927–36.
45. Engin B, Uguz F, Yilmaz E, Ozdemir M, Mevlitoglu I. The levels of depression, anxiety and quality of life in patients with chronic idiopathic urticaria. J Eur Acad Dermatol Venereol. 2008;22:36–40.
46. Ozkan M, Oflaz SB, Kocaman N, Ozseker F, Gelincik A, Buyukozturk S, et al. Psychiatric morbidity and quality of life in patients with chronic idiopathic urticaria. Ann Allergy Asthma Immunol. 2007;99:29–33.
47. Picardi A, Abeni D, Melchi CF, Puddu P, Pasquini P. Psychiatric morbidity in dermatological outpatients: an issue to be recognized. Br J Dermatol. 2000;143:983–91.
48. Staubach P, Eckhardt-Henn A, Dechene M, Vonend A, Metz M, Magerl M, et al. Quality of life in patients with chronic urticaria is differentially impaired and determined by psychiatric comorbidity. Br J Dermatol. 2006;154:294–8.
49. Uguz F, Engin B, Yilmaz E. Quality of life in patients with chronic idiopathic urticaria: the impact of Axis I and Axis II psychiatric disorders. Gen Hosp Psychiatry. 2008;30:453–7.
50. Poon E, Seed PT, Greaves MW, Kobza-Black A. The extent and nature of disability in different urticarial conditions. Br J Dermatol. 1999;140:667–71.
51. Ruft J, Asady A, Staubach P, Casale T, Sussmann G, Zuberbier T, et al. Development and validation of the Cholinergic Urticaria Quality-of-Life Questionnaire (CholU-QoL). Clin Exp Allergy. 2018;48:433–44.
52. Weller K, Zuberbier T, Maurer M. Clinically relevant outcome measures for assessing disease activity, disease control and quality of life impairment in patients with chronic spontaneous urticaria and recurrent angioedema. Curr Opin Allergy Clin Immunol. 2015;15:220–6.
53. Weller K, Zuberbier T, Maurer M. Chronic urticaria: tools to aid the diagnosis and assessment of disease status in daily practice. J Eur Acad Dermatol Venereol. 2015;29(Suppl 3):38–44.
54. U.S. Department of Health and Human Services FDA Center for Drug Evaluation and Research; U.S. Department of Health and Human Services FDA Center for Biologics Evaluation and Research; U.S. Department of Health and Human Services FDA Center for Devices and Radiological Health. Guidance for industry: patient-reported outcome measures: use in medical product development to support labeling claims: draft guidance. Health Qual Life Outcomes. 2006;4:79.
55. Kulthanan K, Chularojanamontri L, Tuchinda P, Rujitharanawong C, Baiardini I, Braido F. Minimal clinical important difference (MCID) of the Thai Chronic Urticaria Quality of Life Questionnaire (CU-Q2oL). Asian Pac J Allergy Immunol. 2016;34:137–45.
56. Baiardini I, Fasola S, Maurer M, Weller K, Canonica GW, Braido F. Minimal important difference of the chronic urticaria quality of life questionnaire (CU-Q2oL). Allergy. 2019;74:2542–4.
57. Hawro T, Ohanyan T, Schoepke N, Metz M, Peveling-Oberhag A, Staubach P, et al. The urticaria activity score-validity, reliability, and responsiveness. J Allergy Clin Immunol Pract. 2018;6:1185–90.e1.
58. Weller K, Groffik A, Church MK, Hawro T, Krause K, Metz M, et al. Development and validation of the urticaria control test: a patient-reported outcome instrument for assessing urticaria control. J Allergy Clin Immunol. 2014;133:1365–72, 1372.e1-6.

59. Weller K, Groffik A, Magerl M, Tohme N, Martus P, Krause K, et al. Development, validation, and initial results of the Angioedema Activity Score. Allergy. 2013;68:1185–92.
60. Weller K, Groffik A, Magerl M, Tohme N, Martus P, Krause K, et al. Development and construct validation of the angioedema quality of life questionnaire. Allergy. 2012;67:1289–98.
61. Weller K, Donoso T, Magerl M, Aygoren-Pursun E, Staubach P, Martinez-Saguer I, et al. Development of the Angioedema Control Test (AECT)—a patient reported outcome measure that assesses disease control in patients with recurrent angioedema. Allergy. 2020;75(5):1165–77.
62. Maurer M, Gimenez-Arnau AM, Sussman G, Metz M, Baker DR, Bauer A, et al. Ligelizumab for chronic spontaneous urticaria. N Engl J Med. 2019;381:1321–32.
63. Stull D, McBride D, Tian H, Gimenez Arnau A, Maurer M, Marsland A, et al. Analysis of disease activity categories in chronic spontaneous/idiopathic urticaria. Br J Dermatol. 2017;177:1093–101.
64. Zhao ZT, Ji CM, Yu WJ, Meng L, Hawro T, Wei JF, et al. Omalizumab for the treatment of chronic spontaneous urticaria: a meta-analysis of randomized clinical trials. J Allergy Clin Immunol. 2016;137:1742–50.e4.
65. Hawro T, Ohanyan T, Schoepke N, Metz M, Peveling-Oberhag A, Staubach P, et al. Comparison and interpretability of the available urticaria activity scores. Allergy. 2018;73:251–5.
66. Hollis K, Proctor C, McBride D, Balp MM, McLeod L, Hunter S, et al. Comparison of Urticaria Activity Score Over 7 Days (UAS7) values obtained from once-daily and twice-daily versions: results from the ASSURE-CSU study. Am J Clin Dermatol. 2018;19:267–74.
67. Mathias SD, Crosby RD, Zazzali JL, Maurer M, Saini SS. Evaluating the minimally important difference of the urticaria activity score and other measures of disease activity in patients with chronic idiopathic urticaria. Ann Allergy Asthma Immunol. 2012;108:20–4.
68. Potter P, Mitha E, Barkai L, Mezei G, Santamaria E, Izquierdo I, et al. Rupatadine is effective in the treatment of chronic spontaneous urticaria in children aged 2-11 years. Pediatr Allergy Immunol. 2016;27:55–61.
69. Brzoza Z, Badura-Brzoza K, Mlynek A, Magerl M, Baiardini I, Canonica GW, et al. Adaptation and initial results of the Polish version of the GA(2)LEN chronic urticaria quality of life questionnaire (CU-Q(2)oL). J Dermatol Sci. 2011;62:36–41.
70. Dias GA, Pires GV, Valle SO, Franca AT, Papi JA, Dortas SD Jr, et al. Cross-cultural adaptation of the Brazilian-Portuguese version of the chronic urticaria quality-of-life questionnaire—CU-Q2oL. Allergy. 2011;66:1487–93.
71. Ferreira PL, Goncalo M, Ferreira JA, Costa AC, Todo-Bom A, Abreu CL, et al. Psychometric properties of the portuguese version of the chronic urticaria quality of life questionnaire (CU-Q2oL). Health Qual Life Outcomes. 2019;17:190.
72. Kessel A, Graif Y, Vadasz Z, Schichter-Konfino V, Almog M, Cohen S, et al. adaptation and validation of the israeli version of the chronic urticaria quality of life questionnaire (CU-Q2oL). Isr Med Assoc J. 2016;18:461–5.
73. Kocaturk E, Weller K, Martus P, Aktas S, Kavala M, Sarigul S, et al. Turkish version of the chronic urticaria quality of life questionnaire: cultural adaptation, assessment of reliability and validity. Acta Derm Venereol. 2012;92:419–25.
74. Tavakol M, Mohammadinejad P, Baiardini I, Braido F, Gharagozlou M, Aghamohammadi A, et al. The Persian version of the chronic urticaria quality of life questionnaire: factor analysis, validation, and initial clinical findings. Iran J Allergy Asthma Immunol. 2014;13:278–85.
75. Valero A, Herdman M, Bartra J, Ferrer M, Jauregui I, Davila I, et al. Adaptation and validation of the Spanish version of the chronic urticaria quality of life questionnaire (CU-Q2oL). J Investig Allergol Clin Immunol. 2008;18:426–32.
76. Ye YM, Park JW, Kim SH, Choi JH, Hur GY, Lee HY, et al. Clinical evaluation of the computerized chronic urticaria-specific quality of life questionnaire in Korean patients with chronic urticaria. Clin Exp Dermatol. 2012;37:722–8.
77. Maurer M, Altrichter S, Bieber T, Biedermann T, Brautigam M, Seyfried S, et al. Efficacy and safety of omalizumab in patients with chronic urticaria who exhibit IgE against thyroperoxidase. J Allergy Clin Immunol. 2011;128:202–9.e5.

78. Metz M, Weller K, Neumeister C, Izquierdo I, Bodeker RH, Schwantes U, et al. Rupatadine in established treatment schemes improves chronic spontaneous urticaria symptoms and patients' quality of life: a prospective, non-interventional trial. Dermatol Ther (Heidelb). 2015;5:217–30.
79. Staubach P, Metz M, Chapman-Rothe N, Sieder C, Brautigam M, Canvin J, et al. Effect of omalizumab on angioedema in H1-antihistamine-resistant chronic spontaneous urticaria patients: results from X-ACT, a randomized controlled trial. Allergy. 2016;71:1135–44.
80. Baiardini I, Braido F, Molinengo G, Caminati M, Costantino M, Cristaudo A, et al. Chronic urticaria patient perspective (CUPP): the first validated tool for assessing quality of life in clinical practice. J Allergy Clin Immunol Pract. 2018;6:208–18.
81. Finlay AY, Khan GK. Dermatology Life Quality Index (DLQI)—a simple practical measure for routine clinical use. Clin Exp Dermatol. 1994;19:210–6.
82. Shikiar R, Harding G, Leahy M, Lennox RD. Minimal important difference (MID) of the Dermatology Life Quality Index (DLQI): results from patients with chronic idiopathic urticaria. Health Qual Life Outcomes. 2005;3:36.
83. Chren MM, Lasek RJ, Quinn LM, Covinsky KE. Convergent and discriminant validity of a generic and a disease-specific instrument to measure quality of life in patients with skin disease. J Invest Dermatol. 1997;108:103–7.
84. Jauregui I, Ortiz de Frutos FJ, Ferrer M, Gimenez-Arnau A, Sastre J, Bartra J, et al. Assessment of severity and quality of life in chronic urticaria. J Investig Allergol Clin Immunol. 2014;24:80–6.
85. Garcia-Diez I, Curto-Barredo L, Weller K, Pujol RM, Maurer M, Gimenez-Arnau AM. Cross-cultural adaptation of the urticaria control test from German to Castilian Spanish. Actas Dermosifiliogr. 2015;106:746–52.
86. Irani C, Hallit S, Weller K, Maurer M, El Haber C, Salameh P. Chronic urticaria in most patients is poorly controlled. Results of the development, validation, and real life application of the Arabic urticaria control test. Saudi Med J. 2017;38:1230–6.
87. Kocaturk E, Kiziltac U, Can P, Oztas Kara R, Erdem T, Kiziltac K, et al. Validation of the Turkish version of the urticaria control test: correlation with other tools and comparison between spontaneous and inducible chronic urticaria. World Allergy Organ J. 2019;12:100009.
88. Kulthanan K, Chularojanamontri L, Tuchinda P, Rujitharanawong C, Maurer M, Weller K. Validity, reliability and interpretability of the Thai version of the urticaria control test (UCT). Health Qual Life Outcomes. 2016;14:61.
89. Lee JH, Bae YI, Lee SH, Kim SC, Lee HY, Ban GY, et al. Adaptation and validation of the Korean version of the urticaria control test and its correlation with salivary cortisone. Allergy Asthma Immunol Res. 2019;11:55–67.
90. Nakatani S, Oda Y, Washio K, Fukunaga A, Nishigori C. The urticaria control test and urticaria activity score correlate with quality of life in adult Japanese patients with chronic spontaneous urticaria. Allergol Int. 2019;68:279–81.
91. Berard F, Ferrier Le Bouedec MC, Bouillet L, Reguiai Z, Barbaud A, Cambazard F, et al. Omalizumab in patients with chronic spontaneous urticaria nonresponsive to H1-antihistamine treatment: results of the phase IV open-label SUNRISE study. Br J Dermatol. 2019;180:56–66.
92. Ghazanfar MN, Holm JG, Thomsen SF. Effectiveness of omalizumab in chronic spontaneous urticaria assessed with patient-reported outcomes: a prospective study. J Eur Acad Dermatol Venereol. 2018;32:1761–7.
93. Maurer M, Staubach P, Raap U, Richter-Huhn G, Bauer A, Rueff F, et al. H1-antihistamine-refractory chronic spontaneous urticaria: it's worse than we thought—first results of the multicenter real-life AWARE study. Clin Exp Allergy. 2017;47:684–92.
94. Ohanyan T, Schoepke N, Bolukbasi B, Metz M, Hawro T, Zuberbier T, et al. Responsiveness and minimal important difference of the urticaria control test. J Allergy Clin Immunol. 2017;140:1710–3.e11.
95. Weller K, Church MK, Metz M, Hawro T, Ohanyan T, Staubach P, et al. The response to treatment in chronic spontaneous urticaria depends on how it is measured. J Allergy Clin Immunol Pract. 2019;7:2055–6.e4.

96. Aygoren-Pursun E, Magerl M, Graff J, Martinez-Saguer I, Kreuz W, Longhurst H, et al. Prophylaxis of hereditary angioedema attacks: A randomized trial of oral plasma kallikrein inhibition with avoralstat. J Allergy Clin Immunol. 2016;138:934–6.e5.
97. Kulthanan K, Chularojanamontri L, Rujitharanawong C, Weerasubpong P, Maurer M, Weller K. Angioedema quality of life questionnaire (AE-QoL)—interpretability and sensitivity to change. Health Qual Life Outcomes. 2019;17:160.
98. Weller K, Magerl M, Peveling-Oberhag A, Martus P, Staubach P, Maurer M. The Angioedema Quality of Life Questionnaire (AE-QoL)—assessment of sensitivity to change and minimal clinically important difference. Allergy. 2016;71:1203–9.
99. Aygoren-Pursun E, Bygum A, Grivcheva-Panovska V, Magerl M, Graff J, Steiner UC, et al. Oral plasma kallikrein inhibitor for prophylaxis in hereditary angioedema. N Engl J Med. 2018;379:352–62.
100. Riedl MA, Aygoren-Pursun E, Baker J, Farkas H, Anderson J, Bernstein JA, et al. Evaluation of avoralstat, an oral kallikrein inhibitor, in a phase 3 hereditary angioedema prophylaxis trial: the OPuS-2 study. Allergy. 2018;73:1871–80.
101. Weller K, Maurer M, Fridman M, Supina D, Schranz J, Magerl M. Health-related quality of life with hereditary angioedema following prophylaxis with subcutaneous C1-inhibitor with recombinant hyaluronidase. Allergy Asthma Proc. 2017;38:143–51.
102. Weller K, Donoso T, Magerl M, Aygören-Pürsün E, Staubach P, Martinez-Saguer I, et al. Validation of the Angioedema Control Test (AECT)—a patient reported outcome instrument for assessing angioedema control. J Allergy Clin Immunol Pract. 2020;8(6):2050–2057.e4.
103. Koch K, Weller K, Werner A, Maurer M, Altrichter S. Antihistamine updosing reduces disease activity in patients with difficult-to-treat cholinergic urticaria. J Allergy Clin Immunol. 2016;138:1483–1485.e9.

Acute Urticaria

5

Torsten Zuberbier and Zuotao Zhao

Core Messages
- Acute urticaria is a frequent disease with spontaneous appearance of wheals or angioedema.
- The lifetime prevalence is estimated to be around 15–20%.
- The majority of cases are of short limited duration.
- Most common causes are viral infections of the upper airways and drugs, especially NSAID.

5.1 Definition

Acute urticaria is defined by a spontaneous appearance of wheals (hives), angioedema or both, which last no more than 6 weeks [1] but the majority of cases present with hives only. Acute urticaria must be distinguished from acute attacks of physical urticaria, special types of urticaria or other diseases related to urticaria, e.g. urticaria pigmentosa, where whealing may also occur. This is of special importance since the term acute urticaria implies a disease which is clearly distinguished from the short occurrence of wheals for less than a few hours as a symptom of other diseases or anaphylactic reactions. According to the EAACI anaphylaxis guideline a frequent and typical sign is the "involvement of the skin-mucosal tissue (e.g. generalised hives, itch-flush, swollen lips-tongue-uvula)" with a sudden appearance after contact with a specific allergic trigger but it is not called urticaria [2]. This distinction is

---

T. Zuberbier (✉)
Institute for Allergology, Charité – Universitätsmedizin, Berlin, Germany

Fraunhofer Institute for Translational Medicine and Pharmacology ITMP,
Allergology and Immunology, Berlin, Germany
e-mail: Torsten.Zuberbier@charite.de

Z. Zhao
Department of Dermatology and Venereology, Peking University First Hospital,
Beijing, China

© Springer Nature Switzerland AG 2021
T. Zuberbier et al. (eds.), *Urticaria and Angioedema*,
https://doi.org/10.1007/978-3-030-84574-2_5

highly relevant for the interpretation of data regarding the epidemiology and causes of acute urticaria where in older literature often both terms were confused.

In addition it is very important to distinguish the wheals with urticaria-like lesions or wheal-like lesions which can occur in many instances [3]. Especially with the disease COVID-19 urticaria has been frequently described among other skin conditions. However, clinicopathological investigations showed that these are not real wheals [4, 5].

5.2 Epidemiology

According to older literature, lifetime prevalence of acute urticaria, based on questionnaires, ranges from 12 to 15% [6, 7] or even 23.5% [8]. In a prospective study from the Charité [for a doctoral thesis [9], a summary of the data has been published in English [10]], in a rural area of Brandenburg, a 1-year incidence of 0.154% was found, which equals a lifetime prevalence of 11.56% based on a life expectancy of 75 years [10]. These data can be considered reliable with regard to the accuracy of the urticaria diagnosis, since all patients were seen by the same dermatologist while still exhibiting symptoms. This was possible because only one dermatologist was working in the area of investigation and all doctors had been asked to refer all patients to him. However, there is no way of estimating the number of patients who believed their possibly mild symptoms to be of minor importance and who did not get in contact with any physician, which is well conceivable in a rural area with a disease that is mostly self-remitting. Thus, the true lifetime prevalence for the area may be estimated to be higher, around 15–20%.

In a retrospective representative study performed at the Charité, for the population of Berlin, a 1-year incidence rate of 0.6% was found, pointing to a possible lifetime prevalence that is four times higher than that observed in the prospective study in the rural area [11]. However, these data are based on a questionnaire only.

The prevalence of acute urticaria is higher in people with atopic diseases; thus hay fever, allergic asthma or atopic dermatitis were found in 50.2% of patients with acute urticaria in the above cited study of Iffländer [9]. Simons [12] reports on a prospective study in more than 800 12–24-month-old children with atopic dermatitis; in the study group not treated with antihistamines ($n = 396$), acute urticaria occurred in 16.2% over a period of 18 months.

Further epidemiological data revealed a female preponderance of 41–59%; 77% of the patients were younger than 40 years, and 37% were younger than 25 years. The average age was 31.4 years. There was an equal distribution of the prevalence throughout the year [10].

5.3 Clinical Aspects

Acute urticaria is mainly characterised by scattered wheals (Fig. 5.1). The colour is usually light red (88%) and the diameter is usually larger than 1 cm (80%). Wheals are accompanied by angioedema in less than 5% of patients. In 18% of patients,

5 Acute Urticaria

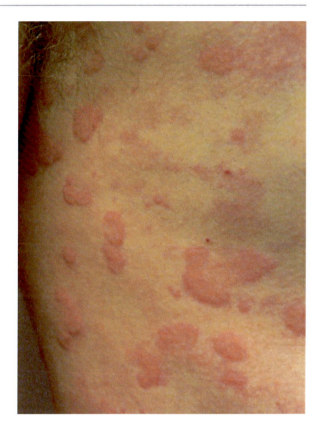

Fig. 5.1 Disseminated wheals in acute urticaria (Courtesy of ©ECARF, All rights reserved)

disease severity is light, with less than 10% of the body area affected; in 42% the disease activity is moderate, with 10–50% of body area affected; in 40% of patients disease activity is severe, with more than 50% of body area affected or systemic symptoms. The reported coexisting systemic symptoms are mild shortness of breath (7.3%), dizziness (2.7%), headache (1.8%), nausea (1.8%) and diarrhoea (0.9%). Full anaphylaxis can occur, but is very rare. In more than 99%, the disease is self-limited and resolves within the first 3 weeks [10].

5.4 Aetiology

In the aforementioned own prospective study in acute urticaria, 63% of the patients suspected food to be the cause, since they had consumed some food items in the 2 h before the onset of urticaria [10]. However, food was shown to be the causing agent upon thorough investigation in only 1 of 109 patients, which shows that patient history, especially in acute urticaria, may be misleading. However, food is more frequently implicated in children, since Legrain et al. [13] reported food, mainly cow's milk, to be relevant for acute urticaria in 10 of 12 children younger than 6 months of age. In older children with urticaria (6 months to 16 years), Kauppinen et al. [14]

observed a 15% prevalence of food intolerance as the eliciting factor for acute urticaria, whereas in an epidemiological study in 50 adult patients by Aoki et al. [15], not a single case of food allergy was found.

Drugs can cause both IgE-mediated and pseudoallergic reactions. While penicillin is the most frequent example of an IgE-mediated drug-induced urticaria, acetyl salicylic acid is the most popular example of a pseudoallergen. The first reaction of urticaria and angioedema after acetyl salicylic acid intake was described by Hirschberg in 1902 [15]. In our own study, mostly non-steroidal analgesic drugs were responsible for 9.2% of the cases with acute urticaria. These were (acetyl salicyl acid 4×, diclofenac 2×, other NSAID 3×, sulphonizide 1×) [10].

The most frequent cause of acute urticaria appears to be infections, mostly acute viral upper respiratory infections. The rate ranges between 28 and more than 60% of patients (Table. 5.1).

A possible explanation for the role of viral infections in acute urticaria is the triggering of mast cells via IgG receptors; however, it is also possible that in addition to the usual IgG response to the viral infection, specific IgE is also being produced under certain conditions. Thus, Grunewald et al. [16] have shown in an experimental model that infection with an influenza A virus can lead to cutaneous anaphylaxis in mice due to the presence of low levels of virus-specific IgE-antibodies. After rechallenge with the antigen, the mice developed virus-specific mast cell degranulation in the skin for more than 48 h.

Regarding the pathophysiology of whealing, similar to other forms of urticaria, the histamine release by mast cells is not the only factor responsible for the symptoms. While the wheal itself is clearly histamine-mediated, release of cytokines either by mast cells or by other inflammatory cells, the endothelia, or even keratinocytes may modulate the clinical appearance. While these additional cytokine effects are probably less important in acute urticaria, they are still not negligible in patients with severe acute urticaria. Fujii et al. [17] have shown that in a group of patients with severe acute urticaria who do not respond to antihistamine treatment, elevated levels of circulating IL-6 could be found, while the other mast cell cytokines IL-8 and TNF-α were not increased. The cytokine increase of IL-6, however, was not consistent in all patients, but limited to 9 of 16 individuals. This shows that as in other forms of urticaria, in acute urticaria the pathophysiological reactions are heterogeneous in different patients, which explains the different response to treatment and underlines the requirements for an individual approach.

Table 5.1 Prevalence of upper respiratory infections in acute urticaria

Study	Prevalence (%)
Kauppinen et al. [11]	28
Zuberbier et al. [7]	39.5
Legrain et al. [10]	50
Simons et al. [9]	54.5
Aoki et al. [12]	62

5.5 Natural Course

There are no epidemiological studies available that have monitored the natural course in patients without any treatment. In our own study, the course of the disease was carefully monitored in a follow-up of acute urticaria patients, divided into two treatment groups. The first group received loratadine 10 mg/day until the remission of symptoms, and the second group prednisolone 50 mg/day for 3 days, followed by loratadine 10 mg/day in case symptoms persisted (Table 5.2) [10]. None of the patients developed chronic urticaria and the disease can be regarded as mostly self-limited. However, 12% of the 109 patients reported solitary episodes of acute urticaria in the last 6 months to 10 years.

5.6 Diagnosis

A thorough examination of patient history is essential and may reveal eliciting factors. However, unless there has been an infection in the last 7 days prior to onset of urticaria or use of drugs (esp. NSAID) on the day of onset, the history is not significant in the majority of cases. According to international consensus, further diagnostic procedures should be limited to cases in which patient history causes suspicion [1]. These may include prick tests (native prick-to-prick) with ingested food as well as provocation tests with drugs at a later time point.

In view of the mostly self-limited disease duration, skin tests or laboratory investigations in patients with suspected reactions to NSAID are not helpful owing to the pseudoallergic nature of these drug reactions, but may be useful for other drugs known to induce IgE-mediated reactions like penicillin. Blood tests for viral antibodies are not helpful, even if viral infections appear to be the most common cause, as they are too unspecific and expensive to warrant their use.

5.7 Treatment

According to international consensus, the first-line treatment for acute urticaria is non-sedating H1-antihistamines, which may be increased in dosage. First generation antihistamines are not recommended to be used due to side effects except if i.v.

Table 5.2 Follow-up of patients with acute urticaria [7]

Cessation of whealing within (days)	Loratadine (10 mg/day) (%)	Prednisolone (50 mg/day for 3 days) (%)
3	65.9	93.8
7	15.9	3.1
14	15.9	1.5
21	2.3	1.5
>21	0	0

After initial treatment with loratadine ($n = 44$) or prednisolone ($n = 65$) for 3 days, all patients were then treated with loratadine (10 mg/day) until remission treatment is required [1]. Depending on severity a short course of corticosteroids, 50 mg/day for 3 days can be considered, is usually sufficient. According to our own study, an initial short course of prednisolone may reduce the duration of the disease, but does not have any influence on the final outcome, since complete remission occurred in all patients (Table 5.2) [10]. However the study was only single blind and currently a new study is planned [18]. Regarding the choice of non-sedating H_1-antihistamines, the general considerations explained in Chap. 11 should be adhered to. Furthermore, in acute urticaria it is important to choose an H_1-antihistamine with a short onset of action at the patient's first visit to guarantee a fast relief of symptoms.

Some of the new H_1-antihistamines are effective as early as 20 min past oral intake and are available as fast-dissolving tablets. Thus, IV emergency treatment is hardly of any benefit, especially since only old sedative H_1-antihistamines are available for parenteral use and require a slow injection over some minutes to avoid side effects like headache. Therefore, IV treatment should be reserved for patients who are at risk for possibly life-threatening systemic reactions or angioedema of the throat or larynx, which is relatively rare.

In a double-blind study by Watson et al. [19], i.m. treatment with famotidine and diphenhydramine has been compared. Both treatments were found to be effective, which is very interesting, but the study was not placebo-controlled. For practical reasons, i.m. treatment has no advantage when compared with oral treatment. It is more expensive and has a higher risk of side effects. It can therefore not be regarded as first choice treatment.

In summary, the overall approach to patients with acute urticaria should start with a reassurance of the usually anxious patient that this type of urticaria is not dangerous and is self-limited in more than 99%, and that symptomatic relief can be achieved and that a thorough diagnosis is only required in the unlikely case that the symptoms persist even if no obvious cause is found in patient history. In case of a viral infection in the past, a comforting explanation for the patient is that the wheals are a sign of an overactive and potent immune system.

Take Home Pearls

In more than 99% of cases, acute urticaria is self-limited.

- Extensive diagnostic procedures are not suggested except that the patient history renders a specific suspicion, e.g. intake of drugs.
- Type I allergy to food is often suspected by patients but rarely the case/course.
- Modern non-sedating H_1 antagonists are the treatment of choice. Dosage can be increased up to fourfold.
- An initial short course of corticosteroids (50 mg prednisolone per day) may shorten the duration.
- First generation antihistamines are not recommended.

References

1. Zuberbier T, et al. The EAACI/GA(2)LEN/EDF/WAO guideline for the definition, classification, diagnosis and management of urticaria. Allergy. 2018;73(7):1393–414.
2. Muraro A, et al. Anaphylaxis: guidelines from the European Academy of Allergy and Clinical Immunology. Allergy. 2014;69(8):1026–45.
3. Örnek S, Zuberbier T, Kocaturk E. And Annular urticarial lesions. 2020.
4. Adelino R, Andres-Cordon JF, De La Cruz Martinez CA. Acute urticaria with angioedema in the setting of coronavirus disease 2019. J Allergy Clin Immunol Pract. 2020;8(7):2386–7.
5. Rodriguez-Jimenez P, et al. Urticaria-like lesions in COVID-19 patients are not really urticaria—a case with clinicopathological correlation. J Eur Acad Dermatol Venereol. 2020;34(9):e459–60.
6. Sheldon JM, Mathews KP, Lovell RG. The vexing urticaria problem: present concepts of etiology and management. J Allergy. 1954;25(6):525–60.
7. Champion RH, et al. Urticaria and angio-oedema. A review of 554 patients. Br J Dermatol. 1969;81(8):588–97.
8. Swinny B. The atopic factor in urticaria. South Med J. 1941;34:855–8.
9. Iffländer J. Akute Urtikaria—Ursachen, Verlauf und Therapie. Humboldt University: Berlin; 1999.
10. Zuberbier T, et al. Acute urticaria: clinical aspects and therapeutic responsiveness. Acta Derm Venereol. 1996;76(4):295–7.
11. Zuberbier T, et al. Epidemiology of urticaria: a representative cross-sectional population survey. Clin Exp Dermatol. 2010;35(8):869–73.
12. Simons FE. Prevention of acute urticaria in young children with atopic dermatitis. J Allergy Clin Immunol. 2001;107(4):703–6.
13. Legrain V, et al. Urticaria in infants: a study of forty patients. Pediatr Dermatol. 1990;7(2):101–7.
14. Kauppinen K, Juntunen K, Lanki H. Urticaria in children. Retrospective evaluation and follow-up. Allergy. 1984;39(6):469–72.
15. Aoki T, Kojima M, Horiko T. Acute urticaria: history and natural course of 50 cases. J Dermatol. 1994;21(2):73–7.
16. Grunewald SM, et al. Infection with influenza a virus leads to flu antigen-induced cutaneous anaphylaxis in mice. J Invest Dermatol. 2002;118(4):645–51.
17. Fujii K, et al. Acute urticaria with elevated circulating interleukin-6 is resistant to anti histamine treatment. J Dermatol. 2001;28(5):248–50.
18. Javaud N, et al. Glucocorticoids for acute urticaria: study protocol for a double-blind non-inferiority randomised controlled trial. BMJ Open. 2019;9(8):e027431.
19. Watson NT, Weiss EL, Harter PM. Famotidine in the treatment of acute urticaria. Clin Exp Dermatol. 2000;25(3):186–9.

Chronic Spontaneous Urticaria

6

Dorothea Terhorst-Molawi and Marcus Maurer

6.1 Definition

Chronic spontaneous urticaria (CSU) is characterized by the rapid and unprompted appearance of itchy weals and/or angio-oedema. Weals are short-lived superficial skin swellings of variable size that are associated with itching or burning (Fig. 6.1). Weals come with flare reactions of the surrounding skin, and they resolve spontaneously (usually within several hours). Angio-oedemas are sudden, deeper, pronounced, and sometimes painful swellings of the lower dermis and subcutis. They are of longer duration and slower resolution than weals (usually several hours to a few days) (Fig. 6.2). The signs and symptoms of CSU occur spontaneously, seemingly "out of the blue," and it is usually impossible to predict when, why, and where they will appear next. This makes CSU unique. In all other forms of chronic urticaria, definite triggers (Table 6.1) induce the signs and symptoms.

6.2 Clinical Picture

Several studies have looked at the patterns of occurrence of weals and angio-oedema in CSU patients. A representative cross-sectional population survey conducted in Germany included 4093 individuals with urticaria. Of the included patients with CSU, 33% had weals and angio-oedema, and 61% and 6%, respectively, exclusively had weals and angio-oedema [1]. A more recent study included 673 patients primarily from hospital-based specialist centers. Within these patients with CSU from

D. Terhorst-Molawi · M. Maurer (✉)
Institute for Allergology, Charité – Universitätsmedizin, Berlin, Germany

Fraunhofer Institute for Translational Medicine and Pharmacology ITMP, Allergology and Immunology, Berlin, Germany
e-mail: Marcus.Maurer@charite.de

Fig. 6.1 Weal and flare type skin reactions in CU patient

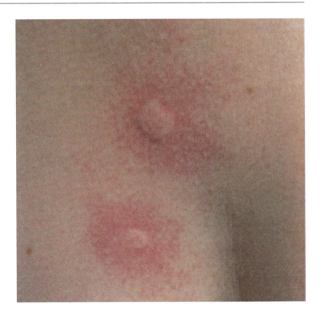

Fig. 6.2 Angio-oedema of the left hand in CU patient

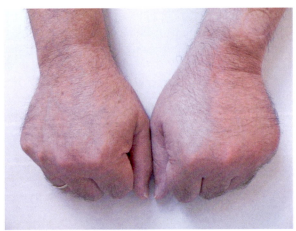

Canada, France, Germany, Italy, Spain, the Netherlands, and the United Kingdom 59% had both weals and angio-oedema [2]. Another recent study found 50% of CSU patients had weals and angio-oedema, about 1 in 3 CSU patients had only weals, and 1 in 10 patients had only angio-oedema [3]. In pediatric patients with CSU, 5–14% were found to have angio-oedema [4].

The signs and symptoms of CSU can occur at anytime and anywhere on the skin. Most often, however, weals develop during the evening hours favoring the arms and legs [5], whereas angio-oedema is most commonly located in the head region (e.g., eye lids, lips, tongue) as well as hands and feet [1]. In most patients with moderate or severe CSU, weals and/or angio-oedema occur every or almost every day [6]. In

Table 6.1 Classification of chronic urticaria

Chronic urticaria	
Chronic spontaneous urticaria	Inducible urticaria
Spontaneous appearance of weals, angio-oedema or both for >6 weeks	Symptomatic dermographism (also called Urticaria factitia/dermographic urticaria)
	Cold urticaria (also called cold contact urticaria)
	Solar urticaria
	Delayed pressure urticaria
	Heat contact urticaria
	Vibratory angio-oedema
	Cholinergic urticaria
	Contact urticaria
	Aquagenic urticaria

Adapted from Zuberbier et al. (2017)

the same patient, disease activity can change markedly over time. Periods of weeks and months, in which no or very few signs and symptoms occur, can alternate with other times, in which disease activity is high. In some patients, unspecific triggers such as stress or infections can sporadically lead to exacerbation of CSU.

CSU is of long duration in most patients, about 50% of patients with CSU are affected for more than 10 years [6, 7] although others show more rapid resolution, and the average duration of CSU is held to range from 4 to 7 years. CSU shows spontaneous remission in virtually all patients [6, 8–10]. It is expected that cases presenting to specialist clinics are likely to be more severe and prolonged than those that are managed in the community.

6.3 Epidemiology

CU is a common condition in all parts of the world. Lifetime prevalence for CSU was found to be around 2% [1]. Women are consistently found to suffer at least twice as often from CSU as men [1]. The peak age bracket of disease onset is 20–60 years in both [6], but CSU can occur at any age. The estimated 1 year interval prevalence of CSU in pediatric patients was 0.75% in a physician-based on-line survey [4] and thus similar to adults. CSU may be more common in Asia and South America as compared to North America and Europe, and the prevalence appears to be increasing [11].

6.4 Etiopathogenesis

The signs and symptoms of CSU are brought about by the activation of cutaneous mast cells [12]. Mast cells are large resident skin cells with characteristic metachromatic cytoplasmic granules that contain preformed mediators such as histamine. Mast cells are preferentially localized in the vicinity of sensory nerves and small

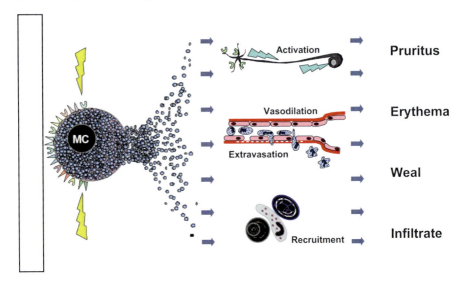

Fig. 6.3 Mast cell degranulation and its effects in CU

blood vessels of the dermis. Their main physiological role is to provide a first line of defense against pathogens and other environmental dangers [13]. Mast cell degranulation and the subsequent release of mediators including histamine induce sensory nerve stimulation (pruritus) and vasodilatation (erythema), increased extravasation (edema) as well the recruitment of eosinophils, basophils, neutrophils, and other immune cells (infiltrate) (Fig. 6.3). Mast cell degranulation and its modulation are a complex process that can involve a large range and number of receptor–ligand interactions (Fig. 6.4). In CSU patients, two different types of autoimmune mechanisms are held to be relevant for the degranulation of skin mast cells, IgE-mediated auto-allergic activation, and IgG-mediated type IIb autoimmune activation [14].

6.4.1 Autoallergy and Autoimmunity, Causes of CSU

Autoallergy describes the phenomenon of type I hypersensitivity to self, in which antigens crosslink IgE autoantibodies bound to the high affinity IgE receptor on mast cells and basophils to cause their degranulation. CSU characterized by functional IgE autoantibodies is referred to as auto-allergic or type I autoimmune CSU. IgE against autoantigens is found and held to contribute to CSU pathogenesis in more than two-thirds of patients with CSU. Half of CSU patients were found to have elevated levels of IgE autoantibodies against thyreoperoxidase [15], and 70% of CSU patients had IgE autoantibodies against interleukin-24 (IL-24) [16]. Recent studies showed that IgE autoantibodies of CSU patients are directed to a wide variety of autoantigens, many of which are expressed in the skin. These include IL-24,

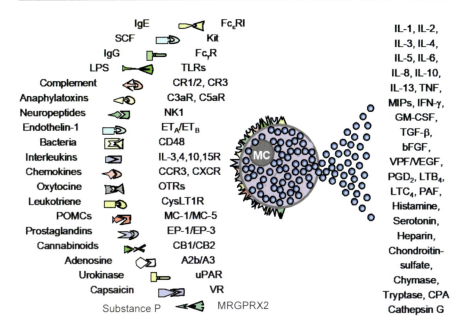

Fig. 6.4 Selection of receptor–ligand interactions resulting in mast cell activation

which is often recognized by IgE of CSU patients and which is functionally relevant. IgE anti-IL-24 and IL-24 together lead to the degranulation of mast cells [16]. The IgE anti-IL-24 levels of urticaria patients correlate with their disease activity. Furthermore, it has been shown that IgE autoantibodies are responsible for the increased total IgE levels in CSU patients and that the overall IgE of CSU patients is mostly directed against autoantigens [16] Recently, the relevance of IgE-anti-TPO in the pathogenesis of auto-allergic CSU has been demonstrated *in vivo*, by adoptive transfer of patient serum [17].

The therapeutic success of omalizumab in CSU provides further evidence for the relevance of IgE autoantibodies for the pathogenesis of CSU. The first ever placebo-controlled multicentric study with omalizumab in CSU showed very rapid improvement and very high rates of response (70% complete responders). Only patients with IgE against thyroid thyreoperoxidase were treated in this study [8].

6.4.2 Autoimmunity

Type IIb autoimmunity describes a hypersensitivity reaction to self in which antibodies, usually IgG or IgM, bind to antigen on a target cell, which then leads to the activation of this target cell. In a subpopulation of CSU patients, type IIb autoimmunity, i.e., IgG autoantibodies to IgE or its high affinity receptor, FceRI, is held to be the underlying cause. Functional IgG autoantibodies to the alpha-chain of FceRI are found in 20–30% of all patients with CSU. The prevalence of IgG autoantibodies to IgE is significantly lower. IgG autoantibodies to IgE or the IgE receptor can be functional and degranulate mast cells, *in vitro* and *in vivo* [18, 19].

About 50% of patients with autoreactivity (a positive autologous serum skin test) have functional autoantibodies as evidence of type IIb autoimmune urticaria. To perform a positive Autologous Serum Skin Test (ASST), serum of the patient is injected intradermally and induces a weal-and-flare response [20]. Other tests such as the Basophil Histamine Release Assay, BHRA, or the Basophil Activation Test, BAT, are more specific than the ASST to screen for type IIb autoimmune CSU. Herein, the serum of CSU patients is incubated with basophils of healthy individuals. If histamine release or activation of basophils occurs, this points to the presence of IgG autoantibodies [21]. Numerous studies suggest that CSU patients with IgG-mediated type IIb autoimmune urticaria have a longer duration of illness, a higher likelihood of developing angio-oedema, increased disease activity, and more frequent autoimmune comorbidities [14, 21, 22]. It has recently been shown that CSU patients with features of type IIb autoimmune CSU have a different and most importantly delayed response to omalizumab therapy [23, 24].

6.4.3 Stress, Infections, and Food Intolerance, Modulators of CSU

Stress, infections, and foods can be relevant modulators of mast cell activation and CSU disease activity. Many CSU patients know that stress makes their disease worse. Several neuropeptides, such as Substance P (SP), released during stress reactions have mast cell modulating effects. SP is upregulated in the serum of patients with CSU patients and is linked to disease activity [25]. Weal reactions to intradermally injected neuropeptides such as SP are larger and longer lasting in CSU patients. SP acts on mast cell via binding to MRGPRX2 [26], which has been reported to be strongly expressed by skin mast cells in CSU.

Clinical experience shows that the treatment of chronic infections can lead to an improvement in CSU. In the context of persistent bacterial infections, bacterial components and components of the immune system (for example, complement factors) act on mast cells. Infections that can modulate CSU activity include bacterial infections, e.g., of the nasopharynx or by Helicobacter pylori of the gastrointestinal tract, and parasite infections, e.g., with Blastocystis hominis [27–29]. Mast cells have been shown in murine models to protect the host from pathogen invasion and from the pathology associated with bacterial infections, and mast cells are equipped with multiple surface receptors that function as sensors for pathogens. These include toll like receptors, complement receptors, and Fc receptors. Which of these mechanisms are relevant for the activation of mast cells in patients with CSU who have infections remains unclear. Also, there are very few controlled trials on the role and relevance of chronic infections in CSU patients. Generally, CSU patients do not exhibit an increased prevalence of infections, and infections should only be regarded as relevant in patients who show CSU improvement or remission upon successful eradication of the infectious pathogen. The most common bacterial infection linked to CSU is *Helicobacter pylori*-gastritis. Parasite infections (e.g., by *Toxocara canis*, *Giardia lamblia*, or *Blastocystis hominis*) rarely contribute to CSU in Northern European countries, but are more frequent in other regions of the world. Intestinal candidosis used to be regarded as a common underlying cause for CSU [30], but more recent findings do not support this view [31]. Nevertheless, it is recommended that symptomatic candidosis is treated, especially in sensitized patients identified by intracutaneous testing.

CSU patients frequently suspect that their symptoms are brought about by the food they eat [32]. This can be indicative of CSU exacerbation due to intolerance, i.e., non-allergic, dose dependent, and delayed (4–12 h) onset hypersensitivity to food pseudoallergens such as food colorants, preservatives, taste intensifiers, and naturally occurring substances, e.g., aromatic compounds, biogenic amines, and salicylic acid. A role of intolerance in patients with CSU is supported by decreased disease activity following a 3–4 week diet low in pseudoallergens and increased disease activity following challenge tests with pseudoallergens. Responder rates vary and range from 50 to 90% following elimination and from 20 to 60% following challenge testing [33]. Many pseudoallergens are known to alter the activation threshold of mast cells for subsequent degranulation, but they themselves have no degranulating effects.

Skin mast cells express numerous G protein-coupled receptors (GPCRs), which are the largest group of membrane receptor proteins and common targets of drug therapy. Many compounds including some neuropeptides, antimicrobial peptides, and drugs activate human skin mast cells through a GPCR known as Mas-related G protein-coupled receptor X2 (MRGPRX2) [34]. MRGPRX2 may play an important role in the pathogenesis of CSU [26].

6.5 Diagnostic Workup

Spontaneously recurring weals and/or angio-oedema occur not only in patients with CSU. Several differential diagnoses need to be ruled out, by a thorough history and follow up diagnostic tests if indicated. Recurrent weals without angio-oedema occur in urticaria vasculitis and autoinflammatory disorders such as Schnitzler syndrome or cryopyrin-associated periodic syndromes (CAPS). Patients who exclusively develop recurrent angio-oedema, but not weals, may have bradykinin-mediated angio-oedema, e.g., angiotensin-converting-enzyme (ACE)-inhibitor induced angio-oedema or hereditary angio-oedema.

Once the diagnosis of chronic urticaria has been established, it is important to determine which form or forms of chronic urticaria the patient is suffering from. Individuals affected by the various forms of chronic inducible urticaria report that they can deliberately trigger weals or angio-oedema by exposing themselves to the relevant triggers, while patients with CSU cannot.

History taking is indispensable in patients with CSU. In addition to ruling out differential diagnoses, the history should explore comorbidities, markers of disease

Table 6.2 Chronic urticaria—Questions that should be asked…

1	When did your urticaria first present? (Life events?)
2	How often do you have weals and how long do they last?
3	When during the day are the weals most itchy?
4	What is the usual shape and size of weals and what skin areas are affected?
5	Do you get angio-oedema? How often? Where? For how long?
6	What problems do the weals/angio-oedema cause? (e.g., itch/pain/burning?)
7	Does or did anyone in your family also suffer from urticaria (or allergies)?
8	Do you have allergies/other diseases? What do you think is the cause?
9	Can you induce the onset of weals/angio-oedema, e.g., rubbing of the skin?
10	What drugs do you use (NSAIDs, hormones, laxatives, alternative remedies)?
11	Do you see a relationship of weal/angio-oedema onset and the food you eat?
12	Do you smoke/drink alcohol? Do you see a relationship?
13	What type of work do you do? Do you see a relationship?
14	What do you do for fun? Do you see a relationship?
15	Does your urticaria change on the weekend/during holidays or vacation?
16	Do you react normally to insect stings/bites (e.g., bees, yellow jackets)?
17	What therapies have you tried and what were the results?
18	Does stress trigger weals?
19	Is your quality of life affected by the urticaria? How?
20	In female patients: do you see a relationship with your menstrual cycle?

course and activity, and predictors of response to treatment. In patients with long-lasting and uncontrolled disease, further diagnostic steps to identify relevant drivers of disease activity should be considered and taken if indicated. These steps should be based on a thorough history, taking the following questions into consideration (Table 6.2).

In all patients with CSU, initial laboratory tests should include erythrocyte sedimentation rate and/or C-reactive protein as well as a differential blood count. While the goal of these tests is to rule out systemic inflammatory events, CSU, by itself, may lead to elevated levels. Depending on the history and the duration and severity of CSU, patients should subsequently undergo further diagnostic workup for causes and associated disorders. Exhaustive and pricy general screening programs for causes of urticaria are strongly advised against.

Whereas type I allergy is hardly ever a cause of CSU, non-allergic hypersensitivity reactions to NSAIDs or food may be more relevant for CSU. Bacterial, viral, parasitic, or fungal infections, e.g., with *H. pylori,* streptococci, staphylococci, *Yersinia, Giardia lamblia, Mycoplasma pneumoniae*, hepatitis viruses, *norovirus, parvovirus B19, Anisakis simplex, Entamoeba* spp, *Blastocystis* spp, have been implicated as potential causes of urticaria [35]. More data on the role of infections in modulating CSU disease activity is needed in order to make definitive recommendations. Ruling out malignancies is necessary if patient history (e.g., sudden loss of weight) points to this, routine screening is not suggested.

Basophil tests (BTs) and the Autologous Serum Skin Test (ASST) are the only generally available tests to screen for autoantibodies against IgE or against the high affinity IgE receptor (FcεR1). Histamine release or activation of donor basophils after stimulation with the serum of CSU patients is measured by BTs. BTs also help to diagnose autoimmune urticaria [36], co-assess disease activity [37], and to predict the response to ciclosporin A or omalizumab [24, 38]. The ASST evaluates the presence of vasoactive factors and a heightened responsiveness of skin during active urticaria to stimulation [20, 21].

In order to guide treatment decisions, to understand and assess the patients' disease burden, and to better document the patient's history, patient-reported outcome (PRO) measures should be used in the diagnostic workup of CSU. As most of CSU patients show a great variability in daily symptoms, the use of these tools is highly recommended. Disease activity should be assessed with the urticaria activity score (UAS) and the angio-oedema activity score (AAS). Patients record and quantify their symptoms (UAS: weals and pruritus, AAS: angio-oedema) on a daily basis. Disease control is assessed by use of the urticaria control test (UCT) and angio-oedema control test (AECT). The UCT and the AECT allow patients and their physicians to rapidly and reliably measure retrospectively disease control with four simple questions each. Quality of life impairment is determined with the chronic urticaria quality of life questionnaire (CU-Q2oL) and the angio-oedema quality of life questionnaire (AE-QoL).

In everyday clinical practice, assessment of disease burden, activity and control simplifies treatment decision making.

6.6 Therapy

CSU in most patients cannot be cured, as no causal treatment is available as of yet to eliminate the underlying autoimmunity or autoallergy. The goal of therapeutic approaches in CSU, therefore, is for patients to gain complete control of all signs and symptoms, to be free of weals and angio-oedema, until spontaneous remission occurs. All patients should avoid known triggers, such as nonsteroidal anti-inflammatory drugs. In addition, prophylactic symptomatic medication is recommended for all patients.

The first line treatment for CSU is a non-sedating H1-antihistamine of the second generation [39]. Patient-reported outcome measures such as the UAS, the AAS, the UCT, and/or the AECT should be used to monitor the response to this treatment. Initially, the antihistamine shall be taken at the approved standard dose of once daily. It is important to explain to patients the benefits of the regular use of antihistamines, so that they do not take them only once symptoms occur. Patients who still develop weals or angio-oedema after two to four weeks of the daily use of a standard-dosed H1-antihistamine should increase their dose of this antihistamine to up to fourfold of the standard dose. For many non-sedating antihistamines, updosing has been shown to be efficient and safe and well tolerated [40].

Patients who still have no control over their CSU with a higher than standard-dosed non-sedating H1-antihistamine should be treated with add on omalizumab. This recombinant humanized anti-IgE antibody is administered by subcutaneous injection at the standard dose of 300 mg every 4 weeks. Safety and efficacy of omalizumab in the treatment of patients with CSU were shown in clinical studies and in everyday use [41, 42]. Several mechanisms have been suggested to add to the therapeutic response of omalizumab in patients with CSU as well as to the heterogeneity of their clinical reactions [24, 43–45].

Most patients show a strong response even before the second dose [46, 47]. Some patients require multiple doses to achieve treatment success [24]. If, after 6 months of treatment, the effects of omalizumab are still limited, off-label treatment with cyclosporine is suggested [39]. Placebo-controlled trials have confirmed the efficacy of cyclosporine in CSU [48]. There is also potential value of low-evidence drugs such as dapsone, sulphasalazine, methotrexate, mycophenolate mofetil, doxepin, montelukast, H2 antihistamines, and others [39]. They are widely used internationally and can be effective even though well-designed double-blind studies may not be available.

Patients who have complete control of their symptoms should be checked for a complete remission of their CSU every 6–12 months.

References

1. Zuberbier T, et al. Epidemiology of urticaria: a representative cross-sectional population survey. Clin Exp Dermatol. 2010;35(8):869–73.
2. Maurer M, et al. The burden of chronic spontaneous urticaria is substantial: real-world evidence from ASSURE-CSU. Allergy. 2017;72(12):2005–16.
3. Sussman G, et al. Angioedema in chronic spontaneous urticaria is underdiagnosed and has a substantial impact: analyses from ASSURE-CSU. Allergy. 2018;73(8):1724–34.
4. Balp MM, et al. Prevalence and clinical characteristics of chronic spontaneous urticaria in pediatric patients. Pediatr Allergy Immunol. 2018;29(6):630–6.
5. Maurer M, Ortonne JP, Zuberbier T. Chronic urticaria: an internet survey of health behaviours, symptom patterns and treatment needs in European adult patients. Br J Dermatol. 2009;160(3):633–41.
6. Maurer M, et al. Unmet clinical needs in chronic spontaneous urticaria. A GA(2)LEN task force report. Allergy. 2011;66(3):317–30.
7. van der Valk PG, Moret G, Kiemeney LA. The natural history of chronic urticaria and angioedema in patients visiting a tertiary referral centre. Br J Dermatol. 2002;146(1):110–3.
8. Maurer M, et al. Efficacy and safety of omalizumab in patients with chronic urticaria who exhibit IgE against thyroperoxidase. J Allergy Clin Immunol. 2011;128(1):202–209.e5.
9. Zuberbier T, et al. Acute urticaria: clinical aspects and therapeutic responsiveness. Acta Derm Venereol. 1996;76(4):295–7.
10. Zuberbier T, et al. Double-blind crossover study of high-dose cetirizine in cholinergic urticaria. Dermatology. 1996;193(4):324–7.
11. Fricke J, et al. Prevalence of chronic urticaria in children and adults across the globe: systematic review with meta-analysis. Allergy. 2020;75(2):423–32.
12. Church MK, et al. The role and relevance of mast cells in urticaria. Immunol Rev. 2018;282(1):232–47.
13. Metz M, Siebenhaar F, Maurer M. Mast cell functions in the innate skin immune system. Immunobiology. 2008;213(3-4):251–60.
14. Kolkhir P, et al. Autoimmune chronic spontaneous urticaria: what we know and what we do not know. J Allergy Clin Immunol. 2017;139(6):1772–1781.e1.
15. Altrichter S, et al. IgE mediated autoallergy against thyroid peroxidase—a novel pathomechanism of chronic spontaneous urticaria? PLoS One. 2011;6(4):e14794.

16. Schmetzer O, et al. IL-24 is a common and specific autoantigen of IgE in patients with chronic spontaneous urticaria. J Allergy Clin Immunol. 2018;142(3):876–82.
17. Sanchez J, Sanchez A, Cardona R. Causal relationship between anti-TPO IgE and chronic urticaria by in vitro and in vivo tests. Allergy Asthma Immunol Res. 2019;11(1):29–42.
18. Maurer M, et al. [Autoreactive urticaria and autoimmune urticaria]. Hautarzt. 2004;55(4):350–6.
19. Schoepke N, et al. Biomarkers and clinical characteristics of autoimmune chronic spontaneous urticaria: results of the PURIST Study. Allergy. 2019;74(12):2427–36.
20. Konstantinou GN, et al. EAACI/GA(2)LEN task force consensus report: the autologous serum skin test in urticaria. Allergy. 2009;64(9):1256–68.
21. Konstantinou GN, et al. EAACI taskforce position paper: evidence for autoimmune urticaria and proposal for defining diagnostic criteria. Allergy. 2013;68(1):27–36.
22. Kolkhir P, et al. Autoimmune comorbidity in chronic spontaneous urticaria: a systematic review. Autoimmun Rev. 2017;16(12):1196–208.
23. Deza G, et al. Basophil FcepsilonRI expression in chronic spontaneous urticaria: a potential immunological predictor of response to omalizumab therapy. Acta Derm Venereol. 2017;97(6):698–704.
24. Gericke J, et al. Serum autoreactivity predicts time to response to omalizumab therapy in chronic spontaneous urticaria. J Allergy Clin Immunol. 2017;139(3):1059–1061.e1.
25. Metz M, et al. Substance P is upregulated in the serum of patients with chronic spontaneous urticaria. J Invest Dermatol. 2014;134(11):2833–6.
26. Fujisawa D, et al. Expression of Mas-related gene X2 on mast cells is upregulated in the skin of patients with severe chronic urticaria. J Allergy Clin Immunol. 2014;134(3):622–633.e9.
27. Barahona Rondon L et al. [Human blastocystosis: prospective study symptomatology and associated epidemiological factors]. Rev Gastroenterol Peru. 2003;23(1):29–35.
28. Cribier B. Urticaria and hepatitis. Clin Rev Allergy Immunol. 2006;30(1):25–9.
29. Federman DG, et al. The effect of antibiotic therapy for patients infected with Helicobacter pylori who have chronic urticaria. J Am Acad Dermatol. 2003;49(5):861–4.
30. Champion RH, et al. Urticaria and angio-oedema. A review of 554 patients. Br J Dermatol. 1969;81(8):588–97.
31. Ergon MC, et al. Candida spp. colonization and serum anticandidal antibody levels in patients with chronic urticaria. Clin Exp Dermatol. 2007;32(6):740–3.
32. Siebenhaar F, et al. Histamine intolerance in patients with chronic spontaneous urticaria. J Eur Acad Dermatol Venereol. 2016;30(10):1774–7.
33. Buhner S, et al. Pseudoallergic reactions in chronic urticaria are associated with altered gastroduodenal permeability. Allergy. 2004;59(10):1118–23.
34. Subramanian H, Gupta K, Ali H. Roles of Mas-related G protein-coupled receptor X2 on mast cell-mediated host defense, pseudoallergic drug reactions, and chronic inflammatory diseases. J Allergy Clin Immunol. 2016;138(3):700–10.
35. Kolkhir P, et al. Chronic spontaneous urticaria and internal parasites—a systematic review. Allergy. 2016;71(3):308–22.
36. Kim Z, et al. Basophil markers for identification and activation in the indirect basophil activation test by flow cytometry for diagnosis of autoimmune urticaria. Ann Lab Med. 2016;36(1):28–35.
37. Curto-Barredo L, et al. basophil activation test identifies the patients with chronic spontaneous urticaria suffering the most active disease. Immun Inflamm Dis. 2016;4(4):441–5.
38. Iqbal K, et al. A positive serum basophil histamine release assay is a marker for ciclosporin-responsiveness in patients with chronic spontaneous urticaria. Clin Transl Allergy. 2012;2(1):19.
39. Zuberbier T, et al. The EAACI/GA(2)LEN/EDF/WAO guideline for the definition, classification, diagnosis and management of urticaria. Allergy. 2018;73(7):1393–414.
40. Staevska M, et al. The effectiveness of levocetirizine and desloratadine in up to 4 times conventional doses in difficult-to-treat urticaria. J Allergy Clin Immunol. 2010;125(3):676–82.

41. Rubini NPM, et al. Effectiveness and safety of Omalizumab in the treatment of chronic spontaneous urticaria: Systematic review and meta-analysis. Allergol Immunopathol (Madr). 2019;47(6):515–22.
42. Zhao ZT, et al. Omalizumab for the treatment of chronic spontaneous urticaria: a meta-analysis of randomized clinical trials. J Allergy Clin Immunol. 2016;137(6):1742–1750.e4.
43. Chang TW, et al. The potential pharmacologic mechanisms of omalizumab in patients with chronic spontaneous urticaria. J Allergy Clin Immunol. 2015;135(2):337–42.
44. Metz M, et al. Clinical efficacy of omalizumab in chronic spontaneous urticaria is associated with a reduction of FcepsilonRI-positive cells in the skin. Theranostics. 2017;7(5):1266–76.
45. Metz M, et al. Omalizumab normalizes the gene expression signature of lesional skin in patients with chronic spontaneous urticaria: a randomized, double-blind, placebo-controlled study. Allergy. 2019;74(1):141–51.
46. Kaplan A, et al. Omalizumab in patients with symptomatic chronic idiopathic/spontaneous urticaria despite standard combination therapy. J Allergy Clin Immunol. 2013;132(1):101–9.
47. Maurer M, et al. Omalizumab for the treatment of chronic idiopathic or spontaneous urticaria. N Engl J Med. 2013;368(10):924–35.
48. Kulthanan K, et al. Cyclosporine for chronic spontaneous urticaria: a meta-analysis and systematic review. J Allergy Clin Immunol Pract. 2018;6(2):586–99.

Chronic Spontaneous Urticaria and Comorbidities

Pavel Kolkhir and Marcus Maurer

7.1 Introduction

Chronic spontaneous urticaria (CSU) affects up to 1% of the population [1, 2] and frequently coexists with other diseases, i.e., comorbidities. Comorbidities, in CSU patients, are important for several reasons.

Firstly, some comorbidities, e.g., autoimmune diseases (AIDs), are more common in CSU patients, and CSU patients may benefit from screening for these conditions [3, 4]. For example, high values of ESR, C-reactive protein (CRP), and/ or antithyroid antibodies may point to the presence of autoimmune thyroid disease (AITD) in a CSU patient [5]. Furthermore, there is increasing evidence that other CSU comorbidities such as metabolic syndrome (MS) and mental disorders are more prevalent and under-recognized in CSU [6]. As of yet, urticaria guidelines do not provide specific diagnostic recommendations on screening for these comorbidities [5].

P. Kolkhir
Institute for Allergology, Charité – Universitätsmedizin, Berlin, Germany

Fraunhofer Institute for Translational Medicine and Pharmacology ITMP, Allergology and Immunology, Berlin, Germany

Division of Immune-mediated Skin Diseases, I.M. Sechenov First Moscow State Medical University (Sechenov University), Moscow, Russian Federation

M. Maurer (✉)
Institute for Allergology, Charité – Universitätsmedizin, Berlin, Germany

Fraunhofer Institute for Translational Medicine and Pharmacology ITMP, Allergology and Immunology, Berlin, Germany
e-mail: Marcus.Maurer@charite.de

© Springer Nature Switzerland AG 2021
T. Zuberbier et al. (eds.), *Urticaria and Angioedema*,
https://doi.org/10.1007/978-3-030-84574-2_7

Secondly, CSU comorbidities, for instance, mental disorders and chronic inducible urticarias (CIndUs), add to the burden of disease and quality of life impairment. Their identification and treatment, in clinical practice, can help to optimize the management of CSU patients.

Thirdly, some diseases, namely CIndUs and AITD, were suggested to be markers of longer CSU duration and progression from acute spontaneous urticaria to CSU [7–13].

Finally, certain diseases are linked, pathogenetically, to CSU, although the mechanisms are yet to be defined. Investigation of these diseases can help to better understand CSU, and their treatment can reduce CSU disease activity. In particular, some case reports supported this notion showing CSU remission or improvement after the treatment of malignancy, infection, and hyper- and hypothyroidism [14–16].

Here, we describe important groups of comorbidities of CSU, their prevalence, and their relevance for clinical practice.

7.2 Chronic Inducible Urticaria

CIndU is characterized by wheals and/or angioedema induced by exposure to external stimuli. CIndUs are classified as physical CIndUs (e.g., due to cold, heat, pressure, and other stimuli) and other types of CIndUs (cholinergic, aquagenic, and contact urticarias). CIndUs have been reported in 1–11% of the general population [17, 18] with symptomatic dermographism being the most prevalent type of physical CIndU (1–5%) and cholinergic urticaria being the most prevalent of other types

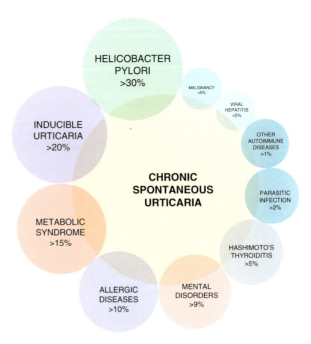

Fig. 7.1 The prevalence of comorbid diseases in CSU

of CIndU (4–11%) [18]. In a meta-analysis, CIndU was observed in 13% among all cases of chronic urticaria [19]. In other studies, 11–75% of CSU patients had comorbid CIndU, with most studies reporting rates of >20% (Fig. 7.1) [7–9, 20–24].

CSU primarily occurs in combination with delayed pressure urticaria (DPU, 2–37%), symptomatic dermographism (SD, 5–75%), cold urticaria (1–13%), and cholinergic urticaria (2–18%). Aquagenic urticaria (0.4%) [7–9, 20, 21, 23, 24], solar urticaria (0.4–0.5%), heat contact urticaria (0.2–4.3%), and vibratory urticaria/angioedema (0.1%) are rare in CSU [17, 24]. Two or more types of CIndU can be present in the same CSU patient [21].

Some CSU patients report that physical and other external stimuli can exacerbate or trigger symptom development. However, CIndU should only be diagnosed when provocation testing is positive. In one study, only half of the 186 patients with CSU, who reported that a physical trigger is relevant, had a positive challenge test result [21]. In the literature, it is not always clear that comorbidity rates reported are based on provocation testing, in fact in some cases it is clear that they are not. Therefore, larger studies of CSU patients subjected to CIndU provocation testing are needed.

Most CIndUs, on average, are of longer duration than CSU [10, 11]. After 10 years, only 26 ± 7% of patients with cold urticaria and 36 ± 10% of patients with cholinergic urticaria exhibited spontaneous remission in comparison to 49 ± 4% of CSU patients [11]. Importantly, CSU is of longer duration when in combination with CIndU [7, 9] (Table 7.1). In one study, rates of remission after 1 year were 21% and 47% for CSU patients with and without CIndU, respectively [7]. SD appears to be an exception. One year spontaneous remission rates of SD patients are similar to those of CSU patients (51 ± 6%), and comorbid SD is not associated with a longer duration of CSU [8, 11].

CSU patients with CIndU may also show higher CSU disease activity as assessed by urticaria activity score, higher rates of a personal history of atopy, and younger age, compared to CSU patients without CIndU [9]. Several studies suggest that CIndU comorbidity is linked to a poor response to antihistamine (AH) treatment. Patients with CSU and CIndU more frequently needed therapy 5 years after the onset of disease and higher doses of second-generation AHs (sgAHs) as compared to patients with CSU only [9]. Moreover, AH-resistant CSU patients show a significantly higher incidence of concomitant CIndU (SD and/or DPU) [27]. In addition, in a multicenter study, CIndU was the most common comorbidity of sgAHs-refractory CSU [24]. In another study, SD and other CIndUs were markers of overall poor treatment control of CSU [28].

In summary, CIndU is a prevalent comorbidity of CSU patients, and SD and DPU appear to be the most common comorbid CIndUs. The presence of CIndU in CSU patients is likely to be linked to a worse prognosis, with the possible exception for SD. If suggested by the patient's history, suspected triggers of CIndU should be assessed for their relevance by challenge tests to diagnose CIndU [17] (Table 7.2). CSU and concomitant CIndU in the same patient can be improved with a similar treatment strategy including antihistamines and omalizumab in refractory cases. A strong body of evidence supports the use of omalizumab in the treatment of patients with CSU as well as difficult-to-treat CIndU [5, 29, 123], although studies that compare the efficacy of omalizumab in patients with CSU vs CIndU vs CSU and CIndU are lacking.

Table 7.1 Comorbid diseases as clinical markers of CSU characteristics and response to treatment

Comorbid disease	Higher prevalence and/or risk of comorbidity in CSU patients vs controls? Response	Level of evidence[1], [Ref]	Marker of progression from acute spontaneous urticaria to CSU? Response	Level of evidence[1], [Ref]	Longer duration of CSU? Response	Level of evidence[1], [Ref]	More severe CSU? Response	Level of evidence[1], [Ref]	A worse response to sgAHs? Response	Level of evidence[1], [Ref]
Chronic inducible urticaria	+	III [21]	+/−	III–IV [9, 25, 26]	+[2]	III [7–11]	+	III [9]	+[2]	III [9, 24, 27–31]
Mental disorders	+	IIb [1, 32–41]	−	IV	−	III [36, 38, 41, 42]	−[3]	III [33, 36, 41, 42]	∅	∅
Autoimmune thyroid diseases	+[4]	IIb [1, 3, 13, 15, 43–46]	+	III [12, 13]	+/−	III [12, 13, 47–51]	+/−	III [49, 50, 52–54]	−	III [28, 31, 52, 55–59]
Other autoimmune diseases	+[4,5]	IIb [3, 43, 44, 60–69]	∅[7]	∅	∅[6]	∅	∅	∅	∅	∅
Helicobacter pylori	+/−	IIb [70–76]	∅	∅	−	III [47, 77–80]	−/+	III [70, 74, 77, 81]	∅	∅
Parasitic infection	+[14]	III [82–86]	∅	∅	∅	∅	∅	∅	∅	∅
Hepatitis B, hepatitis C or HIV infection	−/+[13]	IIb [1, 61, 87–94]	∅	∅	+/−	III–IV[88]	∅	∅	∅	∅
Fungal hypersensitivity	+/−	III [95–101]	∅	∅	−	III [102]	∅	∅	∅	∅

Allergic diseases	+/−	IIb [1, 11, 21, 26, 43–45, 60, 61, 103–106]	+/−	[25, 26, 107, 108]	−	[8, 47, 109, 110]	−	[21, 109]	−/+	[51, 105, 109]
Malignancy	+/−	IIb [1, 44, 111–114]	∅		∅		∅		∅
Metabolic syndrome	+[8]	IIb [1, 6, 45, 60, 115–119]	−[12]	III [26]	+[9]	III [47, 118, 119]	+/−[10]	III [115, 119, 120]	+/−[11]	III [27, 31, 115, 120]

(continued)

+: association is shown in all or all but one study
−: association is not shown in all or all but one study
∅: association is unknown (no data)
+/−: inconsistent evidence with most studies supported the association
−/+: inconsistent evidence with most studies reported against the association
[1]Highest level of evidence of supporting study according to the grading system published by the US Agency for Healthcare Policy and Research Classification (www.ahrq.gov) [121, 122]:
Category of evidence
Ia Evidence from meta-analysis of randomized controlled trials
Ib Evidence from at least one randomized controlled trial
IIa Evidence from at least one well-designed controlled study without randomization
IIb Evidence from at least one other type of quasi-experimental study
III Evidence from nonexperimental descriptive studies, such as comparative studies, correlated studies, and case studies
IV Evidence from expert committee reports or opinions or clinical experience of respected authorities or both
[2]with the possible exception for symptomatic dermographism
[3]however, presence of mental disorder in CSU was associated with a more pronounced reduction of quality of life
[4]in addition, an association of presence of autoimmune diseases with type IIb autoimmune CSU was recently shown [221, 222]
[5]it is primarily true for systemic lupus erythematosus, rheumatoid arthritis, pernicious anemia, insulin-dependent diabetes mellitus, Sjögren's syndrome, celiac disease, psoriasis and vitiligo
[6]CSU linked to higher SLE activity [223]

Table 7.1 (continued)

[7]presence of antinuclear antibodies was not associated with progression from acute urticaria to CSU [12]
[8]in CSU, the risk of metabolic syndrome and its components, hypertension, hyperglycemia/diabetes type II, hyperlipidemia and obesity, is increased. However, in one study, risk of CSU was not increased in patients with type 2 diabetes mellitus, hypertension, or dyslipidemia compared to those without [45]
[9]association with a longer CSU duration was shown for obesity, hypertension and hyperlipidemia
[10]In one study, association between presence of hyperlipidemia and severity of CSU was shown. Another study did not report such association for obesity
[11]no association between obesity and a worse response to AHs was shown
[12]for obesity
[13]in one study, urticaria patients had a higher risk for hepatitis B and C but acute urticaria, inducible urticaria and urticarial vasculitis were not excluded
[14]it is true for protozoa, primarily *Blastocystis hominis*, toxocariasis and fasciolosis seropositivity, *Anisakis simplex* sensitization and strongyloidiasis. These associations are likely to be country-dependent. In some studies, only patients with undefined urticaria were included

7 Chronic Spontaneous Urticaria and Comorbidities

Table 7.2 Management of comorbid diseases in CSU patients

Comorbid disease	Most prevalent types/pathogens	Gender and/or age predisposition	Proposed mechanisms	Personal history, complains and signs of the comorbid disease	Routine diagnostic tests (possible findings)	Extended diagnostic program if indicated by history	Should UV be excluded in the first place?	Treatment of the comorbid disease	CSU remission was shown after treatment of the comorbid disease?
Chronic inducible urticaria	Symptomatic dermographism, DPU	Females	Unknown, might be IgE or IgG autoreactivity	Wheals and/or angioedema due to external stimuli	No	Challenge tests	No	Avoidance of triggers and same treatment strategy as for CSU	Remission is possible because the treatment is the same
Mental disorders	Depression, anxiety	–	–	Specific complains (e.g., depressed mood, past history of a mental disorder	No	Specific questionnaires for mental health evaluation, consultation of a psychiatrist and/or psychologist	No	Psychotropic medications, e.g., doxepin, psychotherapeutic treatments and behavioral interventions	Some psychotropic medications, e.g., doxepin, may be effective in both CSU and a mental disorder
Autoimmune thyroid diseases	Hashimoto's thyroiditis	Adult females	Immune complexes, complement activation, IgE autoantibodies and/or the systemic low-grade inflammation	Complains specific for hyper- or hypothyroidism; can be asymptomatic	No	Antithyroid antibodies, TSH, consultation of an endocrinologist	No	Levothyroxine or antithyroid drugs	Yes, in some patients after treatment of hypo- or hyperthyroidism

(continued)

Table 7.2 (continued)

Comorbid disease	Most prevalent types/pathogens	Gender and/or age predisposition	Proposed mechanisms	Personal history, complaints and signs of the comorbid disease	Routine diagnostic tests (possible findings)	Extended diagnostic program if indicated by history	Should UV be excluded in the first place?	Treatment of the comorbid disease	CSU remission was shown after treatment of the comorbid disease?
Other autoimmune diseases	Vitiligo, pernicious anemia, SLE, insulin-dependent diabetes mellitus, celiac disease	Adult females; children (e.g., celiac disease, type I diabetes)	IgG and IgE-mediated autoreactivity, chronic inflammation, activation of the complement and/or coagulation systems	Complains specific for each autoimmune disease	DBC (leukocytosis), ESR, CRP (increased levels)	ANA, specific autoantibodies, complement, consultation of a rheumatologist	Yes	Immunosuppressive and immunomodulatory therapy, biologics, other specific treatment	CSU may improve due to treatment of comorbid disease
Bacterial infection	Helicobacter pylori	–	Direct activation of MCs by HP proteins, molecular mimicry	Can be asymptomatic	No	Testing for HP only after considering other CSU causes	No	Eradication with antibiotics	Yes, but evidence is inconsistent
Other bacterial infection	Focal infections, e.g., dental infection, streptococcal tonsillitis	–	Chronic inflammation, IgE autoreactivity	Specific for each infection	DBC (leukocytosis), ESR, CRP (increased levels)	Search for infection	No	Antibiotic therapy or other treatment if indicated	Yes, some cases are published

7 Chronic Spontaneous Urticaria and Comorbidities

Parasitic infection	Protozoa, primarily *Gardia spp.* and *Blastocystis hominis*, and helminths, mostly *Anisakis simplex*, *Strongyloides stercoralis* and *Toxocara canis*	–	Presence of the parasite in the skin, IgE-mediated allergy, Th2 cytokine skewing, eosinophils, and/or activation of the complement and/or coagulation	Residence in or recent travel to a parasite-endemic area, dietary habit, GI symptoms	DBC (unexplained eosinophilia)	Consultation of a parasitologist, serologic testing for parasites, stool for parasites, etc.	No	Antiparasitic treatment or fish free-diet (in case of *Anisakis simplex* hypersensitivity)	Yes, especially in patients with previously diagnosed parasitic infection
Viral infection	Chronic hepatitis B and C, HIV	–	Activation of skin MCs by protein Fv produced during viral hepatitis; hyperbilirubinemia; immune complexes; complement activation	Signs and symptoms and/or past history of viral infection	DBC; ESR, CRP (increased levels)	Anti-HCV, HbsAg, anti-HIV, cryoglobulins	Yes	Antiviral treatment if indicated	No, in most CSU patients with viral hepatitis
Fungal infection	*Candida albicans*, *Trichophyton spp.*	–	Hypersensitivity to fungi antigens	Signs of fungal infection	No	Search for fungal infection, allergy tests to fungi	No	Antifungal treatment or avoidance of allergens	Yes, in a few published reports

(continued)

Table 7.2 (continued)

Comorbid disease	Most prevalent types/pathogens	Gender and/or age predisposition	Proposed mechanisms	Personal history, complains and signs of the comorbid disease	Routine diagnostic tests (possible findings)	Extended diagnostic program if indicated by history	Should UV be excluded in the first place?	Treatment of the comorbid disease	CSU remission was shown after treatment of the comorbid disease?
Allergic diseases	Asthma, atopic dermatitis, allergic rhinitis and other allergic diseases	Depends on the disease	IgE-mediated hypersensitivity	Symptoms of allergy	DBC (eosinophilia)	Allergy tests, total IgE	No	Avoidance of allergens, antiallergic therapy, allergen-specific immunotherapy	Yes, if CSU is allergic
Malignancy	Solid tumors (more often), hematologic neoplasms	Adults	Immune dysregulation, chronic inflammation, activation of complement and/or coagulation	Specific signs and symptoms of malignancy	DBC; ESR, CRP (increased levels)	Search for malignancy	Yes	Surgical therapy, chemotherapy and/or radiation therapy	Yes, in most reported cases
Metabolic syndrome	Obesity, dyslipidemia, hyperglycemia, hypertension	Adults	Low-grade inflammation	No or specific symptoms	DBC; ESR, CRP (increased levels)	Measurement of blood pressure, BMI, serum levels of glucose and lipids	No	Specific therapy	Unlikely

UV urticarial vasculitis, *DPU* delayed pressure urticaria, *GI* gastrointestinal symptoms, *MCs* mast cells, *DBC* differential blood count, *ESR* the erythrocyte sedimentation rate, *CRP* C-reactive protein, *TSH* thyroid-stimulating hormone, *SLE* systemic lupus erythematosus, *BMI* Body Mass Index, *ANA* antinuclear antibodies, *HP* Helicobacter pylori

7.3 Mental Disorders

Mental disorders are relatively frequent in the general population with 12–49% affected [124], and they may be more prevalent in CSU patients. In several studies, psychiatric comorbidities were found to be present in 5–60% of patients with CSU. The most frequently recorded diagnoses were depression (3–40%) and anxiety (5–30%) [9, 23, 24, 32, 42, 125]. Other mental disorders included posttraumatic stress disorder (3–34%), somatoform disorder (6–17%), adjustment disorder (4%), harmful use of alcohol (3%), bipolar disorder (2%), hypochondria (2%), obsessive-compulsive disorder (2%), alcohol dependency (1%), and multiple substance abuse (1%) [32, 33, 42]. In one study, 17% of CSU patients had a psychiatric disorder in the past [42].

In several population-based studies, undefined chronic urticaria or CSU was associated with a significantly increased risk of mental disorders [1, 34]. Patients with CSU experienced higher levels of stress, somatization, obsessive-compulsive disorder, depression, and/or anxiety than controls [32, 33, 35–41]. For example, in a nationwide study of 14,859 Italian CSU patients, CSU was statistically significantly associated with anxiety, dissociative and somatoform disorders [1]. Furthermore, CSU patients showed higher scores for hysteria, paranoia, psychasthenia, psychopathic deviation, social introversion personality traits [38], posttraumatic stress disorder, [33] and alexithymia [126] as compared to controls. Urticaria was one of the most common conditions in patients with bipolar disorder (9%) [127]. Increased prevalence of urticaria was found among patients with attention-deficit/hyperactivity disorder as compared to the control group [128]. Patients treated for CSU significantly more often visited psychiatrists and psychologists than controls without CSU [129].

The presence of psychiatric comorbidity in patients with CSU, in two studies, was associated with a more pronounced reduction of quality of life, and the severity of psychiatric disease correlated with quality of life impairment [36, 130]. All but one study reported that the duration of CSU and the presence of psychiatric comorbidity are not linked [36, 38, 41, 42]. Furthermore, no correlations were found between comorbid psychiatric diagnoses and CSU severity [33, 36, 41, 42] (Table 7.1).

In summary, psychiatric disorders, primarily depression and anxiety, are important comorbidities of CSU. They are common, and they significantly contribute to the quality of life impairment of CSU. Exploring CSU patients for comorbid psychiatric diseases can help their management and improve quality of life and reduce emotional distress [32, 38]. Strategies for investigating and approaching mental disease in CSU patients include the use of specific questionnaires for evaluating mental health in routine clinical practice and referral to specialists for diagnosing and treating psychiatric diseases.

7.4 Autoimmune Diseases

CSU is autoimmune in some patients [131], and patients with CSU are known to have higher rates of other AIDs. In a systematic review, the prevalence of individual AIDs in CSU was higher as compared to the general population (≥1% vs ≤1%) [4]. Vice versa, the prevalence of urticarial rash in patients with AIDs was >1% in most studies. Furthermore, in several large population-based studies, patients with chronic urticaria were found to be at higher risk for comorbid AIDs than controls [3, 13, 43, 60].

The most prevalent AIDs in CSU are Hashimoto's thyroiditis (HT, ≥5%), pernicious anemia (≥5%), and vitiligo (≥3%)[4, 15, 24]. On the other hand, chronic urticarial rash was found to be most frequent in eosinophilic granulomatosis with polyangiitis (EGPA ≥10%), AITD (>7%), and systemic lupus erythematosus (SLE, >5%)[4, 15, 132]. In CSU, organ-specific autoimmune comorbidities (most prevalent: HT) were seen more often than systemic AIDs (most prevalent: connective tissue diseases, e.g., SLE). AIDs with high and low prevalence in the general population are also common and rare in CSU patients, respectively [4].

AITD in combination with other AIDs occurs in 1–6% of CSU patients. Interestingly, CSU has been described as a part of "autoimmune polyglandular syndrome" (APS). In fact, more than 2% of CSU patients have AITD and vitiligo (APS type 3C, 1–5%) or AITD and pernicious anemia (APS type 3B, 5–6%). Urticarial rash was reportedly seen in 9% of patients with APS type 1, which includes chronic candidiasis and/or chronic hypoparathyroidism and/or Addison's disease. The prevalence of three or more coexistent AIDs and overlap syndromes appears not be increased in CSU patients (15% of CSU patients [4].

Thyroid autoimmunity was described to be linked to the progression of acute spontaneous urticaria toward CSU [12]. In contrast, evidence regarding the association between levels of antithyroid antibodies and CSU duration or severity/activity, gender and age of patients, autologous serum skin test response, or response to treatment is inconsistent or negative [15] (Table 7.1). Autoimmune comorbidities may, however, be important when it comes to the choice of treatment of CSU patients. In a recently published systematic review, of 285 CSU patients treated with thyroid medication in 22 studies, CSU improved in 42% cases. CSU responded to such treatment in hypothyroid, hyperthyroid, and even in some euthyroid patients [15]. Both CSU and comorbid AIDs may benefit from immunosuppressive treatment. For example, all symptoms of CSU and SLE in a five-year-old female improved after therapy with prednisolone and cyclosporine [133]. However, further research is needed because many previous studies were small, uncontrolled and/or had other limitations of design.

In summary, CSU patients are at risk of developing AIDs, and this is especially true for middle-aged female patients with a positive family history for autoimmune disease [4]. AITD, mostly HT, is the most common autoimmune comorbidity in CSU. In CSU patients with elevated IgG antithyroid antibodies and/or risk for AITD, annual reassessment of thyroid function may be warranted [15]. In hypo- and hyperthyroid CSU patients, treatment with levothyroxine or antithyroid drugs, respectively, can improve CSU. In individual euthyroid patients with difficult-to-treat and long-lasting CSU and presence of antithyroid antibodies, levothyroxine can be regarded as an alternative treatment. Treatment with immunosuppressive drugs and/or biologicals may improve both CSU and comorbid autoimmune disease, e.g., SLE.

7.5 Infection

7.5.1 Bacterial Infection

Chronic infections with various bacteria have been linked to the pathogenesis of CSU including *Helicobacter pylori* (HP), *Staphylococci,* and *Streptococci* [16]. HP is considered responsible for the majority of peptic ulcers, as well as chronic gastritis. The results of studies of the rates of CSU patients with HP infection are controversial. In some studies [70–72], but not in the others [73–75], CSU patients had a higher prevalence of HP infection than controls. A meta-analysis of observational studies involving 965 CSU cases and 1,235 controls suggested that HP infection is significantly, though weakly, associated with an increased risk of CSU [72]. In CSU, the prevalence of HP infection ranged from 10 to 77%, across studies [73, 76, 134–136].

There are studies where HP eradication reduced CSU disease activity [77, 134, 137–139]. On the other hand, many studies did not find that HP eradication leads to CSU improvement [73, 75, 78, 135, 140]. Only three placebo-controlled, double blind trials have been carried out so far [137, 138, 140], two of which linking HP treatment to CSU improvement [137, 138]. In a systematic review of 10 studies, eradication of HP was both quantitatively and statistically associated with remission of CSU [139]. Wedi et al. analyzed pro- and contra-studies and found that the rate of chronic urticaria remission or improvement is nearly doubled when HP is eradicated [16]. In contrast, using the GRADE approach, another review arrived at the conclusion that "evidence that H. pylori eradication leads to improvement of chronic urticaria outcomes is weak and conflicting" [141].

Focal bacterial infections have been reported in 0–50% of CSU patients [25, 136, 142, 143]. These include sinusitis (0.3–32%), dental infection (1–29%), tonsillitis (6–9%), urinary infection (0.5–6%), and lung infection (0–18%) [25, 136, 142–145].

Many reports have linked CSU to dental infection [136, 144, 146–149]. For example, in four cases, CSU cleared or improved after teeth extraction due to periapical abscesses and/or removing caries [146–149]. Of 929 patients with chronic angioedema without wheals, 3% patients had an infection. Appropriate treatment of the infection markedly improved the angioedema in 11 patients with dental granuloma [145]. Of 17 CSU patients with dental or ear-nose-throat infection or yersiniosis, 12 showed remission of their CSU after treatment of the focal infection [136]. Urticaria improved in two cases of sinusitis and in four cases of tooth infection [144]. However, two other studies did not find a significant association between CSU and dental infection [150, 151].

Streptococcus spp. infection occurs as tonsillitis, pharyngitis, cystitis, peritonitis, and rheumatic fever [152]. Levels of antistreptococcal antibodies are reportedly raised in up to 37% of CSU patients [142, 143]. However, in a study by Hellgren and Hersle, no significant difference was found in antistreptolysin antibody titers between patients with chronic urticaria and healthy controls [142]. Evidence for the relevance of streptococcal infection is anecdotal, controlled trials are lacking. Chronic urticaria in some of 16 children in a series by Buckley and Dees went into remission after antibiotic therapy of streptococcal infection [153]. In two patients with CSU and streptococcal tonsillitis, CSU resolved after tonsillectomy. A temporal relationship between CSU exacerbations and tonsillitis was reported [154]. In three out of seven cases with streptococcal infection, improvement of chronic urticaria was seen upon antimicrobial treatment [155]. Bonanni et al. suggested an asymptomatic chronic streptococcal infection in eight of nine CSU patients who benefited from antibiotic treatment [156]. In two patients, antibacterial therapy of urinary tract infection resulted in clearing of chronic urticaria symptoms [25, 157].

Evidence for a link of staphylococcal infection and chronic urticaria is just as weak. Antistaphylolysin antibodies have been detected in 0.3–3% of urticaria patients [143, 158]. Ertam et al. observed statistically higher growth of *Staphylococcus aureus* on cultures prepared from nasal swabs of chronic urticaria patients as compared to the control group [159]. Of 32 chronic urticaria patients with *Staphylococcus aureus* detected in swab specimens from the nasal cavity, 13 patients had complete or partial recovery from urticaria after antimicrobial treatment, whereas the remaining 19 patients (59%) experienced no change of their urticaria [160]. High levels of specific IgE against *Staphylococcus aureus* enterotoxins have been observed in CSU patients [161, 162]. Interestingly, *Staphylococcus* enterotoxin B-IgE levels were strongly correlated with CSU disease activity [161].

In summary, the prevalence and relevance of comorbid bacterial infections in CSU are still ill characterized. Therefore, in CSU, routine screening for HP and other infections is not recommended. In CSU patients with chronic infections with HP, but also *Staphylococcus* or *Streptococcus*, antibiotic therapy can help to reduce CSU symptoms, but should be used only if the infection is properly diagnosed.

7.5.2 Parasitic Infection

In 1895, Duke described two of the first cases of urticaria associated with parasitic infection in Indian soldiers infected by Filaria medinensis [163]. Since then, parasitosis has been reported in up to 75% CSU patients although the prevalence is ≤10% in most studies. Two of three patients with parasitic infection have urticaria including CSU (>10% in most studies) [82]. The most prevalent parasites in CSU reported in the literature are protozoa, mostly *Blastocystis hominis* and *Giardia spp.* [82], whereas helminths are more rarely discovered. For example, CSU was associated with *Enterobius vermicularis* only in 0.1–1.4% of CSU patients [164, 165]. However, in some studies *Toxocara canis* infection was reported in up to 14–29%

of CSU patients [166, 167], and *Anisakis simplex* hypersensitivity had rates of 50–53% [83, 168] compared with 16–20% in the normal population [169].

Anisakis simplex, a nematode, causes IgE-mediated reactions and/or gastrointestinal symptoms, after intake of raw or undercooked fish [169]. CSU patients had significantly higher rates of *Anisakis simplex* sensitization, protozoa infection, and higher risk for *Toxocara canis* seropositivity as compared to healthy controls [170–172]. Patients with undifferentiated urticaria or chronic urticaria more frequently had seropositivity of fasciolosis [166], *Blastocystis hominis,* [173] and Microsporidia [174] infections than controls. Vice versa, patients with strongyloidiasis or *Blastocystis hominis* infection showed increased rates of urticaria as compared to controls [82]. In a cross-sectional Cambodian study including 3,377 participants, urticaria and itching were more frequently reported by patients infected by *Strongyloides stercoralis* [84]. However, Vandenberg and coworkers could not find an association between *Dientamoeba fragilis* infection and urticaria [175].

Peripheral blood eosinophilia is an important sign of both endemic worldwide parasitic infection (e.g., strongyloidiasis, toxocariasis, trichinellosis, hookworm infection) and parasitic infection relevant to certain geographic areas (e.g., filariasis, schistosomiasis). Notably, Giardia and other protozoa generally do not produce eosinophilia, except for *Isospora belli, Dientamoeba fragilis,* and *Sarcocystis species* [176]. Some patients have asymptomatic parasitosis, whereas others can have various manifestations including respiratory and gastrointestinal symptoms [177]. For example, rates of elevated ESR and presence of gastrointestinal symptoms, e.g., abdominal pain and vomiting/nausea, were significantly higher in children with CSU associated with parasites, mostly *Blastocystis hominis*, than in those without [164]. In addition, abdominal pain, diarrhea, itching, and chronic urticaria were frequently seen in patients with *Strongyloides stercoralis* infection [84].

Parasites can be regarded as the underlying cause of CSU if the antiparasitic treatment results in the eradication of the parasite and CSU resolution. In a systematic review, 36% of 269 CSU patients experienced improvement of their urticaria after the treatment of their parasitic infection with antiparasitic drugs. No improvement of CSU was reported in five of 21 studies (64% nonresponders) [82]. Fish-free diet was more effective in patients with chronic urticaria and *Anisakis simplex* sensitization as compared to controls [83, 168]. Interestingly, urticaria improved in 97% of 88 patients with previously diagnosed parasitic infection after treatment with antiparasitic drugs [82]. For example, urticaria and abdominal pain mostly resolved in patients with *Strongyloides stercoralis* infection after treatment with ivermectin [84].

In summary, although parasitic infection is not a frequent comorbidity of CSU in many parts of the world, urticaria including CSU is seen in >10% patients with parasitic infection. Protozoa, primarily *Gardia spp.* and *Blastocystis hominis*, and helminths, mostly *Anisakis simplex, Strongyloides stercoralis* and *Toxocara canis*, are likely to be the most responsible parasites in urticaria but further research is needed. Parasitic infection is an uncommon underlying cause of CSU in nonendemic countries, and routine screening for parasitic infection in CSU patients is not recommended. However, a history of residence in or recent travel to a parasite-endemic area (some parasites are endemic worldwide), relevant dietary habits (e.g., consumption of raw fish), concurrent gastrointestinal symptoms (e.g., diarrhea, abdominal pain), and unexplained eosinophilia may be helpful in suggesting a comorbid parasitic infection. These factors should prompt parasite-specific diagnostic tests in CSU patients. If infection is confirmed, specific treatment of parasitosis can improve CSU. A fish free-diet may be effective for the treatment of CSU due to hypersensitivity to *Anisakis simplex*.

7.5.3 Viral Infection

Viral hepatitis, HIV, herpes, and some other infections have been discussed in the context of CSU. Although acute urticaria or acute recurrent urticaria can appear as a prodromal manifestation of acute viral hepatitis A and B [178, 179], the prevalence of CSU in chronic hepatitis B and C infection or vice versa is not increased (Table 7.1) [87]. In a systematic review of 32 studies, less than 5% and 2% of CSU patients had viral hepatitis B and C, respectively [87]. Urticarial rash including CSU occurred only in ≤3% of patients with chronic hepatitis C infection. Moreover, only two out of nine patients showed improvement of their CSU after antiviral treatment of hepatitis C. In a population-based study, urticaria patients were at higher risk of hepatitis B and C than age- and sex-matched controls [61]. However, in this study, acute urticaria, inducible urticaria, and urticarial vasculitis were not excluded. Urticarial vasculitis is known to be related to chronic hepatitis C and mixed cryoglobulinemia and improved in most patients after antiviral therapy [180].

Only a few studies have looked for a link of HIV infection and CSU [1, 181–183]. For example, Supanaranond et al. reported urticaria in 3–6% of HIV-infected patients [182]. Notably, in a population-based study, the risk of CSU was not associated with HIV infection [1]. In two patients with recurrent genital herpes simplex infection, episodes of genital herpes were associated with exacerbation of CSU. CSU improved after treatment with acyclovir [184] or raltegravir, a retroviral integrase inhibitor [185]. Little is known about the prevalence and relevance of other viruses, e.g., norovirus, parvovirus, HHV-6, in CSU [16].

In summary, viral infections including viral hepatitis, HIV and herpes virus, are unlikely to be linked to CSU and the current evidence does not support that these comorbidities are increased in prevalence or relevant in CSU patients. Routine screening for these infections in patients with CSU is not cost-effective and should not be performed unless risk factors or signs and symptoms of these infections are present, or urticarial vasculitis is suspected.

7.5.4 Fungal Infection

Several fungal agents, namely *Candida albicans*, *Trichophyton spp.*, and *Malassezia furfur*, have been discussed as possible comorbidities of CSU. In a retrospective study, 12% (267/2,221) of patients with urticaria including CSU had concomitant mucocutaneous candidiasis, and this was more than twice as often as compared to control patients [95]. Vice versa, 46% (12/26) of women with recurrent candida infections also had chronic urticaria [186]. However, Ergon and coworkers did not find differences between chronic urticaria patients and controls in intestinal and oral colonization of *Candida spp.* and IgG, IgM, and IgA anti-*Candida* antibodies [96]. Moreover, according to James and Warin, the carriage rate of Candida albicans in the general population is 10–70% [102], which is similar to that in CSU patients.

Five to 36% of patients with chronic urticaria including CSU had positive intradermal tests to *Candida albicans* antigen [97, 102, 187–189]. The rate of over 2+ skin reactions was markedly greater in CSU patients than in controls [97]. Furthermore, CSU patients with positive skin tests to *Candida albicans* had higher rates of positive skin tests to other allergens and positive past and family history of hay fever or asthma [102]. In addition, CSU patients with positive skin tests to *Candida albicans* significantly more often had *Candida albicans* in swab and/or stool tests and exacerbation of their urticaria after challenge tests to *Candida albicans* extract than those with negative skin tests [102]. Increased IgE antibodies to *Candida albicans*, but not to common molds, were detected in 13% of CSU patients [98].

Similar hypersensitivity was demonstrated in CSU patients with fungal infections of the nails, feet, and/or hands after skin tests with *Trichophyton* antigens and passive transfer of patient's serum to a healthy non-hypersensitive subject [99, 100, 190, 191]. 10–29% CSU patients were positive to intradermal testing with *Saccharomyces cerevisiae* antigen [188, 189]. In one study, 61% of CSU patients had a positive response in challenge testing with food yeasts [102].

Candida therapy (nystatin and/or amphotericin B) resolved CSU completely in 8% of skin test positive, but also in 6% of skin test negative patients [102]. In another study, nystatin treatment produced a clinical cure in 55% patients with chronic urticaria, who had immediate skin wheals to *Candida albicans* provocation testing [189]. Gama et al. described four cases of leukorrhea/vulvovaginitis, with improvement of urticaria after the treatment for laboratory-proven candidiasis [155].

In a CSU patient with a positive scratch and intradermal test to *Trichophyton interdigitale* extract [192], both dermatophytosis and CSU promptly relieved after treatment with alcoholic solution of iodine and injections of increasing doses of the diluted fungus extract. In a patient with *Epidermophyton floccosum*-associated dermatophytosis, the dermatophytosis and urticaria healed in 10–14 days after treatment with oral antihistamines and topical clotrimazole [193]. Difficult-to-treat CSU in four Indian patients with tinea infection was successfully resolved with oral antifungal therapy including oral terbinafine, fluconazole, and/or griseofulvin. Clearance of the infection coincided with that of urticaria with no relapse for the next 1–8 weeks [194]. However, in several cases, treatment of proven cases of *Trichophyton* infection did not result in the remission of urticaria [190, 195].

Malassezia furfur infection was found in 65% (82/126) of patients with chronic urticaria, which was significantly more than in normal control subjects. No significant difference was observed between patients treated with AHs or AHs combined with 2% ketoconazole shampoo by the end of treatment [101]. A low-yeast diet reduced CSU symptoms in some patients [102, 188, 189].

In summary, some CSU patients exhibit hypersensitivity to *Candida albicans*, *Trichophyton* spp., or Saccharomyces cerevisiae as shown by positive skin tests and/or IgE antibodies against fungal antigens. However, the clinical relevance of cutaneous and mucosal fungal infection in CSU is still unknown, and antifungal treatment yielded controversial effects on CSU symptoms. As of yet, the search for underlying fungal infection as well as diagnostic tests for fungi allergy in CSU patients is not recommended to be performed routinely [5]. In CSU patients allergic to fungi, avoidance of allergens including a low-yeast diet may help to reduce CSU, and in CSU patients with clinically relevant fungal infection, antifungal treatment might improve CSU.

7.6 Allergic Diseases

On average, 10–40% of the world's population suffers from one or more allergic conditions and the prevalence is increasing worldwide [196]. The prevalence of allergic diseases in CSU is 7–59% [43, 60, 103, 125, 197, 198] and appears to be quite similar to that in the general population [198]. In particular, the rates of asthma in CSU patients were 7–27%, 7–14% for atopic dermatitis, 18–59% for allergic rhinitis, and 19% for other allergies [8, 24, 43, 103, 125, 198–200]. A family history of atopic diseases was reported in 29–57% of CSU patients [197, 198, 201].

Some studies and reviews support the notion that CSU more often affects atopic patients or vice versa [60, 199, 202, 203], whereas other studies argue against a link between chronic urticaria and atopic diseases [197, 204]. A population-based retrospective cohort study including 9,332 patients with chronic urticaria reported a significant association of chronic urticaria with asthma and atopic dermatitis in all age groups [43]. Asthma and atopic dermatitis tended to occur before the onset of chronic urticaria. A cross-sectional study including 11,271 patients with chronic urticaria showed that these patients were much more at risk of allergic rhinitis, atopic dermatitis, and asthma as compared to controls [103]. These studies did not differentiate between CSU and CIndU, unlike another nationwide, population-based, epidemiological study, in which patients with CSU had a 4.7 higher likelihood to develop allergic rhinitis, drug or other allergies, or asthma [44]. Urticaria was significantly more common in children with atopic dermatitis than in children without atopic dermatitis although some cases of urticaria were related to food allergy [104]. In contrast, in another population-based study, acute but not chronic urticaria was significantly associated with allergic diseases and parental history of allergy in pediatric patients [26].

Antihistamines and omalizumab can help to manage the symptoms of both, CSU and allergies, in CSU patients with concomitant allergic asthma [205] and probably other allergic diseases. However, no difference was shown in CSU patients with and without comorbid allergy in terms of the duration and activity of CSU and response to treatment (Table 7.1).

In summary, the results of the studies on the prevalence and relevance of allergic conditions in CSU patients are controversial. Further research is needed to evaluate if CSU patients are at increased risk for developing allergic diseases or vice versa. Unlike acute urticaria, type-I-allergy is a rare cause of CSU in patients who present with daily symptoms but may be considered in CSU patients with intermittent symptoms [5]. Atopy can usually be excluded as a cause of urticaria if there is no temporal relationship to a particular trigger, by either ingestion or contact. Therefore, allergy testing should not be routinely performed in CSU patients, and avoidance of substances is not usually necessary, unless allergic urticaria is suspected. Comorbid allergic diseases should be treated in accordance with clinical guidelines. If allergy is a cause of CSU, then avoidance of relevant type-I-allergens clears urticaria symptoms within 1–2 days. AHs are the first-line treatment of CSU and used widely in many allergic diseases. Omalizumab, an anti-IgE monoclonal antibody, has been shown to be effective in treating resistant CSU as well as asthma and can reduce disease activity in patients with atopic dermatitis or allergic rhinitis.

7.7 Malignancy

Malignant diseases have been reported in 0–9% patients with CSU [111, 112, 136, 206–208]. Among them, 85–92% and 8–15% were nonhematologic and hematologic cancers, respectively [111, 208]. Of the former, the most common were cancers of the hepatogastroenterologic system (46%) and lungs and trachea (16%) in one study [111] and breast cancer (18%) in another study [208]. In a population-based study, the most common cancers in CSU patients were those of the thyroid, liver, and prostate [44]. The frequency of CSU in patients with malignancy is unknown.

In a cohort of 6,913 US adults, a personal history of chronic urticaria was associated with an increased risk of lymphoma, leukemia, or myeloma [113]. A nationwide, population-based Italian study showed a higher risk of developing CSU in patients with a history of malignancies [1]. Another population-based study from Korea reported a 1.4 times higher risk for the concurrence of nonhematological neoplasms in CSU patients than in patients without CSU [44]. Furthermore, a retrospective population-based study of 12,720 Taiwanese patients showed an increased risk of cancer, especially hematologic malignant tumor (the greatest for non-Hodgkin lymphoma) in patients with chronic urticaria. This was true even after excluding patients receiving long-term immunosuppressants [111]. The risk was highest among those aged 20 to 39 years, and neoplasms were mostly detected in the first year following diagnosis of chronic urticaria. In contrast, malignancy was diagnosed only in 3% of 1,155 patients with chronic urticaria in a Swedish study and urticaria was not statistically associated with malignancy in general [112]. Vena et al. reported decreased risk of cancer associated with a history of urticaria [114]. Moreover, Karakelides and coworkers observed that patients with chronic urticaria younger than 43 years were unlikely to have associated monoclonal gammopathy of undetermined significance or malignancy [208]. In a review of case reports, 67% of patients with urticaria and malignancy were ≥35 years [14].

The data from these studies should be analyzed with caution. Two studies from the 1980s defined urticaria as "allergy," so not all of the patients included may have had CSU [113, 114]. Although the Taiwanese and Swedish studies described above involved big cohorts of patients with chronic urticaria, possible confounders, such as smoking or alcohol use, were not investigated [111, 112]. Importantly, some of the patients may have had urticarial vasculitis or Schnitzler syndrome [111–113, 208], which are known to be associated with malignant tumors [180].

In a recent study, virtually all (95%) physicians dealing with urticaria patients worldwide reported that they hold malignancy to be a rare cause of CSU [209]. In 1976, Curth proposed criteria to define a paraneoplastic syndrome, i.e., a strong causal association between dermatosis and tumor [210]. According to these criteria, CSU can be considered to be paraneoplastic if the following two major criteria are met: (1) CSU and malignancy appear at approximately the same time and (2) both conditions follow a parallel course. However, the first criterion is perhaps overly stringent, because tumors are often difficult to detect and the presence of malignancy can be unknown for months or even years. For example, Larenas-Linnemann et al. reviewed 26 cases of urticaria (17 cases of CSU or undefined chronic urticaria) probably causally associated with malignancy [14]. In 68% patients, urticaria appeared 2–8 months before the malignancy was diagnosed. In 75% cases, neoplasms were detected at an early, asymptomatic stage while searching for a cause of urticaria. Carcinomas were found in 68% patients (24% were papillary carcinomas of the thyroid gland) [211], and hematologic neoplasms were reported in 24% cases. On the other hand, Chen et al. observed cancer of the thyroid gland only in 2% among all types of cancer (11/646) in patients with chronic urticaria [111].

In accordance with the second Curth's criterion, resolution of urticaria was reportedly seen in all patients after cure of the tumor (chemotherapy or resection) within days to a few weeks [14]. In some patients, CSU reappeared after relapse of tumor or tapering of specific therapy [212–214]. The main limitations of these reports are publication bias and that spontaneous remission of CSU is common [7]. In a systematic review of 29 studies involving 6,462 patients with chronic urticarial rash [215], 2% ($n = 105$, urticarial vasculitis in 60 cases) patients had internal diseases considered to be the cause of urticaria. Among those, a paraproteinemia, polycythemia vera, and various malignancies were detected as an underlying cause of chronic urticarial rash only in three, four, and five patients, respectively.

In summary, cancer is considered to be a very rare cause of CSU even though CSU can resolve with cure of cancer [14, 209]. Consequently, the association between malignancy and CSU warrants further evaluation. As of yet, malignancy screening should not be performed in CSU patients, unless indicated by the patient's clinical history, physical exam, and/or initial CSU workup [5].

7.8 Metabolic Syndrome

MS is not a disease *per se* but rather a constellation of signs and symptoms that collectively confer an increased risk for developing heart disease and diabetes mellitus. In fact, MS includes central obesity, dyslipidemia, hyperglycemia, and hypertension. The prevalence of MS in the general population is 7–25% [216]. Early recognition and treatment of MS can improve patients' long-term health and quality of life [217].

In CSU, MS has been recorded in 16–30% patients [6, 115]. Among MS components, obesity was observed in 8–52% cases, hypertension in 18–31%, hyperglycemia/diabetes in 5–34%, hyperlipidemia in 7–42%, and low levels of high-density lipoprotein in 28% [6, 24, 60, 115, 116]. Although Egeberg et al. did not report an increased risk of cardiovascular diseases in patients with chronic urticaria [117], several population-based studies demonstrated significantly higher prevalence of MS and/or its components in patients with chronic urticaria including CSU as compared to controls [1, 6, 60, 116].

In a Israeli study with 11,261 patients with undefined chronic urticaria and 67,216 controls, chronic urticaria was significantly associated with higher body mass index (BMI) and a higher prevalence of MS, obesity, diabetes, hyperlipidemia, hypertension, chronic renal failure, and gout [6]. Importantly, this association remained significant after adjustment for steroid treatment. In a Taiwanese study that included 9,798 adults with chronic urticaria and 9,798 sex- and age-matched controls, chronic urticaria patients had a significantly higher prevalence of prior diagnosis of hyperlipidemia and risk of hyperlipidemia than controls. Interestingly, atopic dermatitis, a negative control, was not associated with prior hyperlipidemia [60].

Using the National Health Insurance of Taiwan database, 2,460 patients with CSU were compared to 9,840 age-, sex-, and index year-matched controls. CSU patients had a 1.4-fold greater risk of developing subsequent hypertension than the non-CSU cohort after adjusting for sex, age, comorbidities, and nonsedating AH use [116]. In an Italian study with 14,859 CSU patients, the risk of developing CSU was significantly higher in obese subjects [1]. Interestingly, the risk of CSU was not increased in patients with type 2 diabetes mellitus, hypertension, or dyslipidemia as compared to those without [45].

Four additional smaller cross-sectional or prospective studies looked at the association between CSU and MS components [47, 115, 118, 120]. Severe and uncontrolled urticaria was significantly comorbid with MS in chronic urticaria patients [115]. Nebiolo and coworkers showed that hypertension is associated with long duration of CSU [47]. Zbiciak-Nylec and coauthors described a statistically significant association between CSU and obesity, higher BMI, greater affected body surface area, and older age at disease onset. CSU patients with higher BMI values had a tendency towards longer disease duration [118]. In contrast, no differences were observed in terms of duration of chronic urticaria between patients with and without MS [115]. Moreover, in another study, obesity was not linked to the severity of chronic urticaria [120].

MS is characterized by a systemic pro-inflammatory and procoagulating state. Increased levels of inflammatory and coagulations markers, e.g., CRP, IL-6, TNF-α, D-dimer, have been detected in subjects with MS [218, 219]. Moreover, CRP predicts the development of arterial hypertension on follow-up in normotensive subjects [220]. CSU, a chronic inflammatory disorder, is also accompanied by raised levels of CRP, ESR, IL-6, TNF-α, fibrinogen, D-dimer, and other inflammatory and coagulation markers [115, 207]. In a retrospective multicenter study involving 1,253 German and Russian CSU patients, higher levels of CRP were associated with higher CSU activity and arterial hypertension [207].

In summary, there is an increasing body of evidence that CSU is associated with MS. Further studies are needed to clarify whether obesity, dyslipidemia, hyperglycemia, and hypertension are relevant to CSU characteristics and pathogenesis and whether evaluation of MS should be included in routine diagnostic tests for CSU. Components of MS are considered to be major, modifiable risk factors for atherosclerosis, cardiovascular diseases, and diabetes. Therefore, among the higher risk group of patients with CSU, measurement of blood pressure and BMI, and/or a serum examination for hyperlipidemia and glucose should be performed. With prompt detection and appropriate management, CSU patients' quality of life may be improved and subsequent cardiovascular risks may be reduced.

References

1. Lapi F, et al. Epidemiology of chronic spontaneous urticaria: results from a nationwide, population-based study in Italy. Br J Dermatol. 2016;174(5):996–1004.
2. Fricke J, et al. Prevalence of chronic urticaria in children and adults across the globe: Systematic review with meta-analysis. Allergy. 2020;75(2):423–32.
3. Confino-Cohen R, et al. Chronic urticaria and autoimmunity: associations found in a large population study. J Allergy Clin Immunol. 2012;129(5):1307–13.
4. Kolkhir P, et al. Autoimmune comorbidity in chronic spontaneous urticaria: a systematic review. Autoimmun Rev. 2017;16(12):1196–208.
5. Zuberbier T, et al. The EAACI/GA(2)LEN/EDF/WAO guideline for the definition, classification, diagnosis and management of urticaria. Allergy. 2018;73(7):1393–414.
6. Shalom G, et al. Chronic urticaria and the metabolic syndrome: a cross-sectional community-based study of 11 261 patients. J Eur Acad Dermatol Venereol. 2018;32(2):276–81.
7. Kozel MM, et al. Natural course of physical and chronic urticaria and angioedema in 220 patients. J Am Acad Dermatol. 2001;45(3):387–91.
8. Hiragun M, et al. Prognosis of chronic spontaneous urticaria in 117 patients not controlled by a standard dose of antihistamine. Allergy. 2013;68(2):229–35.
9. Curto-Barredo L, et al. Clinical features of chronic spontaneous urticaria that predict disease prognosis and refractoriness to standard treatment. Acta Derm Venereol. 2018;98(7):641–7.
10. Gregoriou S, et al. Etiologic aspects and prognostic factors of patients with chronic urticaria: nonrandomized, prospective, descriptive study. J Cutan Med Surg. 2009;13(4):198–203.
11. van der Valk PG, Moret G, Kiemeney LA. The natural history of chronic urticaria and angioedema in patients visiting a tertiary referral centre. Br J Dermatol. 2002;146(1):110–3.
12. Magen E, et al. The clinical and laboratory characteristics of acute spontaneous urticaria and its progression to chronic spontaneous urticaria. Allergy Asthma Proc. 2016;37(5):394–9.
13. Eun SJ, et al. Natural course of new-onset urticaria: results of a 10-year follow-up, nationwide, population-based study. Allergol Int. 2018;68(1):52–8.

14. Larenas-Linnemann D, et al. Chronic urticaria can be caused by cancer and resolves with its cure. Allergy. 2018;73(7):1562–6.
15. Kolkhir P, et al. Comorbidity of chronic spontaneous urticaria and autoimmune thyroid diseases: a systematic review. Allergy. 2017;72(10):1440–60.
16. Wedi B, et al. Urticaria and infections. Allergy Asthma Clin Immunol. 2009;5(1):10.
17. Sanchez-Borges M, et al. Review of physical urticarias and testing methods. Curr Allergy Asthma Rep. 2017;17(8):51.
18. Magerl M, et al. The definition, diagnostic testing, and management of chronic inducible urticarias—the EAACI/GA(2) LEN/EDF/UNEV consensus recommendations 2016 update and revision. Allergy. 2016;71(6):780–802.
19. Trevisonno J, et al. Physical urticaria: review on classification, triggers and management with special focus on prevalence including a meta-analysis. Postgrad Med. 2015;127(6):565–70.
20. Barlow RJ, et al. Diagnosis and incidence of delayed pressure urticaria in patients with chronic urticaria. J Am Acad Dermatol. 1993;29(6):954–8.
21. Sanchez J, et al. Prevalence of inducible urticaria in patients with chronic spontaneous urticaria: associated risk factors. J Allergy Clin Immunol Pract. 2017;5(2):464–70.
22. Silpa-archa N, Kulthanan K, Pinkaew S. Physical urticaria: prevalence, type and natural course in a tropical country. J Eur Acad Dermatol Venereol. 2011;25(10):1194–9.
23. Juhlin L. Recurrent urticaria: clinical investigation of 330 patients. Br J Dermatol. 1981;104(4):369–81.
24. Maurer M, et al. H1-antihistamine-refractory chronic spontaneous urticaria: it's worse than we thought—first results of the multicenter real-life AWARE study. Clin Exp Allergy. 2017;47(5):684–92.
25. Sackesen C, et al. The etiology of different forms of urticaria in childhood. Pediatr Dermatol. 2004;21(2):102–8.
26. Lee SJ, et al. Prevalence and risk factors of urticaria with a focus on chronic urticaria in children. Allergy Asthma Immunol Res. 2017;9(3):212–9.
27. Magen E, et al. Clinical and laboratory features of antihistamine-resistant chronic idiopathic urticaria. Allergy Asthma Proc. 2011;32(6):460–6.
28. Amin P, et al. Investigation of patient-specific characteristics associated with treatment outcomes for chronic urticaria. J Allergy Clin Immunol Pract. 2015;3(3):400–7.
29. Kocaturk E, et al. Management of chronic inducible urticaria according to the guidelines: a prospective controlled study. J Dermatol Sci. 2017;87(1):60–9.
30. Humphreys F, Hunter JA. The characteristics of urticaria in 390 patients. Br J Dermatol. 1998;138(4):635–8.
31. Magen E, Mishal J. Possible benefit from treatment of Helicobacter pylori in antihistamine-resistant chronic urticaria. Clin Exp Dermatol. 2013;38(1):7–12.
32. Staubach P, et al. High prevalence of mental disorders and emotional distress in patients with chronic spontaneous urticaria. Acta Derm Venereol. 2011;91(5):557–61.
33. Chung MC, et al. The relationship between posttraumatic stress disorder, psychiatric comorbidity, and personality traits among patients with chronic idiopathic urticaria. Compr Psychiatry. 2010;51(1):55–63.
34. Chu CY, et al. Epidemiology and comorbidities of patients with chronic urticaria in Taiwan: a nationwide population-based study. J Dermatol Sci. 2017;88(2):192–8.
35. Ben-Shoshan M, Blinderman I, Raz A. Psychosocial factors and chronic spontaneous urticaria: a systematic review. Allergy. 2013;68(2):131–41.
36. Engin B, et al. The levels of depression, anxiety and quality of life in patients with chronic idiopathic urticaria. J Eur Acad Dermatol Venereol. 2008;22(1):36–40.
37. Uguz F, Engin B, Yilmaz E. Axis I and Axis II diagnoses in patients with chronic idiopathic urticaria. J Psychosom Res. 2008;64(2):225–9.
38. Pasaoglu G, et al. Psychological status of patients with chronic urticaria. J Dermatol. 2006;33(11):765–71.
39. Barbosa F, Freitas J, Barbosa A. Chronic idiopathic urticaria and anxiety symptoms. J Health Psychol. 2011;16(7):1038–47.

40. Hashiro M, Okumura M. Anxiety, depression, psychosomatic symptoms and autonomic nervous function in patients with chronic urticaria. J Dermatol Sci. 1994;8(2):129–35.
41. Herguner S, et al. Levels of depression, anxiety and behavioural problems and frequency of psychiatric disorders in children with chronic idiopathic urticaria. Br J Dermatol. 2011;164(6):1342–7.
42. Ozkan M, et al. Psychiatric morbidity and quality of life in patients with chronic idiopathic urticaria. Ann Allergy Asthma Immunol. 2007;99(1):29–33.
43. Chiu HY, Muo CH, Sung FC. Associations of chronic urticaria with atopic and autoimmune comorbidities: a nationwide population-based study. Int J Dermatol. 2018;57(7):822–9.
44. Kim BR, et al. Epidemiology and comorbidities of patients with chronic urticaria in Korea: a nationwide population-based study. J Dermatol. 2018;45(1):10–6.
45. Kim YS, et al. Increased risk of chronic spontaneous urticaria in patients with autoimmune thyroid diseases: a nationwide, population-based study. Allergy Asthma Immunol Res. 2017;9(4):373–7.
46. Pan XF, Gu JQ, Shan ZY. The prevalence of thyroid autoimmunity in patients with urticaria: a systematic review and meta-analysis. Endocrine. 2015;48(3):804–10.
47. Nebiolo F, et al. Effect of arterial hypertension on chronic urticaria duration. Ann Allergy Asthma Immunol. 2009;103(5):407–10.
48. Gangemi S, et al. Serum thyroid autoantibodies in patients with idiopathic either acute or chronic urticaria. J Endocrinol Invest. 2009;32(2):107–10.
49. Al-Balbeesi AO. Significance of antithyroid antibodies and other auto-antibodies in Saudi patients with chronic urticaria. Possible parameters in predicting chronic over three years disease. J Saudi Soc Dermatol Dermatol Surg. 2011;15(2):47–51.
50. Toubi E, et al. Clinical and laboratory parameters in predicting chronic urticaria duration: a prospective study of 139 patients. Allergy. 2004;59(8):869–73.
51. Ye Y-M, et al. Prognostic factors for chronic spontaneous urticaria: a 6-month prospective observational study. Allergy Asthma Immunol Res. 2016;8(2):115–23.
52. Eser I, et al. The predictive factors for remission of chronic spontaneous urticaria in childhood: Outcome from a prospective study. Allergol Immunopathol (Madr). 2016;44(6):537–41.
53. Lunge SB, Borkar M, Pande S. Correlation of serum antithyroid microsomal antibody and autologous serum skin test in patients with chronic idiopathic urticaria. Indian Dermatology Online Journal. 2015;6(4):248–52.
54. Kessel A, et al. Elevated serum total IgE—a potential marker for severe chronic urticaria. Int Arch Allergy Immunol. 2010;153(3):288–93.
55. Magen E, Mishal J. The effect of L-thyroxine treatment on chronic idiopathic urticaria and autoimmune thyroiditis. Int J Dermatol. 2012;51(1):94–7.
56. Karagol HI, et al. Association between thyroid autoimmunity and recurrent angioedema in children. Allergy Asthma Proc. 2015;36(6):468–72.
57. Viswanathan RK, Biagtan MJ, Mathur SK. The role of autoimmune testing in chronic idiopathic urticaria. Ann Allergy Asthma Immunol. 2012;108(5):337–341.e1.
58. Nuzzo V, et al. Idiopathic chronic urticaria and thyroid autoimmunity: experience of a single center. Dermatoendocrinol. 2011;3(4):255–8.
59. Verneuil L, et al. Association between chronic urticaria and thyroid autoimmunity: a prospective study involving 99 patients. Dermatology. 2004;208(2):98–103.
60. Chung SD, et al. Hyperlipidemia is associated with chronic urticaria: a population-based study. PLoS One. 2016;11(3):e0150304.
61. Yong SB, et al. Patients with urticaria are at a higher risk of anaphylaxis: a nationwide population-based retrospective cohort study in Taiwan. J Dermatol. 2018;45(9):1088–93.
62. Magen E, et al. Association of alopecia areata with atopic dermatitis and chronic spontaneous urticaria. Allergy Asthma Proc. 2018;39(2):96–102.
63. Lin CH, et al. Clinically diagnosed urticaria and risk of systemic lupus erythematosus in children: a nationwide population-based case-control study. Pediatr Allergy Immunol. 2018;29(7):732–9.

64. Caminiti L, et al. Chronic urticaria and associated coeliac disease in children: a case-control study. Pediatr Allergy Immunol. 2005;16(5):428–32.
65. Gabrielli M, et al. Idiopathic chronic urticaria and celiac disease. Dig Dis Sci. 2005;50(9):1702–4.
66. Ludvigsson JF, et al. Does urticaria risk increase in patients with celiac disease? A large population-based cohort study. Eur J Dermatol. 2013;23(5):681–7.
67. Lindegard B. Diseases associated with psoriasis in a general population of 159,200 middle-aged, urban, native Swedes. Dermatologica. 1986;172(6):298–304.
68. Zhang Z, et al. The analysis of genetics and associated autoimmune diseases in Chinese vitiligo patients. Arch Dermatol Res. 2009;301(2):167–73.
69. Liu JB, et al. Clinical profiles of vitiligo in China: an analysis of 3742 patients. Clin Exp Dermatol. 2005;30(4):327–31.
70. Kohli S, et al. Clinicoepidemiologic features of chronic urticaria in patients with versus without subclinical Helicobacter pylori infection: a cross-sectional study of 150 patients. Int Arch Allergy Immunol. 2018;175(1-2):114–20.
71. Tang L, et al. [A meta-analysis on the relations between Helicobacter pylori infection and chronic urticaria]. Zhonghua Liu Xing Bing Xue Za Zhi. 2014;35(3):317–21.
72. Gu H, et al. Association between Helicobacter pylori infection and chronic urticaria: a meta-analysis. Gastroenterol Res Pract. 2015;2015:486974.
73. Curth HM, et al. Effects of Helicobacter pylori eradication in chronic spontaneous urticaria: results from a retrospective cohort study. Am J Clin Dermatol. 2015;16(6):553–8.
74. Abdou AG, et al. Helicobacter pylori infection in patients with chronic urticaria: correlation with pathologic findings in gastric biopsies. Int J Dermatol. 2009;48(5):464–9.
75. Hook-Nikanne J, et al. Is Helicobacter pylori infection associated with chronic urticaria? Acta Derm Stockholm. 2000;80(6):425–6.
76. Fukuda S, et al. Effect of Helicobacter pylori eradication in the treatment of Japanese patients with chronic idiopathic urticaria. J Gastroenterol. 2004;39(9):827–30.
77. Campanati A, et al. Role of small intestinal bacterial overgrowth and Helicobacter pylori infection in chronic spontaneous urticaria: a prospective analysis. Acta Derm Venereol. 2013;93(2):161–4.
78. Hellmig S, et al. Role of Helicobacter pylori Infection in the treatment and outcome of chronic urticaria. Helicobacter. 2008;13(5):341–5.
79. Moreira A, et al. Is Helicobacter pylori infection associated with chronic idiopathic urticaria? Allergol Immunopathol (Madr). 2003;31(4):209–14.
80. Persechino S, et al. Chronic idiophatic urticaria and Helicobacter pylori: a specific pattern of gastritis and urticaria remission after Helicobacter pylori eradication. Int J Immunopathol Pharmacol. 2012;25(3):765–70.
81. Magen E, et al. Eradication of Helicobacter pylori infection equally improves chronic urticaria with positive and negative autologous serum skin test. Helicobacter. 2007;12(5):567–71.
82. Kolkhir P, et al. Chronic spontaneous urticaria and internal parasites—a systematic review. Allergy. 2016;71(3):308–22.
83. Ventura MT, et al. Anisakis simplex hypersensitivity is associated with chronic urticaria in endemic areas. Int Arch Allergy Immunol. 2013;160(3):297–300.
84. Forrer A, et al. Strongyloides stercoralis is associated with significant morbidity in rural Cambodia, including stunting in children. PLoS Negl Trop Dis. 2017;11(10):e0005685.
85. Rezaei Riabi T, et al. Study of prevalence, distribution and clinical significance of blastocystis isolated from two medical centers in Iran. Gastroenterol Hepatol Bed Bench. 2017;10(Suppl 1):S102–7.
86. Burak Selek M, et al. Toxocara Canis IgG seropositivity in patients with chronic urticaria. Iran J Allergy Asthma Immunol. 2015;14(4):450–6.
87. Kolkhir P, et al. Comorbidity of viral hepatitis and chronic spontaneous urticaria: a systematic review. Allergy. 2018;73(10):1946–53.
88. Kanazawa K, et al. Hepatitis C virus infection in patients with urticaria. J Am Acad Dermatol. 1996;35(2 Pt 1):195–8.

89. Cribier BJ, et al. Chronic urticaria is not significantly associated with hepatitis C or hepatitis G infection: a case-control study. Arch Dermatol. 1999;135(11):1335–9.
90. Tousi P, Rahmati M, Korshid SM. Urticaria and hepatitis C infection: is there a relationship? Int J Dermatol. 2002;41(10):712–3.
91. Maticic M, et al. Lichen planus and other cutaneous manifestations in chronic hepatitis C: pre- and post-interferon-based treatment prevalence vary in a cohort of patients from low hepatitis C virus endemic area. J Eur Acad Dermatol Venereol. 2008;22(7):779–88.
92. Zhong H, et al. Chronic urticaria in Chinese population: a hospital-based multicenter epidemiological study. Allergy. 2014;69(3):359–64.
93. Smith R, Caul EO, Burton JL. Urticaria and hepatitis C. Br J Dermatol. 1997;136(6):980.
94. Doutre MS, Beylot-Barry M, Beylot C. Urticaria and hepatitis C infection. Br J Dermatol. 1998;138(1):194–5.
95. Henseler T. [Mucocutaneous candidiasis in patients with skin diseases]. Mycoses. 1995;38 Suppl 1: 7–13.
96. Ergon MC, et al. Candida spp. colonization and serum anticandidal antibody levels in patients with chronic urticaria. Clin Exp Dermatol. 2007;32(6):740–3.
97. Numata T, Yamamoto S, Yamura T. The role of mite, house dust and Candida allergens in chronic urticaria. J Dermatol. 1980;7(3):197–202.
98. Staubach P, et al. Patients with chronic urticaria exhibit increased rates of sensitisation to Candida albicans, but not to common moulds. Mycoses. 2009;52(4):334–8.
99. Platts-Mills TA, et al. Serum IgE antibodies to Trichophyton in patients with urticaria, angioedema, asthma, and rhinitis: development of a radioallergosorbent test. J Allergy Clin Immunol. 1987;79(1):40–5.
100. Zhang M, et al. Sensitization and cross-reactions of dermatophyte and Candida albicans allergens in patients with chronic urticaria. Int J Dermatol. 2016;55(10):1138–42.
101. Tang XP, et al. [Study of the association of Malassezia furfur with chronic urticaria among the ship crews]. Di Yi Jun Yi Da Xue Xue Bao. 2003;23(8):870–2.
102. James J, Warin RP. An assessment of the role of Candida albicans and food yeasts in chronic urticaria. Br J Dermatol. 1971;84(3):227–37.
103. Shalom G, et al. Chronic urticaria and atopic disorders: a cross-sectional study of 11 271 patients. Br J Dermatol. 2017;177(4):e96–7.
104. Bohme M, et al. Atopic dermatitis and concomitant disease patterns in children up to two years of age. Acta Derm Venereol. 2002;82(2):98–103.
105. Kim JH, et al. Serum clusterin as a prognostic marker of chronic spontaneous urticaria. Medicine (Baltimore). 2016;95(19):e3688.
106. Sanchez Jorge J, Sanchez A, Cardona R. Prevalence of drugs as triggers of exacerbations in chronic urticaria. J Investig Allergol Clin Immunol. 2019;29(2):112–7.
107. Comert S, et al. The general characteristics of acute urticaria attacks and the factors predictive of progression to chronic urticaria. Allergol Immunopathol (Madr). 2013;41(4):239–45.
108. Champion RH, et al. Urticaria and angio-oedema. A review of 554 patients. Br J Dermatol. 1969;81(8):588–97.
109. Lee HC, Hong JB, Chu CY. Chronic idiopathic urticaria in Taiwan: a clinical study of demographics, aggravating factors, laboratory findings, serum autoreactivity and treatment response. J Formos Med Assoc. 2011;110(3):175–82.
110. Kulthanan K, Wachirakaphan C. Prevalence and clinical characteristics of chronic urticaria and positive skin prick testing to mites. Acta Derm Venereol. 2008;88(6):584–8.
111. Chen YJ, et al. Cancer risk in patients with chronic urticaria: a population-based cohort study. Arch Dermatol. 2012;148(1):103–8.
112. Lindelof B, et al. Chronic urticaria and cancer: an epidemiological study of 1155 patients. Br J Dermatol. 1990;123(4):453–6.
113. McWhorter WP. Allergy and risk of cancer. A prospective study using NHANESI followup data. Cancer. 1988;62(2):451–5.
114. Vena JE, et al. Allergy-related diseases and cancer: an inverse association. Am J Epidemiol. 1985;122(1):66–74.

115. Ye YM, et al. Co-existence of chronic urticaria and metabolic syndrome: clinical implications. Acta Derm Venereol. 2013;93(2):156–60.
116. Chang HW, et al. Association between chronic idiopathic urticaria and hypertension: a population-based retrospective cohort study. Ann Allergy Asthma Immunol. 2016;116(6):554–8.
117. Egeberg A, et al. Cardiovascular risk is not increased in patients with chronic urticaria: a retrospective populationbased cohort study. Acta Derm Venereol. 2017;97(2):261–2.
118. Zbiciak-Nylec M, et al. Overweight and obesity may play a role in the pathogenesis of chronic spontaneous urticaria. Clin Exp Dermatol. 2018;43(5):525–8.
119. Maged Amin M, Rushdy M. Hyperlipidemia in association with pro-inflammatory cytokines among chronic spontaneous urticaria: case-control study. Eur Ann Allergy Clin Immunol. 2018;50(6):254–61.
120. Soria A, et al. Obesity is not associated with severe chronic urticaria in a French cohort. J Eur Acad Dermatol Venereol. 2018;32(6):e247–9.
121. US Department of Health and Human Services, Public Health Service, Agency for Health Care and Policy Research. Acute pain management: operative or medical procedures and trauma. Rockville: Agency for Health Care and Policy Research Publications; 1992.
122. Eccles M, Mason J. How to develop cost-conscious guidelines. Health Technol Assess. 2001;5(16):1–69.
123. Maurer M, et al. Omalizumab treatment in patients with chronic inducible urticaria: a systematic review of published evidence. J Allergy Clin Immunol. 2018;141(2):638–49.
124. WHO International Consortium in Psychiatric Epidemiology. Cross-national comparisons of the prevalences and correlates of mental disorders. Bull World Health Organ. 2000;78(4):413–26.
125. Zazzali JL, et al. Cost, utilization, and patterns of medication use associated with chronic idiopathic urticaria. Ann Allergy Asthma Immunol. 2012;108(2):98–102.
126. Hunkin V, Chung MC. Chronic idiopathic urticaria, psychological co-morbidity and post-traumatic stress: the impact of alexithymia and repression. Psychiatr Q. 2012;83(4):431–47.
127. Perugi G, et al. General medical conditions in 347 bipolar disorder patients: clinical correlates of metabolic and autoimmune-allergic diseases. J Affect Disord. 2015;170:95–103.
128. Chen M-H, et al. Comorbidity of allergic and autoimmune diseases among patients with ADHD: a nationwide population-based study. J Attention Disord. 2017;21(3):219–27.
129. Vietri J, et al. Effect of chronic urticaria on US patients: analysis of the National Health and Wellness Survey. Ann Allergy Asthma Immunol. 2015;115(4):306–11.
130. Staubach P, et al. Quality of life in patients with chronic urticaria is differentially impaired and determined by psychiatric comorbidity. Br J Dermatol. 2006;154(2):294–8.
131. Kolkhir P, et al. Autoimmune chronic spontaneous urticaria: what we know and what we do not know. J Allergy Clin Immunol. 2017;139(6):1772–1781.e1.
132. Kolkhir P, et al. Comorbidity and pathogenic links of chronic spontaneous urticaria and systemic lupus erythematosus—a systematic review. Clin Exp Allergy. 2016;46(2):275–87.
133. Spadoni M, et al. Chronic autoimmune urticaria as the first manifestation of juvenile systemic lupus erythematosus. Lupus. 2011;20(7):763–6.
134. Mogaddam MR, et al. Relationship between Helicobacter pylori and idiopathic chronic urticaria: effectiveness of Helicobacter pylori eradication. Adv Dermatol Allergol. 2015;32(1):15–20.
135. Ozkaya-Bayazit E, et al. Helicobacter pylori eradication in patients with chronic urticaria. Arch Dermatol. 1998;134(9):1165–6.
136. Wedi B, et al. Prevalence of Helicobacter pylori-associated gastritis in chronic urticaria. Int Arch Allergy Immunol. 1998;116(4):288–94.
137. Pawłowicz R, Wytrychowski K, Panaszek B. Eradication of Helicobacter pylori, as add-on therapy, has a significant, but temporary influence on recovery in chronic idiopathic urticaria: a placebo-controlled, double blind trial in the Polish population. Adv Dermatol Allergol. 2018;35(2):151–5.

138. Gaig P, et al. Efficacy of the eradication of Helicobacter pylori infection in patients with chronic urticaria. A placebo-controlled double blind study. Allergol Immunopathol (Madr). 2002;30(5):255–8.
139. Federman DG, et al. The effect of antibiotic therapy for patients infected with Helicobacter pylori who have chronic urticaria. J Am Acad Dermatol. 2003;49(5):861–4.
140. Schnyder B, Helbling A, Pichler WJ. Chronic idiopathic urticaria: natural course and association with Helicobacter pylori infection. Int Arch Allergy Immunol. 1999;119(1):60–3.
141. Shakouri A, et al. Effectiveness of Helicobacter pylori eradication in chronic urticaria: evidence-based analysis using the Grading of Recommendations Assessment, Development, and Evaluation system. Curr Opin Allergy Clin Immunol. 2010;10(4):362–9.
142. Hellgren L, Hersle K. Acute and chronic urticaria. A statistical investigation on clinical and laboratory data in 1.204 patients and matched healthy controls. Acta Allergol. 1964;19:406–20.
143. Buss YA, Garrelfs UC, Sticherling M. Chronic urticaria—which clinical parameters are pathogenetically relevant? A retrospective investigation of 339 patients. J Dtsch Dermatol Ges. 2007;5(1):22–9.
144. Liutu M, et al. Etiologic aspects of chronic urticaria. Int J Dermatol. 1998;37(7):515–9.
145. Zingale LC, et al. Angioedema without urticaria: a large clinical survey. CMAJ. 2006;175(9):1065–70.
146. Sonoda T, et al. Chronic urticaria associated with dental infection. Br J Dermatol. 2001;145(3):516–8.
147. Kasperska-Zajac A, et al. Refractory chronic spontaneous urticaria and permanent atrial fibrillation associated with dental infection: mere coincidence or something more to it? Int J Immunopathol Pharmacol. 2016;29(1):112–20.
148. Shelley WB. Urticaria of nine year's duration cleared following dental extraction. A case report. Arch Dermatol. 1969;100(3):324–5.
149. Thyacarajan K, Kamalam A. Chronic urticaria due to abscessed teeth roots. Int J Dermatol. 1982;21(10):606.
150. Büchter A, et al. Odontogenic foci—possible etiology of urticaria? Mund-Kiefer-und Gesichtschirurgie: MKG. 2003;7(6):335–8.
151. Goga D, et al. [The elimination of dental and sinusal infectious foci in dermatologic pathology. A double-blind study in 27 cases confined to chronic urticaria]. Rev Stomatol Chir Maxillofac. 1988;89(5):273–5.
152. Minciullo PL, et al. Urticaria and bacterial infections. Allergy Asthma Proc. 2014;35(4):295–302.
153. Buckley RH, Dees SC. Serum immunoglobulins. 3. Abnormalities associated with chronic urticaria in children. J Allergy. 1967;40(5):294–303.
154. Calado G, et al. Streptococcal tonsillitis as a cause of urticaria: tonsillitis and urticaria. Allergol Immunopathol (Madr). 2012;40(6):341–5.
155. Gama JIS, Perigault PB, Ángeles MB. Chronic urticaria: clinical characteristics of a group of patients of Veracruz, Mexico. Revista Alergia México. 2005;52(5):200–5.
156. Bonanni L, et al. Post-streptococcal nonallergic urticaria? Allergy. 2002;57(6):558–60.
157. Pasricha JS, Gupta R. Urticaria and urinary infection. Indian J Dermatol Venereol Leprol. 1981;47(5):277–8.
158. Kuokkanen K, Sonck CE. Antistreptolysin and antistaphylolysin titres in allergic skin conditions. Observations on 6104 patients suffering from various eczemas and urticaria. Acta Allergol. 1973;28(4):260–82.
159. Ertam I, et al. The frequency of nasal carriage in chronic urticaria patients. J Eur Acad Dermatol Venereol. 2007;21(6):777–80.
160. Sharma AD. Role of nasal carriage of Staphylococcus aureus in chronic urticaria. Indian J Dermatol. 2012;57(3):233–6.
161. Altrichter S, et al. In chronic spontaneous urticaria, IgE against staphylococcal enterotoxins is common and functional. Allergy. 2018;73(7):1497–504.

162. Ye YM, et al. Association of specific IgE to staphylococcal superantigens with the phenotype of chronic urticaria. J Korean Med Sci. 2008;23(5):845–51.
163. Duke J. Note on the symptoms of filaria medinensis or Guinea-worm. Ind Med Gaz. 1895;30(2):64–5.
164. Arik Yilmaz E, et al. Parasitic infections in children with chronic spontaneous urticaria. Int Arch Allergy Immunol. 2016;171(2):130–5.
165. Nettis E, et al. Clinical and aetiological aspects in urticaria and angio-oedema. Br J Dermatol. 2003;148(3):501–6.
166. Demirci M, et al. Tissue parasites in patients with chronic urticaria. J Dermatol. 2003;30(11):777–81.
167. Dal T, et al. Seroprevalence of IgG anti-Toxocara canis antibodies and anti-Fasciola sp. antibodies in patients with urticaria. Clin Ter. 2013;164(4):315–7.
168. Daschner A, Vega de la Osada F, Pascual CY. Allergy and parasites reevaluated: wide-scale induction of chronic urticaria by the ubiquitous fish-nematode Anisakis simplex in an endemic region. Allergol Immunopathol (Madr). 2005;33(1):31–7.
169. Minciullo PL, Cascio A, Gangemi S. Association between urticaria and nematode infections. Allergy Asthma Proc. 2018;39(2):86–95.
170. Dilek AR, et al. The role of protozoa in the etiology of chronic urticaria. Dermatologica Sinica. 2012;30(3):90–2.
171. Frezzolini A, Cadoni S, De Pita O. Usefulness of the CD63 basophil activation test in detecting Anisakis hypersensitivity in patients with chronic urticaria: diagnosis and follow-up. Clin Exp Dermatol. 2010;35(7):765–70.
172. Wolfrom E, et al. Chronic urticaria and toxocara canis infection. A case-control study. Ann Dermatol Venereol. 1996;123(4):240–6.
173. Hameed DM, Hassanin OM, Zuel-Fakkar NM. Association of Blastocystis hominis genetic subtypes with urticaria. Parasitol Res. 2011;108(3):553–60.
174. Karaman U, et al. [Investigation of microsporidia in patients with acute and chronic urticaria]. Mikrobiyol Bul. 2011;45(1):168–73.
175. Vandenberg O, et al. Clinical and microbiological features of dientamoebiasis in patients suspected of suffering from a parasitic gastrointestinal illness: a comparison of Dientamoeba fragilis and Giardia lamblia infections. Int J Infect Dis. 2006;10(3):255–61.
176. Weller P, Klion A Eosinophil biology and causes of eosinophilia. In: Mahoney DH, Rosmarin AG, Feldweg AM, editors. UpToDate. Waltham: UpToDate Inc. http://www.uptodate.com. Accessed 24 July 2018.
177. Khieu V, et al. Strongyloides stercoralis is a cause of abdominal pain, diarrhea and urticaria in rural Cambodia. BMC Res Notes. 2013;6:200.
178. van Aalsburg R, de Pagter AP, van Genderen PJ. Urticaria and periorbital edema as prodromal presenting signs of acute hepatitis B infection. J Travel Med. 2011;18(3):224–5.
179. Lockshin NA, Hurley H. Urticaria as a sign of viral hepatitis. Arch Dermatol. 1972;105(4):570–1.
180. Kolkhir P, et al. Treatment of urticarial vasculitis: a systematic review. J Allergy Clin Immunol. 2019;143(2):458–66.
181. Ranki A, et al. Effect of PUVA on immunologic and virologic findings in HIV-infected patients. J Am Acad Dermatol. 1991;24(3):404–10.
182. Supanaranond W, et al. Cutaneous manifestations in HIV positive patients. Southeast Asian J Trop Med Public Health. 2001;32(1):171–6.
183. Iemoli E, et al. Successful Omalizumab treatment in HIV positive patient with chronic spontaneous urticaria: a case report. Eur Ann Allergy Clin Immunol. 2017;49(2):88–91.
184. Zawar V, Godse K, Sankalecha S. Chronic urticaria associated with recurrent genital herpes simplex infection and success of antiviral therapy—a report of two cases. Int J Infect Dis. 2010;14(6):e514–7.
185. Dreyfus DH. Autoimmune disease: a role for new anti-viral therapies? Autoimmun Rev. 2011;11(2):88–97.

186. Palma-Carlos AG, Palma-Carlos ML. Chronic mucocutaneous candidiasis revisited. Allerg Immunol (Paris). 2001;33(6):229–32.
187. Trachsel C, Pichler WJ, Helbling A. [Importance of laboratory investigations and trigger factors in chronic urticaria]. Schweiz Med Wochenschr. 1999;129(36):1271–9.
188. Serrano H. [Hypersensitivity to "Candida albicans" and other fungi in patients with chronic urticaria]. Allergol Immunopathol (Madr). 1975;3(5):289–98.
189. Holti G. Candida allergy. In: Winner H, Hurley R, editors. Symposium on Candida infections. Edinburgh and London: Livingstone; 1966. p. 249.
190. Shelley WB, Florence R. Chronic urticaria due to mold hypersensitivity: a study in cross-sensitization and autoerythrocyte sensitization. Arch Dermatol. 1961;83(4):549–58.
191. Sulzberger MB, Kerr PS. Trichophytin hypersensitiveness of urticarial type, with circulating antibodies and passive transference. J Allergy. 1930;2(1):11–6.
192. Waldbott GL, Ascher MS. Chronic urticaria, recurring every six weeks, due to a fungous infection. Arch Dermatol Syphilol. 1937;36(2):314–7.
193. Mendez J, Sanchez A, Martinez JC. Urticaria associated with dermatophytosis. Allergol Immunopathol (Madr). 2002;30(6):344–5.
194. Godse KV, Zawar V. Chronic urticaria associated with tinea infection and success with antifungal therapy—a report of four cases. Int J Infect Dis. 2010;14(Suppl 3):e364–5.
195. Doeglas H. Chronic urticaria. Clinical and pathogenetic studies in 141 patients. Groningen: Dijkstra Niemeyer; 1975.
196. Pawankar R, et al. The WAO White Book on Allergy (Update. 2013).
197. Augey F, et al. Is there a link between chronic urticaria and atopy? Eur J Dermatol. 2008;18(3):348–9.
198. Sibbald RG, et al. Chronic urticaria. Evaluation of the role of physical, immunologic, and other contributory factors. Int J Dermatol. 1991;30(6):381–6.
199. Nassif A. Is chronic urticaria an atopic condition? Eur J Dermatol. 2007;17(6):545–6.
200. Lee N, et al. Epidemiology of chronic urticaria in Korea using the Korean Health Insurance Database, 2010–2014. Allergy Asthma Immunol Res. 2017;9(5):438–45.
201. Chansakulporn S, et al. The natural history of chronic urticaria in childhood: a prospective study. J Am Acad Dermatol. 2014;71(4):663–8.
202. Bingefors K, et al. Self-reported lifetime prevalence of atopic dermatitis and co-morbidity with asthma and eczema in adulthood: a population-based cross-sectional survey. Acta Derm Venereol. 2013;93(4):438–41.
203. Olze H, Zuberbier T. Comorbidities between nose and skin allergy. Curr Opin Allergy Clin Immunol. 2011;11(5):457–63.
204. Augey F, et al. Chronic spontaneous urticaria is not an allergic disease. Eur J Dermatol. 2011;21(3):349–53.
205. Normansell R, et al. Omalizumab for asthma in adults and children. Cochrane Database Syst Rev. 2014;1:CD003559.
206. Kozel MM, et al. The effectiveness of a history-based diagnostic approach in chronic urticaria and angioedema. Arch Dermatol. 1998;134(12):1575–80.
207. Kolkhir P, et al. C-reactive protein is linked to disease activity, impact, and response to treatment in patients with chronic spontaneous urticaria. Allergy. 2018;73(4):940–8.
208. Karakelides M, et al. Monoclonal gammopathies and malignancies in patients with chronic urticaria. Int J Dermatol. 2006;45(9):1032–8.
209. Kolkhir P, et al. Management of chronic spontaneous urticaria: a worldwide perspective. World Allergy Organ J. 2018;11(1):14.
210. Curth H. Skin lesions and internal carcinoma. In: Andrade R, et al., editors. Cancer of the skin. Philadelphia: WB Saunders; 1976. p. 1308–9.
211. Manganoni AM, et al. Chronic urticaria associated with thyroid carcinoma: report of 4 cases. J Investig Allergol Clin Immunol. 2007;17(3):192–5.
212. Reinhold U, Bruske T, Schupp G. Paraneoplastic urticaria in a patient with ovarian carcinoma. J Am Acad Dermatol. 1996;35(6):988–9.

213. Hill A, Metry D. Urticarial lesions in a child with acute lymphoblastic leukemia and eosinophilia. Pediatr Dermatol. 2003;20(6):502–5.
214. De P, et al. Urticaria and large cell undifferentiated carcinoma of lung. Dermatol Online J. 2005;11(3):45.
215. Kozel MM, et al. Laboratory tests and identified diagnoses in patients with physical and chronic urticaria and angioedema: a systematic review. J Am Acad Dermatol. 2003;48(3):409–16.
216. Alberti KG, Zimmet P, Shaw J. Metabolic syndrome—a new world-wide definition. A consensus statement from the International Diabetes Federation. Diabet Med. 2006;23(5):469–80.
217. Hoffman EL, VonWald T, Hansen K. The metabolic syndrome. S D Med. 2015;Spec No:24–8.
218. Devaraj S, Rosenson RS, Jialal I. Metabolic syndrome: an appraisal of the pro-inflammatory and procoagulant status. Endocrinol Metab Clin North Am. 2004;33(2):431–53.
219. Gyawali P, Richards RS. Association of altered hemorheology with oxidative stress and inflammation in metabolic syndrome. Redox Rep. 2015;20(3):139–44.
220. Hage FG. C-reactive protein and hypertension. J Hum Hypertens. 2014;28(7):410–5.
221. Schoepke N, et al. Allergy. 2019;74(12):2427–36.
222. Kolkhir P, et al. Allergy Asthma Immunol Res. 2021;13(4):545–59.
223. Ferriani MP, et al. Chronic spontaneous urticaria: a survey of 852 cases of childhood-onset systemic lupus erythematosus. Int Arch Allergy Immunol. 2015;167(3):186–92.

Inducible Urticarias

8

Sabine Altrichter, Markus Magerl, and Martin Metz

8.1 Introduction

Chronic inducible urticaria (CINDU) is a group of diseases that are characterized by the appearance of itchy wheals, angioedema or both, upon exposure to a specific triggering stimulus. Depending on the type of stimulus, CINDU can be classified as physical urticaria (symptomatic dermographism, cold urticaria, heat urticaria, delayed pressure urticaria, solar urticaria, and vibratory angioedema) or nonphysical urticaria (cholinergic urticaria, contact and aquagenic urticaria; Table 8.1) [1]. In most cases, CINDU is a very chronic disease lasting for many years. Overall, CINDU is common, but the prevalence of the individual physical and nonphysical urticarias is very different, from very common (i.e. symptomatic dermographism) to extremely rare (i.e. aquagenic urticaria). Most patients suffer from one CINDU, but some may have two or more CINDUs, and many patients with chronic spontaneous urticaria (CSU) have been reported to also have at least one concomitant CINDU. The diagnosis of CINDU is based on the patient history and a positive provocation test to the offending trigger. In all patients with a history suggestive of CINDU, respective provocation testing should, if possible, be performed to confirm the diagnosis. Many patients with CINDU suffer severely from the disease, and the correct diagnosis is required to inform the patient about the nature of the disease and to provide an optimal treatment.

S. Altrichter
Institute for Allergology, Charité – Universitätsmedizin, Berlin, Germany

Department of Dermatology and Venerology, Kepler University Hospital, Linz, Austria
e-mail: sabine.altrichter@charite.de

M. Magerl (✉) · M. Metz
Institute for Allergology, Charité – Universitätsmedizin, Berlin, Germany
e-mail: Markus.Magerl@charite.de; Martin.Metz@charite.de

Table 8.1 Classification of CINDU subtypes

Physical urticaria	Nonphysical urticaria
Symptomatic dermographism	Cholinergic urticaria
Cold urticaria	Contact urticaria
Delayed pressure urticaria	Aquagenic urticaria
Solar urticaria	
Heat urticaria	
Vibratory angioedema	

8.2 Symptomatic Dermographism

8.2.1 Definition and Clinical Picture

Symptomatic dermographism (SD), also called urticaria factitia or dermographic urticaria, is the most common inducible urticaria. The pruritus associated with this condition is often severe and disabling. The development of itchy wheals (and in rare cases angioedema) is due to shearing forces on the skin, which may be brought about by friction from clothes or by rubbing and scratching the skin. Wheals thus produced are characteristically linear, last 30 min to a few hours and fade without leaving a mark (Fig. 8.1). SD can last for years, exact data on the average duration are, however, missing.

8.2.2 Pathogenesis

The pathogenesis of SD is, as of yet, largely unknown. There is however evidence that, at least in a subgroup of patients, a soluble transferable serum factor, presumably IgE, is responsible for the activation of mast cells in the skin of SD patients. In passive sensitization experiments, the intracutaneous injection of five out of nine sera or plasma from SD patients was able to sensitize skin of healthy subjects for a wheal and flare response after scratching [2]. After heating two of the sera to 56 °C, and thus destroying the IgE, the sensitivity to scratching was no longer transferable. Furthermore, depletion of IgE by immunoabsorption also removed the activity of the serum, indicating that indeed IgE was the relevant serum factor in these patients.

8.2.3 Diagnosis and Differential Diagnosis

The patient's medical history often provides a clear indication of the diagnosis SD. Patients who report pruritus without visible signs on the skin, which is followed by mostly linear, itchy wheals with a surrounding erythema should be evaluated for SD. Some patients suffer from chronic itch or a "skin crawling" sensation that leads to scratching. Other patients report no itching on normal skin, but the development of severely itching wheals after any shear forces to the skin, sometimes only by a light touch or mild brushing [3].

Fig. 8.1 Symptomatic dermographism elicited by FricTest® (©ECARF)

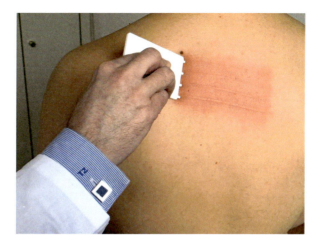

The diagnosis of SD should then be confirmed through provocation testing. Most commonly, this is done by stroking of the skin on the volar forearm or upper back with a smooth blunt object, for example, wooden spatula or a dermographometer. A normal (i.e. negative) response in a healthy individual is a red line lasting less than 10 min (red dermographism). The provocation test is considered positive if an itchy, palpable wheal occurs within 10 min after provocation. For confirmation of the diagnosis, but also to assess trigger strength thresholds, FricTest® can be used. FricTest® is a plastic comb with four tips of different lengths, which induce a graded shearing force to the skin, allowing for determination of trigger thresholds [4].

In atopic patients, white dermographism can occur, which is unrelated to SD. Furthermore, SD needs to be differentiated from the "simple" dermographism, a common physiological variant where whealing, but not pruritus, occurs after firm stroking of the skin.

8.2.4 Treatment and Prognosis

Patients with SD must be informed about the disease and its trigger factor. As complete avoidance of the trigger is not possible, symptomatic treatment is required in most patients. The first line treatment for SD is a non-sedating second-generation H1 antihistamines at the licensed dose [4]. The second line treatment for patients who are not completely controlled is up to fourfold increase of the dose of a second-generation antihistamine. The 2016 consensus recommendations for the management of CINDU recommend, as third line treatment options, omalizumab and ciclosporin [4]. Since then, a randomized, placebo-controlled clinical trial with omalizumab has been performed in SD patients who were unresponsive to antihistamine treatment. Here, both 150 mg and 300 mg omalizumab every 4 weeks were shown to be an effective treatment in SD [5]. It has to be noted that standard-dosed antihistamines are currently the only approved treatment option for patients with SD.

8.3 Cold Urticaria

8.3.1 Definition and Clinical Picture

In cold urticaria (also called acquired cold urticaria or cold contact urticaria), wheals, and sometimes angioedema, appear after skin contact with cold air, liquids, or solid objects. Depending on the critical temperature threshold, i.e. the highest temperature sufficient to induce a whealing response, and the duration and surface area of cold contact, systemic symptoms are common and range from mild fatigue and headache to bronchospasm and anaphylaxis. [6]. There is concern that cold water swimming could be potentially fatal [7]. Some patients can have oropharyngeal symptoms related to drinking chilled drinks and eating ice cream. Cold urticaria is potentially life threatening and especially in patients with outdoor occupations in colder climates very disabling. The estimated annual incidence of cold urticaria is 0.05% [8], but exact numbers are missing. Cold urticaria is often of long disease duration, reportedly 4–8 years [8–10].

8.3.2 Pathogenesis

The pathogenesis of cold urticaria is largely unknown. Similar to some other CINDU diseases, it has been shown that, in a subgroup of patients, the sensitivity to the triggering stimulus, i.e. cold, can be passively transferred. These transferable serum factors may be IgE of unknown specificity. IgG and/or IgM directed against IgE were identified *in vitro* in cold urticaria sera, but only one patient with IgM anti-IgE showed functionality [11, 12]. Furthermore, the excellent efficacy of anti-IgE treatment in patients with cold urticaria points towards an important pathogenetic role for IgE in cold urticaria. This could be a specific IgE that is directed against a skin-derived protein that gets released or has confirmatory changes upon stimulation by cold [13].

8.3.3 Diagnosis and Differential Diagnosis

In classical cold urticaria, itchy wheals occur within minutes of contact with cold. Therefore, a clinical history showing an association of cold contact and the development of signs and symptoms is indicative of the diagnosis of cold urticaria. Other, rare forms of cold urticaria exist [14, 15] and are characterized by negative immediate cold stimulation tests. These rare forms include delayed cold urticaria, where whealing only takes place hours after stimulation, cold-dependent dermographism, where urticarial lesions are elicited by stroking precooled skin, and cold-induced cholinergic urticaria, elicited by exercising in cold environments. Furthermore, there are very rare hereditary (autosomal dominant) conditions such as familial delayed cold urticaria, where affected family members develop delayed reactions resolving with hyperpigmentation, and familial cold auto-inflammatory syndrome, characterized by urticarial rash together with conjunctivitis and fever, eventually leading to deafness and lymphadenopathy [15].

To confirm the diagnosis of cold urticaria, skin provocation tests should be performed by applying localized cold to the skin. This can be done by applying a melting ice cube together with some water within a plastic bag to the skin to avoid cold damage and to prevent direct water contact, which can result in false positive reactions in patients with aquagenic urticaria [3]. Determination of the patient's skin threshold, i.e. detection of the highest temperature able to induce a whealing response, is possible using TempTest® (Courage & Khazaka, Cologne, Germany), which enables skin provocation with a continuous temperature gradient from 4–44 °C [3]. Besides determining the threshold levels for whealing, which in most symptomatic cases is around 16–23 °C [16], the system can also be used for monitoring treatment response. Cold provocation should be performed for 5 min and the skin should be inspected 10 min after provocation testing. The test is considered positive if the test site shows a palpable and clearly visible wheal and flare-type skin reaction [3].

8.3.4 Treatment and Prognosis

To avoid potentially life-threatening situations, for example, jumping into a lake, patients have to be aware of their diagnosis of cold urticaria and ideally know their critical temperature threshold. However, cold avoidance is rarely efficient or even possible as sole therapy, and quality of life is often additionally impaired in the patients because of their efforts in trying to avoid cold objects. Therefore, symptomatic pharmacological therapy is necessary in most patients. The first line treatment of cold urticaria is a non-sedating H1 antihistamine in standard dosing. Although several controlled studies support this recommendation, many patients are not sufficiently treated by standard-dosed antihistamines. It has been shown in controlled clinical trials in patients with cold urticaria that increasing the dose to up to fourfold is more effective than standard doses [17–19]. In cold urticaria patients who are resistant to antihistamine treatment, anti-IgE treatment with omalizumab, both 150 mg and 300 mg, has been shown to be effective in a randomized, placebo-controlled clinical trial [20]. Other treatment options that have been described to have at least some effects on cold urticaria include treatment with antibiotics and cold desensitization [4]. Treatment with antibiotics has been shown to be especially helpful early after onset of disease as reported in early trials but the level of evidence is low as they have not been placebo controlled [8]. The principle of cold desensitization is the induction of tolerance to cold by repeated daily cold exposures. Although this treatment has been reported to protect from symptom development, it is potentially dangerous as it can induce anaphylactic shock during induction and should therefore only be performed under expert physician supervision. Furthermore, maintenance of tolerance requires daily cold showers, which results in very poor compliance over a longer time period [4].

8.4 Delayed Pressure Urticaria

8.4.1 Definition and Clinical Picture

Delayed pressure urticaria (DPU) is defined by the appearance of a skin swelling response after the application of a sustained static pressure stimulus to the skin. The pressure required to trigger urticaria is comparatively high— and on one spot for a longer period of time. Simply scratching the skin does not trigger pressure urticaria. DPU is different from most other forms of CINDU in several ways. The application of the stimulus does not result in a typical superficial, well defined wheal but rather in an erythematous swelling of the deeper skin layers, in which pruritus is not a feature but patients usually report tenderness and a burning or painful sensation [21]. Bullous forms are very rare [22]. The skin lesions develop with a delay of approximately 4–8 h after the stimulus and last for 12–72 h [23, 24]. The size of the lesions fits the area of application of pressure. Although the lesions remain locally, extracutaneous symptoms like malaise, fatigue, fever, chills, headache, or generalized arthralgia are frequent [24, 25].

Approximately two-thirds of the patients with DPU are males, many of them employed in occupations requiring physical work. DPU onset is seen, on average, in the first half of the fourth decade of life [23, 24, 26, 27]. In the majority of the cases, DPU is associated with one or more other forms CU, including spontaneous and inducible. The co-occurrence of DPU in CSU seems to be one of the major drivers of QoL-impairment [28]. DPU patients report more pain and more problems concerning physical ability compared to patients with other forms of CU.

8.4.2 Pathogenesis

Although dermal and subcutaneous mast cells in the deep are believed to be the key cellular drivers, evidence supports not histamine, but a group of proinflammatory cytokines to be responsible for the symptoms, such as interleukin (IL)-1, IL-3, IL-6, and tumor necrosis factor (TNF), as well as leukotriene B4, thus leading to a transient inflammatory infiltrate consisting mainly of eosinophils, T-lymphocytes, and a few neutrophils [27, 29–32]. Histamine as the main mast cell mediator may play a role. However, when taking into account the clinical characteristics of DPU and the poor response to antihistamines, other mediators, and mechanisms seem to be predominant. Which mechanisms in the skin, blood vessels, or nerves lead to the above described response of the immune system after the impact of static pressure remains completely unclear.

8.4.3 Diagnosis and Differential Diagnosis

As DPU is often associated with other forms of CU, it might be overseen in many cases. Therefore, a thorough medical history is essential. To this end, patients need to understand the difference between spontaneous and induced symptoms. In particular, the delay of several hours between impact of pressure and onset of symptoms can cause misunderstandings during history taking. The occurrence of recurrent swellings and uncomfortable skin alterations at sites of predilection hours after certain activities should be asked specifically and in detail, e.g. soles of the feet after standing on a ladder, knees after kneeling work, buttocks after sitting on a hard chair or cycling, hands after crafting or using screwdrivers, shoulder after wearing a heavy bag with a shoulder strap. The principle of testing is to imitate the real-world situation by applying a sustained pressure to the skin to then evaluate the skin reaction [4]. Test methods include the suspension of weights over the shoulder (7 kg on a 3 cm shoulder strap), the application of rods, lowered vertically onto the skin and supported in a frame, on the back, thigh, or forearm. In the literature, different weighted rods are described, their diameter vary between 1.5 and 5.5 cm, the weights between 2.29 and 5 kg, resulting in pressures between 20.7 and 266 kPa, usually they are applied for 15 min on the skin. Alternatively, a dermographometer can be applied statically at 100 g/mm^2 (981 kPa) for 70 s on the upper back. After testing, the test site should be marked with a pen to avoid ambiguities at the evaluation of the test. The reading of the test result should be performed approximately 6 h after the testing procedure, and a palpable erythematous swelling at the site of the test stands for a positive outcome. If the test response is documented by the patient, she/he should be instructed clearly about the expected skin reaction and how to document it.

8.4.4 Treatment and Prognosis

Substantial relief can be achieved by relieving pressure, which unfortunately cannot be achieved in all situations. Patients need to be aware about the fact that static pressure is the trigger in DPU. Patients should understand that pressure is defined as a certain force applied to a certain area, and reducing the force, as well as increasing the area on which this force acts, reduces the applied pressure. It should be advised to wear wide and soft shoes, use padded straps on bags and backpacks and similar measures to prevent the skin symptoms from developing in the first place. In most patients, DPU is difficult to treat and often insufficiently responsive to high doses of antihistamines. The combination with montelukast or theophylline may be more effective than treatment with antihistamines alone [33, 34]. Many other drugs, such as leukotriene antagonists, nonsteroidal anti-inflammatory drugs, corticosteroids, ciclosporin, colchicine, sulphasalazine, dapsone, intravenous immunoglobulin (IVIG), omalizumab have been reported to be beneficial in some patients with DPU, however, high quality studies (prospective, randomized, controlled, sample size calculation) are very rare. The best available evidence favours the use of omalizumab and, if not available, dapsone [35].

As in other forms of CU, DPU shows spontaneous remission, the reported duration of DPU ranges from 6 to 9 years [24]. The remission of DPU may occur independently from other concomitant forms of CU.

8.5 Solar Urticaria

8.5.1 Definition and Clinical Picture

In solar urticaria, itchy wheals occur within minutes of exposure to sunlight. Depending on the wavelength responsible for the elicitation of the symptoms, windshields or window glasses may not be sufficient to avoid the trigger. Solar urticaria is a rare, but very debilitating disease. True solar urticaria always presents as immediate onset of an itch and wheal response following exposure to sunlight, which subsides within a couple of hours (Fig. 8.2). Systemic symptoms in solar urticaria are rare, but possible. Many patients referred with the diagnosis solar urticaria actually suffer from polymorphic light eruption—a relatively common photosensitivity. Polymorphic light eruption develops several hours after sun exposure and lasts for several days even if sunlight is avoided.

8.5.2 Pathogenesis

The exact pathogenesis of solar urticaria is not entirely understood, but a transferable serum factor, presumably IgE, has been thought for a long time to play an important role. The intradermal injection of serum from solar urticaria patients into healthy subjects has been shown to result in a transferred reactivity to UV irradiation [36–38], and the irradiation of serum from solar urticaria patients has been shown to be sufficient to induce a wheal and flare response after intradermal injection into the patient's own skin, suggesting that autologous photoallergens participate in the pathogenesis [36, 39–41]. The responsible photoallergens, however, are not identified so far.

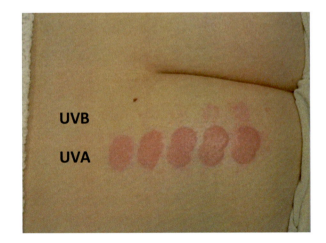

Fig. 8.2 Solar urticaria. Whealing response in the UVA range 10 min after provocation with Saalmann multitester

Patients develop wheals by exposure to specific wavelengths of light, called action spectra, which variably include the broad or narrow spectra distributing among visible light, UV-A, and UV-B. It has been described that whealing induced by the action spectrum can be inhibited by exposure to a longer wavelength light, which is called the inhibition spectrum [42]. This inhibition spectrum suppresses wheal and flare response when it is irradiated before, during, and immediately after the irradiation of the action spectrum [42–46].

8.5.3 Diagnosis and Differential Diagnosis

The diagnosis of solar urticaria is based on the medical history and the results of a provocation test. In the case of solar urticaria, signs and symptoms (i.e. itchy wheals) generally occur within minutes of exposure of the skin with light of the triggering wavelength and intensity. All other theoretically possible differential diagnoses usually show a significantly delayed (hours or days) and/or different skin reaction. In the much more frequent polymorphic light eruption for example (which is, similar to solar urticaria, commonly often called "sun allergy"), papules, vesicles or plaques usually appear after 1–2 days. In the very rare erythropoietic protoporphyria, patients usually describe a burning pain shortly after sun exposure and swelling with urticarial symptoms may also occur in the course of the disease.

Provocation should be performed by exposure to UV radiation and, if necessary, visible light, using solar simulators with filters (UV-A and UV-B) or a monochromator (UV-A and UV-B, visible light). The test should be performed on non-light exposed areas such as the buttocks separately in the UV-A, broadband UV-B wavelength spectrum and in the visible light range. In patients with a negative reaction, sensitivity to visible light can be tested using a projector (e.g. slide projector) at a distance of 10 cm. The test is considered positive if a clearly visible wheal occurs after 10 min (Fig. 8.2). In patients with a positive test reaction, threshold testing should be performed by varying the radiation dose, e.g. by changing the exposure time. This threshold test can identify a minimal urticarial dose and can thus help in determining disease activity and response to therapy.

8.5.4 Treatment and Prognosis

Epidemiological data on solar urticaria is sparse, but current data indicate that solar urticaria is, compared to chronic spontaneous urticaria, a long-lasting disease. For example, in a series of 87 patients with solar urticaria, the disease resolved in only one out of four patients within 10 years after diagnosis [47].

The recommended treatment for solar urticaria is a non-sedating H1-antihistamine in standard or increased dosing. Symptomatic treatment of solar urticaria is, however, often difficult as most patients are not sufficiently controlled by antihistamines. Patients with solar urticaria are therefore advised to avoid the sun, wear protective clothing, and use broad-spectrum sunscreens, especially when the threshold is in the UV spectrum. Complete avoidance of the sun is, however, neither possible nor can it be considered healthy for the patients [4].

Tolerance to UV light can be achieved in some patients by phototherapeutic irradiation of UV-A, broadband UV-B, or narrowband UV-B [41, 48–52]. This hardening effect lasts only for a few days [53], and irradiation therefore needs to be repeated regularly, making it not only a logistic challenge, but also increasing the risk of long-term UV-induced skin damage for the patients. Other potential treatment options with limited evidence include omalizumab [54], cyclosporine [55], intravenous immunoglobulin [56], afamelanotide, an alpha-MSH analogue [57], photopheresis [58], and plasmapheresis [41].

8.6 Heat Urticaria

8.6.1 Definition and Clinical Picture

Unlike cold urticaria, heat urticaria (HeatU) is a very rare disease. HeatU is characterized by the appearance of wheals after passive warming of the skin, e.g. due to hot baths, blow-drying of the hair and sunbathing. Systemic involvement is frequent. The triggering temperature is generally above 38 °C, the average reported threshold temperature is 44 °C. HeatU affects more women than men [59].

8.6.2 Pathogenesis

The pathogenesis of HeatU is largely unknown. In a study from 2002, a patient with localized heat urticaria was found to have a positive reaction on intradermal testing with heated autologous serum, but not after injection of the untreated serum. Further investigation suggested that the trigger is a heat-modified but heat-stable protein [60].

8.6.3 Diagnosis and Differential Diagnosis

The diagnostic workup includes a thorough history, heat provocation and, if positive, threshold testing. The above mentioned TempTest® can be helpful for diagnosis, however, additional testing in patients with a clear history who test negative with TempTest® is recommended [61]. Heat should be applied for 5 min (metal/glass bath, TempTest®) at a temperature of up to 44 °C. The testing site should be assessed 10 min after provocation [4]. HeatU must be differentiated from the much more common entities cholinergic urticaria, solar urticaria, and exercise-induced anaphylaxis.

8.6.4 Treatment and Prognosis

H1-antihistamines are effective in around 60% of patients with HeatU, but less than 20% of patients achieve complete symptom control, even at four times the licensed dose. In antihistamine-resistant HeatU, omalizumab was repeatedly reported to be successful [61, 62]. As most other forms of CINDU, HeatU shows spontaneous remission [59].

8.7 Vibratory Angioedema

8.7.1 Definition and Clinical Picture

Vibratory angioedema (VA) is defined by the presence of itching and swelling within a few minutes at the site of skin exposure to vibration. Typical stimuli include motorcycling, using an electric lawnmower or pneumatic hammer, playing instruments like trumpet or saxophone, or snoring [63–65]. VA is considered to be a rare disease, however, mild forms might be more frequent than thought [66, 67]. Both hereditary autosomal dominant (familial) and acquired sporadic variants were described [68].

8.7.2 Pathogenesis

It has been shown repeatedly that VA is histamine-mediated, and this seems to be true for non-familial as well as for familial forms of VA [66, 69, 70]. Recently, an autosomal dominant variant of VA with hives with a missense variant ADGRE2 (Adhesion G Protein-Coupled Receptor E2) on mast cells has been described. The authors found a gain of function mutation in ADGRE2, which presumably destabilizes the inhibitory interaction between the α and β subunits of its receptor, thereby sensitizing mast cells to vibration-induced degranulation [70]. In non-familial types of VA this mechanism could not be confirmed [66].

8.7.3 Diagnosis and Differential Diagnosis

As in all forms of CINDU, careful and thorough history taking is essential. Symptomatic dermographism and DPU should be ruled out. Symptoms of VA can be induced using a laboratory vortex mixer. The forearm is held on the vortex mixer for 5 min. The reading should be assessed for swelling 10 min after testing. It is helpful to measure the circumference of the forearm at the testing site before and after the challenge.

8.7.4 Treatment and Prognosis

Antihistamines have been described to be effective in VA in some cases. In one case low doses of amitriptyline and bromazepam were effective. Montelukast, ranitidine, dapsone, ciclosporin, methotrexate, prednisolone, and omalizumab failed to produce any improvement (n = 1) [71–73]. Little is known about the prognosis of VA.

8.8 Cholinergic Urticaria

8.8.1 Definition and Clinical Picture

Cholinergic Urticaria (CholU) is a frequent form of inducible urticaria [74–78]. The clinical picture consists of multiple pin-point-sized wheals and often large surrounding flare reactions with severe itch, sometimes even associated with pain (Fig. 8.3). Co-occurrence of angioedema has been described as frequent [79, 80]. Here, symmetrical mild swellings in the face (eyelids, lips) or hand and feet are common. Abortive forms without the development of wheals have been reported and termed cholinergic pruritus [81].

Typical triggers are exercise, hot environment (e.g. sauna, hot climate), overwarm clothing, but also hot and spicy food or psychological stress. In short, patients get their symptoms when sweating is involved. CholU can range from very mild symptoms upon severe physical exercise to severe symptoms upon easy daily activities, like walking or household duties resulting in severe disability and poor quality of life [82]. Wheals predominately occur on the trunk, but also the upper arms and legs. Lower arms and legs can be involved, but the face is rarely affected. Wheals usually last 30 min to an hour and fade without leaving a mark. CholU usually affects young adults, but also patients with advanced age, here predominantly females, have been described [76, 78, 83]. The disease can last for years and decades, but exact data on the mean duration is missing.

Some patients report refractory states following a strong outbreak of symptoms that can last up to 24 h, where usual triggers then do not elicit symptoms. Repetitive exercise could therefore limit symptoms [84]. Furthermore more severe symptoms have been reported in cold seasons [85, 86], and repetitive sweating was suggested as beneficial for reducing the symptoms.

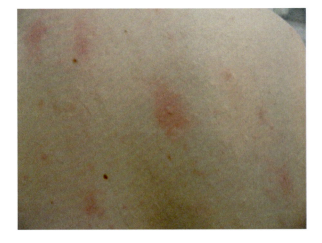

Fig. 8.3 Cholinergic Urticaria. Small wheals with large surrounding flares reaction during pulse controlled ergometry

8.8.2 Pathogenesis

The pathogenesis of CholU is not completely understood. Several concepts had been developed in the past [74, 87–90]. A rise of body temperature has been proposed as the main trigger of symptoms, but detailed reading of the literature as well as follow-up studies did not show a correlation of body temperature rise and the onset of symptoms [91, 92]. More clearly the process of sweating is associated with symptoms. In some patients, hypohidrosis or anhidrosis [93] has been reported, and blockage of the sweat gland duct possibly leading to sweat reflux and maybe leakage into the dermis has been suggested as cause of the symptoms [94]. Another hypothesis suggested the combination of hypohidrosis and a positive autologous serum test as indicating autoimmune destruction of the sweat gland, leading to hypohidrosis and CholU symptoms [95–97]. Hypohidrosis has also been associated with reduced expression of the muscarinic receptor M3 on the sweat glands of the patients, and acetylcholine excess in the synaptic cleft has been proposed as an activator of nearby mast cells [98–101]. This theory is supported by the fact that acetylcholine provokes a wheal and flare-type skin reaction in about one-third of the patients [102] and that omalizumab therapy can fail [103]. Lastly, the following theory currently has the most evidence in the literature. Here, sensitization to sweat and sweat components (i.e. Malassezia globosa antigen) has been seen in Asian patients with CholU [90, 104]. Finding specific IgE to Malassezia globosa in some patients, functional relevance of Malassezia globosa antigen in basophil activation tests and the successful use of anti-IgE therapy (omalizumab) strengthens the idea of true type I allergic mast cell activation in these patients [105, 106]. This is also supported by the fact that a predisposition to allergies has been more frequently reported than in other forms of chronic urticaria [107, 108].

8.8.3 Diagnosis and Differential Diagnosis

The typical clinical picture with multiple small wheals and the description of provoking situations usually point towards the diagnosis of CholU. It must be confirmed using provocation testing [4]. The current guideline recommends exercise provocation until induction of sweating and 10 more minutes before reading or using the pulse controlled ergometry with incremental exercise over a time period of 30 min and a cool-down phase of 10 min before symptom check [109]. The latter has the advantage of individual reproducibility and use in clinical trials. Passive warming in climate chambers or hot water immersion (42 °C, full body immersion, 10 min) is a second possibility for provocation testing [91]. Treatment should be withdrawn before testing and patients should be tested outside a possible refractory period.

If the test is unexpectedly negative, the patient should be retested or the diagnosis should be reconsidered. The differential diagnosis with other forms of urticaria includes heat contact urticaria and aquagenic urticaria. Of note, a combination with other forms of urticaria is common, most often chronic spontaneous urticaria [83] or cold urticaria [12, 110–113]. The delimitation from adrenergic urticaria is unclear [114, 115].

An important differential diagnosis is exercise induced anaphylaxis [116] or food and exercise induced anaphylaxis where patients have a sensitization to allergens, most commonly to wheat (also known as wheat and exercise induced anaphylaxis, most commonly sIgE to omega-5-gliadin) that only becomes manifest after exercise exposure [117–119]. Here, the symptoms usually only occur sporadically (when the food has been consumed within 30 min to a few hours before exercise). Aspirin intake before exercise can be an additional augmenting factor [117, 120]. These patients usually develop larger wheals and can develop severe extracutaneous symptoms like asthma, cramps, hypotonia, and fainting. In such cases, allergological workup including skin prick testing, analysis of specific IgE, and food- and exercise provocation is needed to establish the exact diagnosis.

8.8.4 Treatment and Prognosis

CholU patients have to be informed about the trigger factor and course of the disease. Very mildly affected patients can avoid triggers and might not require specific treatment. For more severely affected patients, complete avoidance of the trigger is usually not possible, and symptomatic treatment is required. According to the current guideline the first line treatment for CholU is a non-sedating second-generation H1 antihistamine at the licensed dose [4]. The second line treatment for patients who are not completely controlled is up to a fourfold increase of the dose of a second-generation antihistamine. The 2016 consensus recommendations for the management of CINDU recommend, as third line treatment options, omalizumab and ciclosporin [4]. However, standard-dosed antihistamines are currently the only approved treatment option for CholU. Dose escalation has minimal benefit [121] and is an off-label treatment, as well as all other alternatives. Omalizumab has shown to be effective in case series [122–124]. In a randomized, placebo-controlled clinical trial with omalizumab, the primary endpoint of complete symptom control was missed, but the treatment showed some efficacy after several months of treatment [125]. As further treatment options in case reports, the successful use of H2-antihistamines [126], anticholinergic drugs [127, 128], beta blockers [129, 130], danazol [131–133], steroids [134], tannic acid [135], sweating therapy [136] or botox have been described. However, clinical trials using these treatments are missing.

CholU usually lasts several years, up to two to three decades, but is eventually self-limiting. Data on exact disease duration or symptom cessation are missing.

8.9 Contact Urticaria

8.9.1 Definition and Clinical Picture

Contact urticaria is characterized by the development of palpable and clearly visible wheal and flare-type skin reaction within a few minutes after skin or mucous membrane contact to an exogenous urticariogenic substance. The lesions usually resolve within 2 h. Systemic involvement and even anaphylaxis can occur. The prevalence of contact urticaria has been calculated to be <0.4% in a cohort of dermatology/allergy/anaphylaxis patients, a lower frequency in the general population has to be assumed [137].

8.9.2 Pathogenesis

Two subtypes of contact urticaria are recognized: immunological contact urticaria and non-immunological contact urticaria. The immunological contact urticaria is an IgE-mediated reaction requiring previous sensitization, it is mainly induced by proteins or hapten-forming molecules, and the reaction can spread beyond the area of contact into generalized urticaria and even evolve into systemic symptoms. Non-immunological contact urticaria does not require previous sensitization and can occur at the very first contact to the eliciting agent, e.g. plants like stinging nettles, animals like jelly fish, or chemicals like cinnamon aldehyde. The lesions are strictly limited to the areas of direct contact of the eliciting agent [4].

8.9.3 Diagnosis and Differential Diagnosis

After taking a thorough history with particular attention on potential causative agents in food, home/work environment, and personal care products, provocation testing should be performed to confirm contact urticaria, using open controlled application testing, skin prick test, or closed patch tests for 20 min. It should be taken in account that systemic anaphylaxis may be provoked in highly sensitized cases. No in-vivo provocation tests are necessary, when the eliciting agent is obvious, for example, stinging nettles or jellyfish. In immunological contact urticaria, measurement of total and specific IgE can be confirmative in the diagnostic workup. Virtually all other forms of urticaria need to be considered as differential diagnoses to contact urticaria, first of all CINDUs like symptomatic dermographism, cold urticaria, solar, and aquagenic urticaria [138].

8.9.4 Treatment and Prognosis

The management of contact urticaria includes identification of the eliciting substance, its avoidance, and patient education. Antihistamines are usually helpful in IgE-mediated immunological contact urticaria, if given before exposure to the elicitor. Occupational contact urticaria should be managed as other occupational skin diseases, by eliminating the allergen from the direct work environment and other measures to reduce levels of allergen exposure [139]. In a 6-month follow-up study of 1048 patients diagnosed with occupational skin disease, the prognosis was best in the 155 patients with occupational CU, of whom 35% were cured [140].

8.10 Aquagenic Urticaria

8.10.1 Definition and Clinical Picture

Aquagenic Urticaria (AqU) is an extremely rare form of inducible urticaria. Typically, small extremely itchy wheals are provoked by skin contact with water. Most commonly, patients develop wheals on the trunk, especially on the décolleté, but can also have symptoms elsewhere [141]. Wheals last 30 min to a few hours and disappear without leaving a mark (Fig. 8.4). AqU can last for years, but there is hardly any data on disease duration available.

Some patients report provocation of symptoms only to sweat or salty water [142–145], the majority react regardless of the type of water. Swimming, bathing, or showering is extremely problematic for the patients, and systemic reactions had been reported [146]. Some also report sweating as symptom trigger and combined forms of cholinergic and aquagenic urticaria have been reported [147]. Overall, the patients have extremely poor quality of life and are very restricted in their daily life. More women than men had been reported, and the condition typically presents for the first-time during puberty, but can also start in infancy [148].

8.10.2 Pathogenesis

The pathogenesis of AqU is unclear. Interaction between water and a component in or on the skin or sebum has been suggested. This theory suggests that a substance is formed by this interaction, the absorption of which causes perifollicular mast cell degranulation with release of histamine [149]. Another hypothesis suggests a mechanism in which AqU has to do with sudden changes in osmotic pressure surrounding

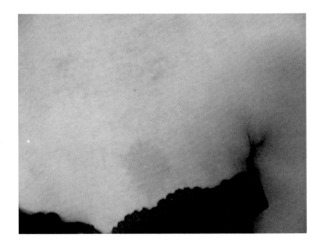

Fig. 8.4 Aquagenic Urticaria. Small wheal with large surrounding flare reaction, 10 min after water provocation

hair follicles, leading to increased passive diffusion of water [150]. Another proposed mechanism involves existence of water-soluble antigens in the epidermis, which dissolve and diffuse across the dermis with resulting histamine release from mast cells [151]. On the other hand, some evidence exists, that the mechanism may be completely independent of histamine release [152]. This is supported by the observation that pretreatment with scopolamine (an anticholinergic drug) prior to water contact can suppress wheal formation [153].

Single reports of familiar AqU can be found in the literature [154–157], but most cases are sporadic.

8.10.3 Diagnosis and Differential Diagnosis

The patient's history and reported triggers usually hint to this diagnosis. Water provocation tests are performed on the trunk of the patients, where wet cloth, preimmersed in 37 °C warm water, is applied for 10 up to 30 min. Evoked symptoms usually occur within 10 min after stop of the water test [158].

As differential diagnoses, other forms of urticaria must be excluded such as cold and heat urticaria, as well as cholinergic urticaria. Itching after contact with water, without the development of physical hives, is known as aquagenic pruritus [159–162] and aquadynia is a variant of aquagenic pruritus, characterized by a widespread burning pain that lasts 15–45 min after water exposure [163–165]. If these are abortive forms of AqU or distinct diagnosis is not clear as of yet [160, 166, 167].

8.10.4 Treatment and Prognosis

Complete avoidance of water contact is not possible or healthy. Accordingly, complete avoidance of the trigger is not possible. Oil in water emulsion creams [168], or petrolatum [153, 169], applied as barrier agents prior to a shower or bath may control symptoms, but cannot really be used practically, especially if cleaning of the skin is the reason for water contact. The recommended treatment for AqU is the same as in other forms of chronic urticaria: non-sedating H1-antihistamines in standard or increased dosing [4]. It has been shown to be effective in some cases [170], but limited knowledge is available on the overall efficacy of the treatment.

Omalizumab has been reported to be effective in single cases [171, 172], but this or other treatments like anticholinergic treatment [153], stanozolol [173], or selective serotonin reuptake inhibitors (SSRIs) [174] are not licensed in this indication [175]. Also, knowledge on the efficacy of UV-therapy is very limited [176, 177].

AqU often lasts for several years. Data on mean duration of the disease or resolution are not available from the literature.

References

1. Zuberbier T, et al. The EAACI/GA(2)LEN/EDF/WAO guideline for the definition, classification, diagnosis and management of urticaria. Allergy. 2018;73(7):1393–414.
2. Newcomb RW, Nelson H. Dermographia mediated by immunoglobulin E. Am J Med. 1973;54(2):174–80.
3. Maurer M, Fluhr JW, Khan DA. How to approach chronic inducible urticaria. J Allergy Clin Immunol Pract. 2018;6(4):1119–30.
4. Magerl M, et al. The definition, diagnostic testing, and management of chronic inducible urticarias—The EAACI/GA(2) LEN/EDF/UNEV consensus recommendations 2016 update and revision. Allergy. 2016;71(6):780–802.
5. Maurer M, et al. Omalizumab is effective in symptomatic dermographism-results of a randomized placebo-controlled trial. J Allergy Clin Immunol. 2017;140(3):870–873.e5.
6. Alangari AA, et al. Clinical features and anaphylaxis in children with cold urticaria. Pediatrics. 2004;113(4):e313–7.
7. Mazarakis A, et al. Kounis syndrome following cold urticaria: the swimmer's death. Int J Cardiol. 2014;176(2):e52–3.
8. Möller A, et al. [Epidemiology and clinical aspects of cold urticaria]. Hautarzt. 1996;47(7):510–4.
9. Krause K, Zuberbier T, Maurer M. Modern approaches to the diagnosis and treatment of cold contact urticaria. Curr Allergy Asthma Rep. 2010;10(4):243–9.
10. Neittaanmaki H. Cold urticaria. Clinical findings in 220 patients. J Am Acad Dermatol. 1985;13(4):636–44.
11. Gruber BL, et al. Prevalence and functional role of anti-IgE autoantibodies in urticarial syndromes. J Invest Dermatol. 1988;90(2):213–7.
12. Kaplan AP, Garofalo J. Identification of a new physically induced urticaria: cold-induced cholinergic urticaria. J Allergy Clin Immunol. 1981;68(6):438–41.
13. Kaplan AP, et al. Idiopathic cold urticaria: in vitro demonstration of histamine release upon challenge of skin biopsies. N Engl J Med. 1981;305(18):1074–7.
14. Siebenhaar F, et al. Acquired cold urticaria: clinical picture and update on diagnosis and treatment. Clin Exp Dermatol. 2007;32(3):241–5.
15. Wanderer AA, Hoffman HM. The spectrum of acquired and familial cold-induced urticaria/urticaria-like syndromes. Immunol Allergy Clin North Am. 2004;24(2):259–86, vii.
16. Mlynek A, et al. Results and relevance of critical temperature threshold testing in patients with acquired cold urticaria. Br J Dermatol. 2010;162(1):198–200.
17. Abajian M, et al. Rupatadine 20 mg and 40 mg are effective in reducing the symptoms of chronic cold urticaria. Acta Derm Venereol. 2016;96(1):56–9.
18. Krause K, et al. Up-dosing with bilastine results in improved effectiveness in cold contact urticaria. Allergy. 2013;68(7):921–8.
19. Siebenhaar F, et al. High-dose desloratadine decreases wheal volume and improves cold provocation thresholds compared with standard-dose treatment in patients with acquired cold urticaria: a randomized, placebo-controlled, crossover study. J Allergy Clin Immunol. 2009;123(3):672–9.
20. Metz M, et al. Omalizumab is effective in cold urticaria-results of a randomized placebo-controlled trial. J Allergy Clin Immunol. 2017;140(3):864–867.e5.
21. Ryan TJ, Shim-Young N, Turk JL. Delayed pressure urticaria. Br J Dermatol. 1968;80(8):485–90.
22. Weins AB, et al. Delayed bullous pressure urticaria: the puzzling role of eosinophils. J Dtsch Dermatol Ges. 2018;16(10):1253–5.
23. Sussman GL, Harvey RP, Schocket AL. Delayed pressure urticaria. J Allergy Clin Immunol. 1982;70(5):337–42.
24. Dover JS, et al. Delayed pressure urticaria. Clinical features, laboratory investigations, and response to therapy of 44 patients. J Am Acad Dermatol. 1988;18(6):1289–98.

25. Dortas SD, Jr et al. [Delayed pressure urticaria with systemic manifestations: case report]. An Bras Dermatol. 2009;84(6):671–4.
26. Warin RP. Clinical observations on delayed pressure urticaria. Br J Dermatol. 1989;121(2):225–8.
27. Czarnetzki BM, et al. Clinical, pharmacological and immunological aspects of delayed pressure urticaria. Br J Dermatol. 1984;111(3):315–23.
28. Poon E, et al. The extent and nature of disability in different urticarial conditions. Br J Dermatol. 1999;140(4):667–71.
29. Czarnetzki BM, et al. Morphology of the cellular infiltrate in delayed pressure urticaria. J Am Acad Dermatol. 1985;12(2 Pt 1):253–9.
30. Hermes B, et al. Upregulation of TNF-alpha and IL-3 expression in lesional and uninvolved skin in different types of urticaria. J Allergy Clin Immunol. 1999;103(2 Pt 1):307–14.
31. Haas N, Hermes B, Henz BM. Adhesion molecules and cellular infiltrate: histology of urticaria. J Investig Dermatol Symp Proc. 2001;6(2):137–8.
32. Kasperska-Zajac A, et al. Markers of systemic inflammation in delayed pressure urticaria. Int J Dermatol. 2013;52(3):309–10.
33. Nettis E, et al. Efficacy of montelukast, in combination with loratadine, in the treatment of delayed pressure urticaria. J Allergy Clin Immunol. 2003;112(1):212–3.
34. Kalogeromitros D, et al. Theophylline as "add-on" therapy in patients with delayed pressure urticaria: a prospective self-controlled study. Int J Immunopathol Pharmacol. 2005;18(3):595–602.
35. Kulthanan K, et al. Delayed pressure urticaria: a systematic review of treatment options. J Allergy Clin Immunol Pract. 2020;8(6):2035–2049.e5.
36. Kojima M, et al. Solar urticaria. The relationship of photoallergen and action spectrum. Arch Dermatol. 1986;122(5):550–5.
37. Harber LC, et al. Immunologic and biophysical studies in solar urticaria. J Invest Dermatol. 1963;41:439–43.
38. Torinuki W, Tagami H. Solar urticaria without inhibitory spectrum: demonstration of both circulating photoallergen and reaginic antibodies. Dermatologica. 1986;173(3):116–9.
39. Ng JC, et al. Changes of photosensitivity and action spectrum with time in solar urticaria. Photodermatol Photoimmunol Photomed. 2002;18(4):191–5.
40. Danno K, Mori N. Solar urticaria: report of two cases with augmentation spectrum. Photodermatol Photoimmunol Photomed. 2000;16(1):30–3.
41. Collins P, et al. Plasma exchange therapy for solar urticaria. Br J Dermatol. 1996;134(6):1093–7.
42. Hasei K, Ichihashi M. Solar urticaria. Determinations of action and inhibition spectra. Arch Dermatol. 1982;118(5):346–50.
43. Uetsu N, et al. The clinical and photobiological characteristics of solar urticaria in 40 patients. Br J Dermatol. 2000;142(1):32–8.
44. Horio T, Yoshioka A, Okamoto H. Production and inhibition of solar urticaria by visible light exposure. J Am Acad Dermatol. 1984;11(6):1094–9.
45. Ichihashi M, Hasei K, Hayashibe K. Solar urticaria. Further studies on the role of inhibition spectra. Arch Dermatol. 1985;121(4):503–7.
46. Leenutaphong V. Solar urticaria induced by UVA and inhibited by visible light. J Am Acad Dermatol. 1993;29(2 Pt 2):337–40.
47. Beattie PE, et al. Characteristics and prognosis of idiopathic solar urticaria: a cohort of 87 cases. Arch Dermatol. 2003;139(9):1149–54.
48. Addo HA, Sharma SC. UVB phototherapy and photochemotherapy (PUVA) in the treatment of polymorphic light eruption and solar urticaria. Br J Dermatol. 1987;116(4):539–47.
49. Beissert S, Ständer H, Schwarz T. UVA rush hardening for the treatment of solar urticaria. J Am Acad Dermatol. 2000;42(6):1030–2.
50. Dawe RS, Ferguson J. Prolonged benefit following ultraviolet A phototherapy for solar urticaria. Br J Dermatol. 1997;137(1):144–8.

51. Keahey TM, et al. Studies on the mechanism of clinical tolerance in solar urticaria. Br J Dermatol. 1984;110(3):327–38.
52. Ramsay CA. Solar urticaria treatment by inducing tolerance to artificial radiation and natural light. Arch Dermatol. 1977;113(9):1222–5.
53. Horio T. Solar urticaria-idiopathic? Photodermatol Photoimmunol Photomed. 2003;19(3):147–54.
54. Morgado-Carrasco D, et al. Clinical response and long-term follow-up of 20 patients with refractory solar urticaria under treatment with omalizumab. J Am Acad Dermatol. 2019.
55. Edstrom DW, Ros AM. Cyclosporin A therapy for severe solar urticaria. Photodermatol Photoimmunol Photomed. 1997;13(1–2):61–3.
56. Puech-Plottova I, et al. [Solar urticaria: one case treated by intravenous immunoglobulin]. Ann Dermatol Venereol. 2000;127(10):831–5.
57. Haylett AK, et al. Systemic photoprotection in solar urticaria with alpha-melanocyte-stimulating hormone analogue [Nle4-D-Phe7]-alpha-MSH. Br J Dermatol. 2011;164(2):407–14.
58. Mang R, et al. Successful treatment of solar urticaria by extracorporeal photochemotherapy (photopheresis)—a case report. Photodermatol Photoimmunol Photomed. 2002;18(4):196–8.
59. Pezzolo E, et al. Heat urticaria: a revision of published cases with an update on classification and management. Br J Dermatol. 2016;175(3):473–8.
60. Fukunaga A, et al. Localized heat urticaria in a patient is associated with a wealing response to heated autologous serum. Br J Dermatol. 2002;147(5):994–7.
61. Bonnekoh H, et al. Treatment of severe heat urticaria with omalizumab - Report of a case and review of the literature. J Eur Acad Dermatol Venereol. 2020;34(9):e489–91.
62. Bullerkotte U, et al. Effective treatment of refractory severe heat urticaria with omalizumab. Allergy. 2010;65(7):931–2.
63. Patruno C, et al. Vibratory angioedema in a saxophonist. Dermatitis. 2009;20(6):346–7.
64. Sarmast SA, Fang F, Zic J. Vibratory angioedema in a trumpet professor. Cutis. 2014;93(2):E10–1.
65. Kalathoor I. Snoring-induced vibratory angioedema. Am J Case Rep. 2015;16:700–2.
66. Zhao Z, et al. Ordinary vibratory angioedema is not generally associated with ADGRE2 mutation. J Allergy Clin Immunol. 2019;143(3):1246–1248.e4.
67. Vergara-de-la-Campa L, et al. Vibratory urticaria-angioedema: further insights into the response patterns to vortex provocation test. J Eur Acad Dermatol Venereol. 2020;34(11):e699–701.
68. Kulthanan K, et al. Vibratory angioedema subgroups, features, and treatment: results of a systematic review. J Allergy Clin Immunol. 2020;S2213-2198(20):30955–7.
69. Metzger WJ, et al. Hereditary vibratory angioedema: confirmation of histamine release in a type of physical hypersensitivity. J Allergy Clin Immunol. 1976;57(6):605–8.
70. Boyden SE, et al. Vibratory urticaria associated with a missense variant in ADGRE2. N Engl J Med. 2016;374(7):656–63.
71. Guarneri F, Guarneri C, Marini HR. Amitriptyline and bromazepam in the treatment of vibratory angioedema: which role for neuroinflammation? Dermatol Ther. 2014;27(6):361–4.
72. Lawlor F, et al. Vibratory angioedema: lesion induction, clinical features, laboratory and ultrastructural findings and response to therapy. Br J Dermatol. 1989;120(1):93–9.
73. Pressler A, et al. Failure of omalizumab and successful control with ketotifen in a patient with vibratory angio-oedema. Clin Exp Dermatol. 2013;38(2):151–3.
74. Fukunaga A, et al. Cholinergic urticaria: epidemiology, physiopathology, new categorization, and management. Clin Auton Res. 2018;28(1):103–13.
75. Kumaran MS, Arora AK, Parsad D. Cholinergic urticaria: clinicoepidemiological paradigms from a tertiary care center in North India. Indian J Dermatol Venereol Leprol. 2017;83(5):599–601.
76. Kim JE, et al. Clinical characteristics of cholinergic urticaria in Korea. Ann Dermatol. 2014;26(2):189–94.
77. Godse K, et al. Prevalence of cholinergic urticaria in Indian adults. Indian Dermatol Online J. 2013;4(1):62–3.

78. Zuberbier T, et al. Prevalence of cholinergic urticaria in young adults. J Am Acad Dermatol. 1994;31(6):978–81.
79. Mellerowicz EJ, et al. Angioedema frequently occurs in cholinergic urticaria. J Allergy Clin Immunol Pract. 2019;7(4):1355–1357.e1.
80. Washio K, et al. Clinical characteristics in cholinergic urticaria with palpebral angioedema: report of 15 cases. J Dermatol Sci. 2017;85(2):135–7.
81. Haustein UF. Adrenergic urticaria and adrenergic pruritus. Acta Derm Venereol. 1990;70(1):82–4.
82. Ruft J, et al. Development and validation of the Cholinergic Urticaria Quality-of-Life Questionnaire (CholU-QoL). Clin Exp Allergy. 2018;48(4):433–44.
83. Asady A, et al. Cholinergic urticaria patients of different age groups have distinct features. Clin Exp Allergy. 2017;47(12):1609–14.
84. Abajian M, et al. Physical urticarias and cholinergic urticaria. Immunol Allergy Clin North Am. 2014;34(1):73–88.
85. Ramam M, Pahwa P. Is cholinergic urticaria a seasonal disorder in some patients? Indian J Dermatol Venereol Leprol. 2012;78(2):190–1.
86. Shoenfeld Y, et al. Cholinergic urticaria. A seasonal disease. Arch Intern Med. 1981;141(8):1029–30.
87. Nakamizo S, et al. Cholinergic urticaria: pathogenesis-based categorization and its treatment options. J Eur Acad Dermatol Venereol. 2012;26(1):114–6.
88. Bito T, Sawada Y, Tokura Y. Pathogenesis of cholinergic urticaria in relation to sweating. Allergol Int. 2012;61(4):539–44.
89. Horikawa T, Fukunaga A, Nishigori C. New concepts of hive formation in cholinergic urticaria. Curr Allergy Asthma Rep. 2009;9(4):273–9.
90. Fukunaga A, et al. Responsiveness to autologous sweat and serum in cholinergic urticaria classifies its clinical subtypes. J Allergy Clin Immunol. 2005;116(2):397–402.
91. Illig L, et al. Experimental investigations on the trigger mechanism of the generalized type of heat and cold urticaria by means of a climatic chamber. Acta Derm Venereol. 1980;60(5):373–80.
92. Koch K, et al. Antihistamine updosing reduces disease activity in patients with difficult-to-treat cholinergic urticaria. J Allergy Clin Immunol. 2016;138(5):1483–1485.e9.
93. Oda Y, et al. Combined cholinergic urticaria and cold-induced cholinergic urticaria with acquired idiopathic generalized anhidrosis. Allergol Int. 2015;64(2):214–5.
94. Kobayashi H, et al. Cholinergic urticaria, a new pathogenic concept: hypohidrosis due to interference with the delivery of sweat to the skin surface. Dermatology. 2002;204(3):173–8.
95. Iwasaki A, et al. A case of cholinergic urticaria with localized hypohidrosis showing sweat gland eosinophilic infiltration. Allergol Int. 2017;66(3):495–6.
96. Kim JE, et al. The significance of hypersensitivity to autologous sweat and serum in cholinergic urticaria: cholinergic urticaria may have different subtypes. Int J Dermatol. 2015;54(7):771–7.
97. Winkelmann RK. Cholinergic urticaria shows neutrophilic inflammation. Acta Derm Venereol. 1985;65(5):432–4.
98. Tokura Y. New etiology of cholinergic urticaria. Curr Probl Dermatol. 2016;51:94–100.
99. Sawada Y, et al. Decreased expression of acetylcholine esterase in cholinergic urticaria with hypohidrosis or anhidrosis. J Invest Dermatol. 2014;134(1):276–9.
100. Nakamizo S, et al. A case of cholinergic urticaria associated with acquired generalized hypohidrosis and reduced acetylcholine receptors: cause and effect? Clin Exp Dermatol. 2011;36(5):559–60.
101. Sawada Y, et al. Cholinergic urticaria: studies on the muscarinic cholinergic receptor M3 in anhidrotic and hypohidrotic skin. J Invest Dermatol. 2010;130(11):2683–6.
102. Kiistala R, Kiistala U. Local cholinergic urticaria at methacholine test site. Acta Derm Venereol. 1997;77(1):84–5.
103. Sabroe RA. Failure of omalizumab in cholinergic urticaria. Clin Exp Dermatol. 2010;35(4):e127–9.

104. Takahagi S, Tanaka A, Hide M. Sweat allergy. Allergol Int. 2018;67(4):435–41.
105. Altrichter S, et al. Sensitization against skin resident fungi is associated with atopy in cholinergic urticaria patients. Clin Transl Allergy. 2020;10:18.
106. Hiragun M, et al. Elevated serum IgE against MGL_1304 in patients with atopic dermatitis and cholinergic urticaria. Allergol Int. 2014;63(1):83–93.
107. Altrichter S, et al. Atopic predisposition in cholinergic urticaria patients and its implications. J Eur Acad Dermatol Venereol. 2016;30(12):2060–5.
108. Hirschmann JV, et al. Cholinergic urticaria. A clinical and histologic study. Arch Dermatol. 1987;123(4):462–7.
109. Altrichter S, et al. Development of a standardized pulse-controlled ergometry test for diagnosing and investigating cholinergic urticaria. J Dermatol Sci. 2014;75(2):88–93.
110. Tanaka M, et al. A case of cold-induced cholinergic urticaria accompanied by cholinergic urticaria showing a positive ice cube test. Allergol Int. 2020;69(1):150–1.
111. Abraham T, et al. Pure cold-induced cholinergic urticaria in a pediatric patient. Case Reports Immunol. 2016;2016:7425601.
112. Geller M. Cold-induced cholinergic urticaria—case report. Ann Allergy. 1989;63(1):29–30.
113. Ormerod AD, et al. Combined cold urticaria and cholinergic urticaria—clinical characterization and laboratory findings. Br J Dermatol. 1988;118(5):621–7.
114. Hogan SR, Mandrell J, Eilers D. Adrenergic urticaria: review of the literature and proposed mechanism. J Am Acad Dermatol. 2014;70(4):763–6.
115. Shelley WB, Shelley ED. Adrenergic urticaria: a new form of stress-induced hives. Lancet. 1985;2(8463):1031–3.
116. Montgomery SL. Cholinergic urticaria and exercise-induced anaphylaxis. Curr Sports Med Rep. 2015;14(1):61–3.
117. Li PH, et al. Differences in omega-5-gliadin allergy: East versus West. Asia Pac Allergy. 2020;10(1):e5.
118. Foong RX, Giovannini M, du Toit G. Food-dependent exercise-induced anaphylaxis. Curr Opin Allergy Clin Immunol. 2019;19(3):224–8.
119. Xu YY, et al. Wheat allergy in patients with recurrent urticaria. World Allergy Organ J. 2019;12(2):100013.
120. Christensen MJ, et al. Wheat-dependent cofactor-augmented anaphylaxis: a prospective study of exercise, aspirin, and alcohol efficacy as cofactors. J Allergy Clin Immunol Pract. 2019;7(1):114–21.
121. Mellerowicz E, et al. Real-life treatment of patients with cholinergic urticaria in German-speaking countries. J Dtsch Dermatol Ges. 2019;17(11):1141–7.
122. Altrichter S, et al. Real-life treatment of cholinergic urticaria with omalizumab. J Allergy Clin Immunol. 2019;143(2):788–791.e8.
123. Maurer M, et al. Omalizumab treatment in patients with chronic inducible urticaria: a systematic review of published evidence. J Allergy Clin Immunol. 2018;141(2):638–49.
124. Metz M, et al. Successful treatment of cholinergic urticaria with anti-immunoglobulin E therapy. Allergy. 2008;63(2):247–9.
125. Gastaminza G, et al. Efficacy and safety of omalizumab (Xolair) for cholinergic urticaria in patients unresponsive to a double dose of antihistamines: a randomized mixed double-blind and open-label placebo-controlled clinical trial. J Allergy Clin Immunol Pract. 2019;7(5):1599–1609.e1.
126. Alsamarai AM, Hasan AA, Alobaidi AH. Evaluation of different combined regimens in the treatment of cholinergic urticaria. World Allergy Organ J. 2012;5(8):88–93.
127. Altrichter S, Wosny K, Maurer M. Successful treatment of cholinergic urticaria with methantheliniumbromide. J Dermatol. 2015;42(4):422–4.
128. Tsunemi Y, et al. Cholinergic urticaria successfully treated with scopolamine butylbromide. Int J Dermatol. 2003;42(10):850.
129. Ammann P, Surber E, Bertel O. Beta blocker therapy in cholinergic urticaria. Am J Med. 1999;107(2):191.

130. Feinberg JH, Toner CB. Successful treatment of disabling cholinergic urticaria. Mil Med. 2008;173(2):217–20.
131. La Shell MS, England RW. Severe refractory cholinergic urticaria treated with danazol. J Drugs Dermatol. 2006;5(7):664–7.
132. Berth-Jones J, Graham-Brown RA. Cholinergic pruritus, erythema and urticaria: a disease spectrum responding to danazol. Br J Dermatol. 1989;121(2):235–7.
133. Wong E, et al. Beneficial effects of danazol on symptoms and laboratory changes in cholinergic urticaria. Br J Dermatol. 1987;116(4):553–6.
134. Chin YY, Chang TC, Chang CH. Idiopathic pure sudomotor failure and cholinergic urticaria in a patient after acute infectious mononucleosis infection. Clin Exp Dermatol. 2013;38(2):156–9.
135. Hiragun T, Hide M. Sweat Allergy. Curr Probl Dermatol. 2016;51:101–8.
136. Minowa T, et al. Regular sweating activities for the treatment of cholinergic urticaria with or without acquired idiopathic generalized anhidrosis. Dermatol Ther. 2020;33(4):e13647.
137. Suss H, et al. Contact urticaria: frequency, elicitors and cofactors in three cohorts (Information Network of Departments of Dermatology; Network of Anaphylaxis; and Department of Dermatology, University Hospital Erlangen, Germany). Contact Dermatitis. 2019;81(5):341–53.
138. Vethachalam S, Persaud Y. Contact urticaria. In: StatPearls. Treasure Island; 2020.
139. Bensefa-Colas L, et al. Occupational contact urticaria: lessons from the French National Network for Occupational Disease Vigilance and Prevention (RNV3P). Br J Dermatol. 2015;173(6):1453–61.
140. Malkonen T, et al. A 6-month follow-up study of 1048 patients diagnosed with an occupational skin disease. Contact Dermatitis. 2009;61(5):261–8.
141. Wassef C, Laureano A, Schwartz RA. Aquagenic urticaria: a perplexing physical phenomenon. Acta Dermatovenerol Croat. 2017;25(3):234–7.
142. Vieira M, et al. Localized salt-dependent aquagenic urticaria, a rare subtype of urticaria: a case report. Eur Ann Allergy Clin Immunol. 2018;50(3):141–4.
143. Napolitano M, et al. Salt-dependent aquagenic urticaria in children: report of two cases. Pediatr Allergy Immunol. 2018;29(3):324–6.
144. Gallo R, et al. Localized salt-dependent aquagenic urticaria: a subtype of aquagenic urticaria? Clin Exp Dermatol. 2013;38(7):754–7.
145. Gallo R, et al. Localized aquagenic urticaria dependent on saline concentration. Contact Dermatitis. 2001;44(2):110–1.
146. Fukumoto T, et al. Aquagenic urticaria: severe extra-cutaneous symptoms following cold water exposure. Allergol Int. 2018;67(2):295–7.
147. Davis RS, et al. Evaluation of a patient with both aquagenic and cholinergic urticaria. J Allergy Clin Immunol. 1981;68(6):479–83.
148. Wasserman D, Preminger A, Zlotogorski A. Aquagenic urticaria in a child. Pediatr Dermatol. 1994;11(1):29–30.
149. Shelley WB, Rawnsley HM. Aquagenic urticaria. Contact sensitivity reaction to water. JAMA. 1964;189:895–8.
150. Tkach JR. Aquagenic urticaria. Cutis. 1981;28(4):454–63.
151. Czarnetzki BM, Breetholt KH, Traupe H. Evidence that water acts as a carrier for an epidermal antigen in aquagenic urticaria. J Am Acad Dermatol. 1986;15(4 Pt 1):623–7.
152. Luong KV, Nguyen LT. Aquagenic urticaria: report of a case and review of the literature. Ann Allergy Asthma Immunol. 1998;80(6):483–5.
153. Sibbald RG, et al. Aquagenic urticaria: evidence of cholinergic and histaminergic basis. Br J Dermatol. 1981;105(3):297–302.
154. Kai AC, Flohr C. Aquagenic urticaria in twins. World Allergy Organ J. 2013;6(1):2.
155. Seize MB, et al. [Familial aquagenic urticaria: report of two cases and literature review]. An Bras Dermatol. 2009;84(5):530–3.
156. Pitarch G, et al. Familial aquagenic urticaria and bernard-soulier syndrome. Dermatology. 2006;212(1):96–7.

157. Treudler R, et al. Familial aquagenic urticaria associated with familial lactose intolerance. J Am Acad Dermatol. 2002;47(4):611–3.
158. Seol JE, et al. Aquagenic urticaria diagnosed by the water provocation test and the results of histopathologic examination. Ann Dermatol. 2017;29(3):341–5.
159. Murphy B, Duffin M, Tolland J. Aquagenic pruritus successfully treated with omalizumab. Clin Exp Dermatol. 2018;43(7):858–9.
160. Heitkemper T, et al. Aquagenic pruritus: associated diseases and clinical pruritus characteristics. J Dtsch Dermatol Ges. 2010;8(10):797–804.
161. Bircher AJ, Meier-Ruge W. Aquagenic pruritus. Water-induced activation of acetylcholinesterase. Arch Dermatol. 1988;124(1):84–9.
162. Lubach D. [Aquagenic pruritus sine materia]. Hautarzt. 1984;35(11):600–1.
163. Lehman JS, Kuntz NL, Davis DM. Localized aquadynia responsive to clonidine in a 13-year-old girl. Pediatr Dermatol. 2010;27(6):646–9.
164. Misery L, et al. [Aquadynia: a role for VIP?]. Ann Dermatol Venereol. 2003;130(2 Pt 1):195–8.
165. Shelley WB, Shelley ED. Aquadynia: noradrenergic pain induced by bathing and responsive to clonidine. J Am Acad Dermatol. 1998;38(2 Pt 2):357–8.
166. Wang F, et al. Aquagenic cutaneous disorders. J Dtsch Dermatol Ges. 2017;15(6):602–8.
167. Frances AM, Fiorenza G, Frances RJ. Aquagenic urticaria: report of a case. Allergy Asthma Proc. 2004;25(3):195–7.
168. Bayle P, et al. Localized aquagenic urticaria: efficacy of a barrier cream. Contact Dermatitis. 2003;49(3):160–1.
169. McGee JS, et al. An adolescent boy with urticaria to water: review of current treatments for aquagenic urticaria. Pediatr Dermatol. 2014;31(1):116–7.
170. Park H, et al. Aquagenic urticaria: a report of two cases. Ann Dermatol. 2011;23(Suppl 3):S371–4.
171. Damiani G, et al. Omalizumab in chronic urticaria: an Italian survey. Int Arch Allergy Immunol. 2019;178(1):45–9.
172. Rorie A, Gierer S. A case of aquagenic urticaria successfully treated with omalizumab. J Allergy Clin Immunol Pract. 2016;4(3):547–8.
173. Fearfield LA, Gazzard B, Bunker CB. Aquagenic urticaria and human immunodeficiency virus infection: treatment with stanozolol. Br J Dermatol. 1997;137(4):620–2.
174. Baptist AP, Baldwin JL. Aquagenic urticaria with extracutaneous manifestations. Allergy Asthma Proc. 2005;26(3):217–20.
175. Rothbaum R, McGee JS. Aquagenic urticaria: diagnostic and management challenges. J Asthma Allergy. 2016;9:209–13.
176. Martinez-Escribano JA, et al. Treatment of aquagenic urticaria with PUVA and astemizole. J Am Acad Dermatol. 1997;36(1):118–9.
177. Parker RK, Crowe MJ, Guin JD. Aquagenic urticaria. Cutis. 1992;50(4):283–4.

Angioedema

L. Bouillet

Core Message

Recurrent isolated AEs are a diagnostic and therapeutic challenge. Only a rigorous clinical approach can eliminate the most obvious diagnoses. The major clinical sign to look for is the presence or absence of recurrent hives, concomitant or distant from the AE flare. The hives then point to a mast cell origin.

In the majority of cases, AEs are secondary to non-specific activation of mast cells. In these cases, they are mild and spontaneous. They require treatment with antihistamines at 2 or 3 times the authorized dose. Allergic AE are exceptionally isolated. They are almost always associated with extra-cutaneous signs (digestive and respiratory disorders, collapse) and associated with acute urticaria or generalized erythema.

You have to keep in mind that some AEs may reveal a life-threatening bradykinin disease which does not respond to usual treatment. The most frequent bradykinin AEs are drug induced AE mainly converting enzyme inhibitors, angiotensin receptor antagonist. When the diagnosis is confirmed the drug is contraindicated for life. In the event of a strong suspicion of bradykinin AE, specific treatment with C1Inh concentrate or icatibant (bradykinin receptor antagonist) should be administered.

The key laboratory test is the functional dosage of C1Inh. Only this test can exclude a C1Inh deficiency. The C4 assay can be useful in the diagnostic process.

L. Bouillet (✉)
French National Reference Center for Angioedema (CREAK), Internal Medicine/Clinical Immunology Department, Grenoble University Hospital, Grenoble, France
e-mail: LBouillet@chu-grenoble.fr

© Springer Nature Switzerland AG 2021
T. Zuberbier et al. (eds.), *Urticaria and Angioedema*,
https://doi.org/10.1007/978-3-030-84574-2_9

9.1 Introduction

Angioedema (AE) is a clinical syndrome characterized by localized, sudden, and transient swelling. It is not inflammatory. It is cold, skin-colored, and not itchy. It disappears without sequelae. It can be located in subcutaneous or submucosal tissues. It can be recurrent with different frequencies. When it occurs in areas where the tissues are loose (face, genitals …), it is very deforming (Photo 9.1).

AE is secondary to localized fluid infiltration of the subcutaneous and / or submucosal tissues. This does not concern the infiltration of inert substance (tophus, amyloidosis, myxedema …), granulomatous infiltrations (sarcoidosis, Miescher syndrome …), and malignant cells (lymphoma, …). It is caused by the sudden and localized increase in vascular permeability. This increase is secondary to the release of various substances, most of which are derived from mast cells: histamine, leukotrienes … In some cases, it may be bradykinin. These proteins, by binding to specific vascular receptors, dissociate tight junctions between endothelial vascular cells (for

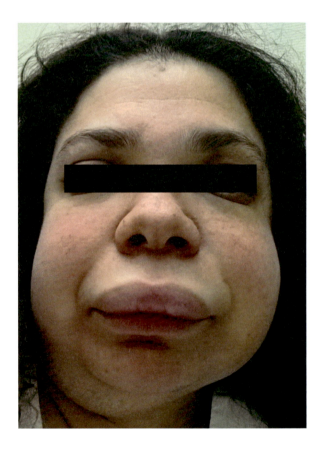

Photo 9.1 Distorting edema of the face; the color of the skin; without pruritus. Typical appearance of angioedema. This aspect does not prejudge anything of the cause of angioedema

example, VE-cadherin….) and promote the passage of fluid from the blood to adjacent tissues.

The word "angioedema" is not synonymous with an etiology. In most of the cases, AE is secondary to non-specific activation (non-IgE dependent) or specific activation (allergic-dependent IgE) of mast cells (Fig. 9.1). Then, mast cell AE (MC-AE) includes histaminergic AE (Hi-AE) and others (leukotrienes AE…). In rare cases, AE is secondary to activation of the kallikrein–kinin pathway. It is bradykinin, a powerful vasodilator, which then mediates AE (BK-AE).

Diagnosis of BK-AE is important because this type does not respond to treatments usually given in case of MC-AE. In addition, life-threatening is more engaged in the case of localization to the upper airways. A French study showed that the risk of death by BK-AE was 45 times higher than that of MC-AE [1].

The prevalence of angioedema (all causes) is estimated at 0.05% in the general population. In the USA, it is a cause of consultation in emergencies in about 1 case out of 1000 [2].

9.2 Differential Diagnosis

9.2.1 Pseudo Angioedema (Figs. 9.2 and 9.3)

Some clinical syndromes may mimic it. But by carefully examining the patient and collecting all the anamnestic elements, the diagnostic trap can be avoided. The main mimics are the superior vena cava syndromes (extensive and permanent swelling but which can be modified by the position of the patient), the granulomatous edema of the face and/or the tongue which can be fluctuating but which never disappears completely (syndrome of Miescher, Melkersson Rosenthal disease, Crohn's disease), subacute edematous polyarthritis of the elderly, lymphoedema … [3].

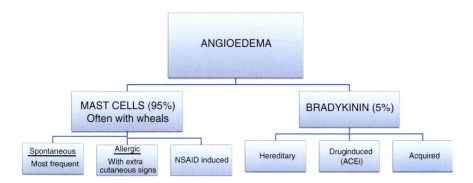

Fig. 9.1 Angioedema causes

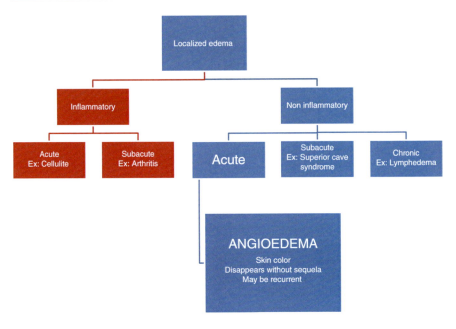

Fig. 9.2 Differential diagnosis of angioedema

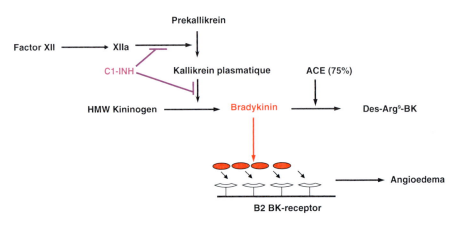

Fig. 9.3 Kallikrein–kinin system. *ACE* angiotensin converting enzyme, *BK* bradykinin, *HMW* high-molecular weight

9.2.2 Angioedema Associated with Systemic Syndromes

- Gleich syndrome: this syndrome is characterized by febrile recurrent angioedema associated with eosinophilia and polyclonal elevation of IgM. It is very steroid responsive.
- Schnitzler syndrome: this auto inflammatory syndrome is characterized by superficial hive flare-ups (rarely angioedema), associated with monoclonal gammopathy (often IgM).

9 Angioedema

Table 9.1 Characteristics of AE

Angioedema	Bradykinin	Mast cell
Hives	None	Frequent
Duration	More than 24 h	Some hours or some days
Abdominal localization	Sub-occlusive attacks very painful	Abdominal discomfort
Family context	Frequent But 30% *de novo* mutation.	Atopic familial context
Favoring factors	ACE I Contraceptive pill Pregnancy	NSAID Physic factors
Long-term prophylaxis with high dose of anti-histamine	Inefficient	Improvement

9.2.3 Diagnostic Strategy for Isolated Angioedema (Table 9.1)

In the case of isolated AE (without hives), the most common pathology, MC-AE (95% of cases), should be mentioned first (Fig. 9.1) [4]. The short duration, the context of atopy, the frequent intake of non-steroid anti-inflammatory drugs (NSAID) are strongly suggestive. The BK-AE are rare but do not miss their diagnosis because they do not respond to anti-histamine and adrenaline treatments. Different elements refer to BK-AE: the existence of sub-occlusive abdominal episodes, consumption of an angiotensin-converting enzyme (ACE) inhibitor, worsening of symptoms with birth control pills or during pregnancy, familial context….But this last point can be misleading. Indeed, it is common to have an atopic family context with MC-AE attacks. In contrast, in BK-AE, family history may be missed because (1) it may be a de novo mutation (30% of cases); (2) people with a *SERPING1* (C1Inh gene) mutation may be totally asymptomatic (10% of cases) [5].

In the presence of an isolated and recurrent AE with no obvious sign for MC-AE, C1Inh explorations (concentration and activity level) should be performed. If this is normal, 2 options:

- There are strong clinical arguments for a hereditary BK-AE with normal C1Inh: women, aggravation with contraceptive pill or during pregnancies, strong family context. You must then look for mutations on *F12, PLG, ANGPT1* genes. You can also try long-term prophylaxis with tranexamic acid in case of frequent attack.
- There are very few arguments for a BK-AE. A long-term antihistamine treatment at 2 or 4 times the recommended dose should be attempted in case of frequent attack. In case of failure, anti-IgE (omalizumab) could be proposed.

9.3 Mast Cell Angioedema (Histaminergic, …)

They are often associated with hives but in 10% they are isolated [6]. This is most often AE rapid onset and will disappear in a few hours. Sometimes, however, they can last a few days

9.3.1 Isolated Allergic Angioedema

They are linked to specific activation of mast cells, IgE mediated [7]. This is called anaphylactic reaction. Diagnosis is easy because they are almost never isolated. They are often associated with a sensation of discomfort, a general erythema, respiratory, and digestive signs (vomiting, abdominal pains, and diarrhea). They often occur within minutes of contact (food, drug, sting…). Tryptase level is very high during the attack and makes it possible to do the diagnosis a posteriori.

9.3.2 Spontaneous MC-AE (More Frequent)

Spontaneous MC-AE are secondary to non-specific (non-allergic) activation of mast cells. When they are recurrent over a period of at least 6 weeks, they are treated as spontaneous chronic urticaria (CSU [8]. Para-clinical assessment of these AEs should be limited as for CSU [9]. C1Inh exploration must be done and also tests for thyroid dysimmunity as recommended for UCS. In some cases, AE may be a symptom of inducible urticaria. It is then especially associated with cold urticaria.

The presence of AE in CSU is a serious factor: CSU is more severe and responds less well to antihistamines [10]. The MC-AE are often associated with atopy context as CSU [11].

In a case series of 31 patients, the median duration of MC-AE was 24 h and frequency 24 attacks per year. Fifty-five percent of patients had present at least one attack in the upper respiratory tract. In 42% of attack, a factor facilitating was identified, mainly a drug: morphine derivatives, antibiotic, NSAID… [12].

9.3.3 Non-steroid Anti-inflammatory Drugs Induced AE (NSAID-AE)

NSAID can induce several types of hypersensitivity and / or allergic reactions. In the case of isolated AE, it is important to question patients about taking NSAID / aspirin and about the time between taking them and the occurrence of AE. The examination must be careful because there are several types of reactions [13]:

- NSAID exacerbated chronic spontaneous AE and/or CSU: Sensitivity to some or all COX-1–inhibiting NSAIDs (pharmacologic effect of COX-1 inhibition). Avoidance is advised but is not final. Celecoxib (anti COX2) can be an alternative [14].
- NSAID-induced AE: These patients have no underlying chronic AE and /or urticaria, but experience cutaneous symptoms with COX-1–inhibiting NSAIDs. Avoidance is advised but is not final. Celecoxib (anti COX2) can be an alternative [14].

– NSAID allergy: Patients experience cutaneous and/or systemic anaphylactic reactions isolated to a single NSAID. The removal of the identified NSAID is essential and definitive.

9.4 Bradykinin Mediated AE (Fig. 9.4)

9.4.1 Clinical Description

The BK-AE are never accompanied by hives. They are isolated, recurrent and last at least 24 h (between 2 and 5 days on average). These AE are marked by three particular signs.

9.4.1.1 Abdominal Localization

It concerns the majority of the patients: 93% of them with hereditary C1Inh deficiency [15]. This localization results in very painful sub-occlusive attacks (EVA at 10 in 69% of patients) with vomiting and diarrhea at the end of the crisis [16]. It lasts an average of three days with almost constant bed rest. In some patients, the crisis may be inaugural. Abundant ascites can be present (transudate).

Ultrasound (and CT) images show edema of the digestive walls, sometimes signs of volvulus [17, 18]. The symptoms and images disappear spontaneously at the end of the crisis, without any sequelae. There is no fever. C-reactive protein and blood count are usually normal [19]. In some cases, the hematocrit level may be high (sign

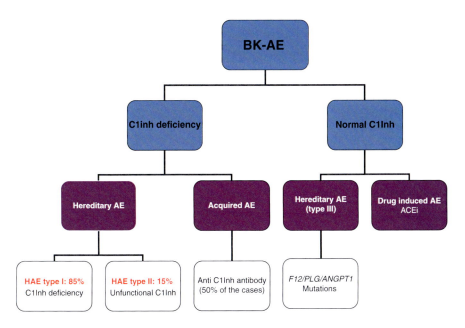

Fig. 9.4 Bradykinin AE

of hemoconcentration). The intensity of pain and hypovolemia may result in hypotensive discomfort. These attacks may simulate a surgical emergency. Some patients have had multiple useless laparotomies before the diagnosis of BK-AE [20].

9.4.1.2 Upper Airways Localization
This location threatens the vital prognosis. Before the arrival of specific treatments, it was associated with death by asphyxiation in 25% of cases. The fatal laryngeal attack happens in three phases [21]:

– The pre-dyspnea phase which lasts on average 4 h (sometimes only a few minutes).
– The dyspnea phase lasts an average of 41 min (sometimes 2 min).
– The loss of consciousness that precedes death on average 9 min.

There have been reports of fatal asphyxia within minutes and others more than 15 h after the onset of symptoms. Upper airways edema is so large that intubation is often impossible to do. It is recommended to try a cricothyroidotomy or a tracheostomy instead [22]. Some situations favor this type of attack: dental care, intubation, endoscopy ... [23].

9.4.1.3 Erythema Marginatum (Photo 9.2)
More than one in two patients have this erythema [24]. This can precede the AE attack by a few hours or even a few days. Sometimes erythema is not followed by AE. It can be mistaken for hives by the patients. But, it is a serpiginous, non-pruritic, non-inflammatory rash that is often located on the trunk.

9.4.2 Pathophysiology (Fig. 9.2)

BK-AE are secondary to the localized vascular release of bradykinin and its binding to specific B2 receptors constituting vessels [25]. Bradykinin has a very short half (a few minutes) because it is rapidly degraded by kininases including the angiotensin-converting enzyme (65%) [26]. Bradykinin is released following activation of the kallikrein–kinin pathway. This can be activated by the factor of Hageman (or factor XII) or directly via the kallikrein [27]. This proteolytic cascade is controlled by C1Inhibitor (C1Inh). It controls 90% of the proteolytic activity of Hageman's factor and 60% of kallikrein and plasmin [28].

9.4.3 BK-AE with C1Inh Deficiency (Fig. 9.4)

9.4.3.1 Hereditary Angioedema (HAE Type I/II)
It is a rare disease whose prevalence is estimated at 1 case per 50,000 inhabitants [29]. Transmission is autosomal dominant. The C1Inh gene is located on chromosome 11. More than 250 mutations have been reported [30]. The heterozygous

Photo 9.2 Erythema marginatum

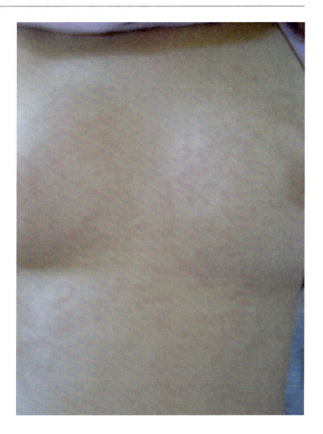

forms are the majority. Cases of homozygous have been reported in Spain [21, 31, 32]. Thirty percent of the mutations are *de novo*. The absence of family context does not therefore exclude the diagnosis. There is great inter- and intra-familial phenotypic variability. HAE type I is related to the lack of production of C1Inh protein (85% of cases). HAE type II is associated with production of a non-functional C1Inh (15% of cases) [33]. The biological diagnosis is therefore based on the concentration and the function evaluation of C1Inh (Table 9.2). The C4 level is almost always lowered and can be a good screening exam. The analysis can be done in children from the 6th month of life (physiologically lowered rate before) [34]. In case of normal C1Inh function, HAE type I/II can be excluded.

The diagnostic criteria of HAE with C1Inh deficiency are defined by a low level of C1Inh (<50%) identified by 2 separate samples and/or a pathological mutation on the C1Inh gene, associated with clinical signs [35]. When a patient is the index case of his family, all members of it should be screened even those asymptomatic. Indeed, nearly 10% of patients with C1Inh deficiency are asymptomatic. The average age of the first attack is 12 years old but very young children (from 6 months of life) can present one that can be atypical [36, 37].

Women are more often symptomatic than men [15]. In 50% of cases, the disease worsens during pregnancy [38]. Estrogens are a precipitating factor and it is

Table 9.2 Biologic profiles of bradykinin angioedema

	Hereditary AE			Acquired AE	
	HAE type I	HAE type II	HAE with C1Inh normal (type III)	Acquired AE type I/II	ACE induced AE
C1Inh	< 50 %	Normal	Normal	< 50%	Normal
C1inh Function	< 50%	< 50%	Normal	< 50%	Normal
C4	Low	Low	Normal	Low	Normal
C1q	Normal	Normal	Normal	Low	Normal
Ac anti C1Inh	Absent	Absent	Absent	Positive in 50% of cases	Absent
Mutation	SERPING1	SERPING1	F12 PLG ANGPT1, KNG1	None	None

advisable to avoid contraceptive pill in these patients [39]. The evolution of the pathology is unpredictable: long asymptomatic periods can follow very intense periods. The frequency of attacks can range from less than one crisis per year to more than 2 a week. All patients will experience at least one abdominal crisis. Fifty percent will have at least one upper airway involvement.

9.4.3.2 Acquired AE (Type I/II)

AE acquired with C1Inh deficiency are rare [40]. The symptomatology is comparable to that of hereditary forms but without family context and with a later start. These are typically patients over 50 years of age but forms in young adults have been described. The diagnosis is evoked on the lowering of C1Inh, C1q (90% of cases), and the presence of an anti-C1Inh antibody (present in 50% of cases) (Table 9.2) [41]. It is associated with 40% of cases with a monoclonal gammopathy of indeterminate origin (often of the same isotype as the anti-C1Inh antibody). It may be the first symptom of a malignant hematological pathology [42]. In this case, it improves when the hematology is treated. Sometimes it is associated with an autoimmune disease such as rheumatoid arthritis or lupus [43].

9.4.4 BK-AE with Normal C1Inh (Fig. 9.4)

9.4.4.1 Hereditary AE with Normal C1Inh (Previously Type III) [44]

Described since 2000, this pathology is mainly expressed in women and begins later than HAE with C1Inh deficiency [45, 46]. The first symptoms often appear after 20 years when the patient starts contraceptive pill and/or a pregnancy. This form is much related to female hormones [47]. This pathology can lead to serious obstetric problems (children died in utero). It is therefore necessary to be vigilant when these women carry out pregnancies [48]. In France, there is a predominance of women from North Africa. The diagnosis is based on the clinic (and family context) and must be confirmed by a specialist in pathology. In case of suspicion, and after checking the normality of C1Inh, genetic investigation must be done: *F12* (Hageman factor), *PLG* (plasminogen), KNG1 (Kininogen) and ANGPT1 (angiopoietin 1) genes are the main candidates [49–52].

9.4.4.2 Drug Induced BK-AE (Mainly Angiotensin-Converting Enzyme Inhibitor (ACEi))

These are the most common BK-AE [53]. They concern 0.7%–1% of IEC consumers [54, 55]. AE may occur a few days or years after initiation of treatment. It is a side effect neither dose nor time dependent. The risk factors are black American origin, the occurrence of cough under ACE inhibitors and the association of ACEi with gliptins and/or mTor inhibitors [56, 57]. These AE have a predilection for the face, tongue, and upper airways which is life-threatening (Photo 9.3) [58]. Its occurrence involves the discontinuation and the definitive contraindication of this treatment.

BK-AE may occur at a lower frequency under angiotensin II receptor antagonists [59].

Cases are also described with a new treatment for heart failure: the combination of sacubitril (inhibitor of neprilysin) and valsartan [60]. Incidence of BK-AE may be the same than ACEi.

Alteplase thrombolysis for ischemic stroke can induced BK-AE. The incidence is high: 1.3%–5.9%. In a study of 530 patients, the AE occurred within 5–189 min after the injection (median 65 min) [61]. Thirty-three percent of these patients took an ACEi.

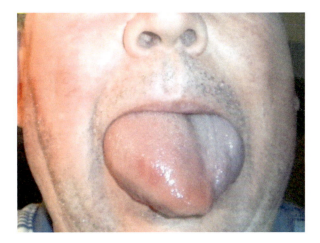

Photo 9.3 ACEi induced BK-AE of the tongue

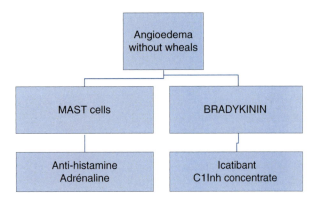

Fig. 9.5 Treatments of angioedema

9.5 Conclusion

Isolated and recurrent angioedema are a diagnostic challenge. Careful history taking is essential. The description of the crisis if it is not seen by the doctor must be detailed. Indeed, outside the clinic, the doctor has few biological elements to identify the etiological framework. First of all, it is important to exclude life-threatening AE: allergic angioedema and bradykinin AE. Spontaneous MC-AE are the most common and the most benign. But it is sometimes difficult to differentiate them from BK-AE with normal C1Inh (Fig. 9.5).

References

1. Crochet J, Lepelley M, Yahiaoui N, Vermorel C, Bosson JL, Pralong P, Leccia MT, Bouillet L. Bradykinin mechanism is the main responsible for death by isolated asphyxiating angioedema in France. Clin Exp Allergy. 2019;49(2):252–4.
2. Kelly M, Donnelly JP, McAnnally JR, Wang HE. National estimates of emergency department visits for angioedema and allergic reactions in the United States. Allergy Asthma Proc. 2013;34:150–4.
3. Miest R, Bruce A, Rogers RS 3rd. Orofacial granulomatosis. Clin Dermatol. 2016;34:505–13.
4. Wu MA, Perego F, Zanichelli A, Cicardi M. Angioedema phenotypes: disease expression and classification. Clin Rev Allergy Immunol. 2016;51:162–9.
5. Longhurst H, Cicardi M. Hereditary angioedema. Lancet. 2012;379:474–81.
6. Maurer M, Weller K, Bindslev-Jensen C, Gimenez-Arnau A, Bousquet PJ, Bousquet J, et al. Unmet clinical needs in chronic spontaneous urticaria. A GA2LEN task force report. Allergy. 2011;66:317–30.
7. Soria A, Francès C. Urticaria: diagnosis and treatment. Rev Med Interne. 2014;35:586–94.
8. Zuberbier T, Aberer W, Asero R, Bindslev-Jensen C, Brzoza Z, Canonica GW, et al. The EAACI/GA2LEN/EDF/WAO Guideline for the definition, classification, diagnosis, and management of urticaria: the 2013 revision and update. Allergy. 2014;69:868–87.
9. Bouillet L, Boccon-Gibod I, Berard F, Nicolas JF. Recurrent angioedema: diagnosis strategy and biological aspects. Eur J Dermatol. 2014;24:293–6.
10. Boccon-Gibod I, Bouillet L. Angioedema and urticaria. Ann Dermatol Venereol. 2014;141:S586–95.
11. Gimenez-Arnau A, Toubi E, Marsland A, Maurer M. Clinical management of urticaria using omalizumab: the first licensed biological therapy available for chronic spontaneous urticarial. J Eur Acad Dermatol Venereol. 2016;30:25–32.

12. Faisant C, Boccon-Gibod I, Mansard C, Dumestre Perard C, Pralong P, Chatain C, Deroux A, Bouillet L. Idiopathic histaminergic angioedema without wheals: a case series of 31 patients. Clin Exp Immunol. 2016;185:81–5.
13. Modena B, White AA, Woessner KM. Aspirin and nonsteroidal antiinflammatory drugs hypersensitivity and management. Immunol Allergy Clin North Am. 2017;37:727–49.
14. Liccardi G, Cazzola M, De Giglio C, Manfredi D, Piscitelli E, D'Amato M, D'Amato G. Safety of celecoxib in patients with adverse skin reactions to acetaminophen (paracetamol) and other non-steroidal anti-inflammatory drugs. J Invest Allergol Clin Immunol. 2005;15:249–53.
15. Bork K, Meng G, Staubach P, Hardt J. Hereditary angioedema: new findings concerning symptoms, affected organs, and course. Am J Med. 2006;119:267–74.
16. Bork K, Staubach P, Eckardt AJ, Hardt J. Symptoms, course, and complications of abdominal attacks in hereditary angioedema due to C1 inhibitor deficiency. Am J Gastroenterol. 2006;101:1–9.
17. Courtier J, Kamri A. Hereditary angioedema in the duodenum. Radiology. 2009;253:564–9.
18. Farkas H, Harmat G, Kaposi PN, Karadi I, Fekete B, Fust G, Fay K, Vass A, Varga L. Ultrasonography in the diagnosis and monitoring of ascites in acute abdominal attacks of hereditary angioneurotic oedema. Eur J Gastroenterol Hepatol. 2001;13:1225–30.
19. Jalaj S, Scolapio J. Gastrointestinal manifestations, diagnosis, and management of hereditary angioedema. Clin Gastroenterol. 2013;47:817–23.
20. Patel N, Suarez L, Kapur S, Bielory L. Hereditary angioedema and gastrointestinal complications: an extensive review of the literature. Case Reports Immunol. 2015;2015:925861.
21. Bork K, Hardt J, Witzke G. Fatal laryngeal attacks and mortality in hereditary angioedema due to C1-INH deficiency. J Allergy Clin Immunol. 2012;130:692–7.
22. Floccard B, Javaud N, Crozon J, Rimmelé T. Emergency management of bradykinin-mediated angioedema. Presse Med. 2015;44:70–7.
23. Bork K, Hardt J, Schicketanz K, Ressel N. Clinical studies of sudden upper airway obstruction in patients with hereditary angioedema due to C1 esterase inhibitor. Arch Intern Med. 2003;163:1229–35.
24. Martinez-Saguer I, Farkas H. Erythema marginatum as an early symptom of hereditary angioedema: case report of 2 newborns. Pediatrics. 2016;137:e2015241.
25. Davis AE III. The physiopathology of hereditary angioedema. Clin Immunol. 2005;114:3–9.
26. Maurer M, Bader M, Bas M, Bossi F, Cicardi M, Cugno M, et al. New topics in bradykinin research. Allergy. 2011;66:1397–406.
27. Joseph K, Tholanikunnel B, Bygum A, Ghebrehiwet B, Kaplan A. Factor XII–independent activation of the bradykinin-forming cascade: implications for the pathogenesis of hereditary angioedema types I and II. J Allergy Clin Immunol. 2013;132:470–5.
28. Kaplan A. Complement, kinins, and hereditary angioedema: mechanisms of plasma instability when C1 inhibitor is absent. Clin Rev Allergy Immunol. 2016;51:207–15.
29. Bygum A. Hereditary angioedema in Denmark: a nationwide survey. Br J Dermatol. 2009;161:1153–8.
30. Germenis A, Speletas M. Genetics of hereditary angioedema revisited. Clin Rev Allergy Immunol. 2016;51:170–82.
31. Blanch A, Roche O, Urrutia I, Gamboa P, Fontán G, Lopez-Trascasa M. First case of homozygous C1 inhibitor deficiency. J Allergy Clin Immunol. 2006;118:1330–5.
32. López-Lera A, Favier B, de la Cruz RM, Garrido S, Drouet C, López-Trascasa M. A new case of homozygous C1-inhibitor deficiency suggests a role for Arg378 in the control of kinin pathway activation. J Allergy Clin Immunol. 2010;126:1307–10.
33. Farkas H, Veszeli N, Kajdácsi E, Cervenak L, Varga L. Nuts and bolts of laboratory evaluation of angioedema. Clin Rev Allergy Immunol. 2016;51:140–51.
34. Nielsen EW, Johansen HT, Holt J, Mollnes TE. C1 inhibitor and diagnosis of hereditary angioedema in newborns. Pediatr Res. 1994;35:184–7.
35. Cicardi M, Zanichelli A. Functional C1Inhibitor diagnsotics in hereditary angioedema: assay evaluation and recommendations. Angioedema. 2010;1:8–12.

36. Bouillet L, Launay D, Fain O, Boccon-Gibod I, Laurent J, Martin L, et al. Hereditary angioedema with C1 inhibitor deficiency: clinical presentation and quality of life of 193 French patients. Ann Allergy Asthma Immunol. 2013;111:290–4.
37. Agostoni A, Cicardi M. Hereditary and acquired C1-inhibitor deficiency: biological and clinical characteristics in 235 patients. Medicine. 1992;71:206–15.
38. Caballero T, Farkas H, Bouillet L, Bowen T, Gompel A, Fagerberg C. International consensus and practical guidelines on the gynecologic and obstetric management of female patients with hereditary angioedema caused by C1 inhibitor deficiency. J Allergy Clin Immunol. 2012;129:308–2.
39. Bork K, Fischer B, Dewald G. Recurrent episodes of skin angioedema and severe attacks of abdominal pain induced by oral contraceptives or hormone replacement therapy. Am J Med. 2003;114:294–8.
40. Fain O, Gobert D, Khau CA, Mekinian A, Javaud N. Acquired angioedema. Presse Med. 2015;44:48–51.
41. Cicardi M, Zingale LC, Pappalardo E, Folcioni A, Agostoni A. Autoantibodies and lymphoproliferative diseases in acquired C1-inhibitor deficiencies. Medicine. 2003;82:274–81.
42. Castelli R, Zanichelli A, Cicardi M, Cugno M. Acquired C1-inhibitor deficiency and lymphoproliferative disorders: a tight relationship. Crit Rev Oncol Hematol. 2013;7:323–32.
43. Cacoub P, Frémeaux-Bacchi V, De Lacroix I, Guillien F, Kahn MF, Kazatchkine MD, et al. A new type of acquired C1 inhibitor deficiency associated with systemic lupus erythematosus. Arthritis Rheum. 2001;44:1836–4.
44. Bork K, Barnstedt S, Koch P, Traupe P. Hereditary angioedema with normal C1-inhibitor activity in women. Lancet. 2000;356:213–7.
45. Vitrat-Hincky V, Gompel A, Dumestre-Perard C, et al. Type III hereditary angioedema: clinical and biological features in a French cohort. Allergy. 2010;65:1331–6.
46. Deroux A, Boccon-Gibod I, Fain O, Pralong P, Ollivier Y, Pagnier A, et al. Hereditary angioedema with normal C1 inhibitor and factor XII mutation: a series of 57 patients from the French National Center of Reference for Angioedema. Clin Exp Immunol. 2016;185:332–7.
47. Bork K, Wulff K, Witzke G, Hardt J. Hereditary angioedema with normal C1-INH with versus without specific F12 gene mutations. Allergy. 2015;70:1004–12.
48. Picone O, Donnadieu AC, Brivet FC, Boyer-Neumann C, Fremeaux-Bacchi V, Frydman R. Obstetrical complications and outcome in two families with hereditary angioedema due to mutation in the F12 gene. Obstet Gynecol Int. 2010;2010:957507.
49. Firinu D, Bafunno V, Vecchione G, Barca MP, Manconia ME, Santacroce R, Margaglione R, Del Giacco SR. Characterization of patients with angioedema without wheals: the importance of F12 gene screening. Clinical Immunology. 2015;157:239–48.
50. Bork K, Wulff K, Steinmüller-Magin L, Braenne I, Staubach-Renz P, Witzke G, Hardt J. Hereditary angioedema with a mutation in the plasminogen gene. Allergy. 2018;73:442–50.
51. Belbézier A, Hardy G, Marlu R, Defendi F, Dumestre Perard C, Boccon-Gibod I, Launay D, Bouillet L. Plasminogen gene mutation with normal C1 inhibitor hereditary angioedema: three additional French families. Allergy. 2018;73:2237–9.
52. Bafunno V, Firinu D, D'Apolito M, Cordisco G, Loffredo S, Leccese A, Bova M, Barca MP, Santacroce R, Cicardi M, Del Giacco S, Margaglione M. Mutation of the angiopoietin-1 gene (ANGPT1) associates with a new type of hereditary angioedema. J Allergy Clin Immunol. 2018;141:1009–17.
53. Nosbaum A, Bouillet L, Floccard B, Javaud N, Launay D, Boccon-Gibod I, et al. Management of angiotensin-converting enzyme inhibitor-related angioedema: recommendations from the French National Center for Angioedema. Rev Med Interne. 2013;34:209–1.
54. Miller D, Oliveria S, Berlowitz D, Fincke B, Stang P, Lillienfeld D. Angioedema incidence in US veterans initiating angiotensin converting enzyme inhibitors. Hypertension. 2008;51:1–2.
55. Weber M, Messerli F. Angiotensin converting enzyme inhibitors and angioedema estimating the risk. Hypertension. 2008;51:1465–7.

56. Brown N, Byiers S, Carr D, Maldonado M, Warner B. Dipeptidyl peptidase IV inhibitor use associated with increased risk of ACE inhibitor- associated angioedema. Hypertens. 2009;54:516–23.
57. Duerr M, Glander P, Diekmann F, Dragun D, Neumayer H, Budde K. Increased Incidence of angioedema with ACE inhibitors in combination with mTOR inhibitors in kidney transplant recipients. Clin J Am Soc Nephrol. 2010;5:703–8.
58. Roberts J, Lee J, Marthers D. Angiotensin-converting enzyme (ACE) inhibitor angioedema: the silent epidemic. Am J Cardiol. 2012;109:774–7.
59. Haymore BR, Yoon J, Mikita CP, Klote MM, DeZee KJ. Risk of angioedema with angiotensin receptor blockers in patients with prior angioedema associated with angiotensin converting enzyme inhibitors: a meta-analysis. Ann Allergy Asthma Immunol. 2008;101:495–9.
60. Bas M, Greve J, Strassen U, Khosravani F, Hoffmann TK, Kojda G. Angioedema induced by cardiovascular drugs: new players join old friends. Allergy. 2015;70:1196–200.
61. Hurford R, Rezvani S, Kreimei M, Herbert A, Vail A, Parry-Jones AR, Douglass C, Molloy J, Alachkar H, Tyrrell PJ, Smith CJ. Incidence, predictors and clinical characteristics of orolingual angio-oedema complicating thrombolysis with tissue plasminogen activator for ischaemic stroke. J Neurol Neurosurg Psychiatry. 2015;86:520–3.

Management Principles in Urticaria

10

Torsten Zuberbier, Marcus Maurer, and Clive Grattan

Core Messages
- Basic principles in the management of patients with urticaria include the identification and elimination of the underlying causes as causal treatment.
- Induction of tolerance can be tried in patients with CINDU where trigger avoidance is not practical.
- Symptomatic pharmacological treatment comprises a step-wise approach of different agents and should be regularly reassesed.

Management of patients with urticaria should follow some basic principles and should be based on a Shared-Decision-Making concept including the patient's participation and encouraging self-management.

Since to date there is no causal treatment option available in urticaria, the treatment aims at complete symptom alleviation.

This goal may be achieved using different approaches, including the identification and subsequent elimination of the underlying cause, avoidance of eliciting and aggravating factors, induction of tolerance and pharmacological interventions inhibiting mast cell mediator release and/or effect of these mediators. Not all approaches are feasible in each patient and should be evaluated based on clinical presentation, history and diagnostic results.

T. Zuberbier (✉) · M. Maurer
Institute for Allergology, Charité – Universitätsmedizin, Berlin, Germany

Fraunhofer Institute for Translational Medicine and Pharmacology ITMP,
Allergology and Immunology, Berlin, Germany
e-mail: Torsten.Zuberbier@charite.de

C. Grattan
St John's Institute of Dermatology, Guy's Hospital, London, UK

© Springer Nature Switzerland AG 2021
T. Zuberbier et al. (eds.), *Urticaria and Angioedema*,
https://doi.org/10.1007/978-3-030-84574-2_10

10.1 Identification and Elimination of Underlying Causes

Acute as well as chronic urticaria may be attributed to or associated with distinct causes. Linking urticaria to a cause is not easily achievable since factors, e.g. infections, have been described as causative as well as aggravating factors, but can also be entirely unrelated to the urticarial symptoms. Additionally, spontaneous remission of urticaria can occur any time and the elimination of a factor suspected to be causative or aggravating can be coincidental.

Conducting a detailed medical history and a careful examination are the basic approach. It is not only prerequisite for accurate diagnosis but also essential for the detection of comorbidities such as infections, allergic conditions, autoimmune disorders or malignancy which may be associated as eliciting or aggravating factor but should certainly also be treated independent of the presence of urticaria.

In the management of urticaria, the following factors should be taken into consideration as being of possible causative or aggravating nature:

10.2 Drugs

If pharmacological agents are suspected they should be omitted completely or substituted by agents of another pharmacological class. Frequent suspects are NSAIDs although case reports linking urticaria to many different substance categories have been published.

10.3 Infection

If suggested by medical history or examination results, the diagnosis of bacterial, viral or fungal infection should be treated and/or followed-up.

10.4 Food Intolerance

Although extremely rare as cause of urticaria, IgE-mediated food allergy and non-IgE-mediated food hypersensitivity should be considered if strongly indicated by patient's history.

10.5 Physical Stimuli

Primarily in CIndU exposure to the respective stimulus should be investigated and patients should be trained to recognize and control the exposure, e.g. broadening the handle of heavy bags in delayed pressure urticaria or soft suspension for bikes in vibratory angioedema.

10.6 Lifestyle Adjustments

Regardless of the search for an underlying cause the patient's social and occupational situation should be investigated. Not only can urticaria impair the patient's quality of life, but can also interfere with the ability to work. Patients with physical urticaria may not be able to avoid the respective trigger in their work environment and the disease may cause psychological stress. On the other hand, psychological as well as physical stress has been described to induce exacerbations and stress-reducing lifestyle adjustments can be helpful in the management of urticaria.

10.7 Inducing Tolerance

Tolerance induction protocols are available for some forms of inducible urticarias and normally consist of an induction phase where tolerance is obtained and the maintenance phase in which the patient needs to expose him- or herself regularly to the trigger at the obtained threshold. For example in solar urticaria therapy with UV-A has been proven to induce tolerance in 3 days, but constant exposure to UV light is necessary afterwards. As this can be difficult at times in most climates, specialized lamps may become necessary. Similar protocols for cold urticaria require the patient to take cold baths or showers on a daily basis and frequently encounter adherence problems.

10.8 Pharmacological Treatment

Pharmacotherapy should comply with the principle to use as much as needed but as little as possible. The adequacy of pharmacological treatment should be evaluated regularly, extent and selection of medication may vary in the course of the disease.

According to the current guideline evidence-based pharmacological therapy should include second-generation antihistamines as first-line-therapy and their updosing as second-line-therapy. As third-line treatment option the add-on of monoclonal anti-IgE-antibody omalizumab is recommended, fourth-line treatment includes ciclosporin A instead of omalizumab (Fig. 10.1). Other treatment options where evidence of efficacy is inconclusive are available and are discussed further in this chapter.

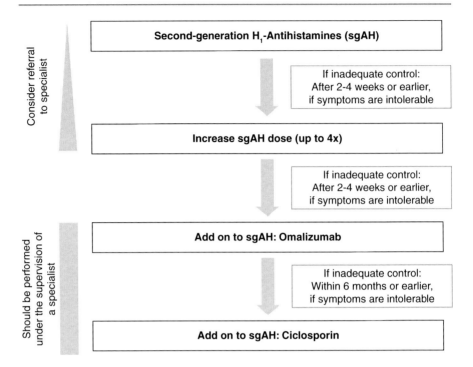

Fig. 10.1 Treatment algorithm according to the International Guideline for the Definition, Classification, Diagnosis, and Management of Urticaria (REF)

Antihistamines

11

Martin K. Church

Core Messages

This chapter traces the development of H_1-antihistamines from first generation drugs with marked sedative and other unwanted effects, through second generation drugs with minimal sedation, to the most recent drugs which do not penetrate the brain.

11.1 Introduction

To understand the strengths and weaknesses of H_1-antihistamines, it is necessary to appreciate how they were developed in the 1930s. In his review about his own work [1] Daniel Bovet wrote 'Three naturally occurring amines, acetylcholine, epinephrine, and histamine, may be grouped together because they have a similar chemical structure, are all present in the body fluids, and exert characteristically strong pharmacologic activities. There are alkaloids that interfere with the effects of acetylcholine. Similarly, there are sympatholytic poisons that neutralize or reverse the effects of epinephrine. It seemed possible to me, therefore, that some substance might exist which exerts a specific antagonism toward histamine'. It was against this background that Bovet, who was looking for antagonists of acetylcholine, asked his student, Anne-Marie Staub, to test some of these compounds against histamine. Anne-Marie Staub, who was preparing her doctorate thesis in his laboratory, used three types of laboratory methods for the evaluation of the degree of activity of the various compounds [1]. In the first test, they determined the action against the lethal

---

M. K. Church (✉)
Department of Dermatology and Allergy, Allergie-Centrum-Charité/ECARF, Charité-Universitätsmedizin Berlin, Berlin, Germany
e-mail: mkc@southampton.ac.uk

© Springer Nature Switzerland AG 2021
T. Zuberbier et al. (eds.), *Urticaria and Angioedema*,
https://doi.org/10.1007/978-3-030-84574-2_11

effects of histamine in guinea pigs. This test they believed to be 'perfectly specific'. In the second test, they determined the protection against histamine administered in the form of an aerosol. Here, they believed that symptoms similar to asthma were produced. In the third test for determining antihistaminic activity, which they believed to be the least specific one, they ascertained the effect of compounds on histamine-induced spasm of the isolated guinea pig ileum. These tests led to the discovery of the first H_1-antihistamine, thymoxyethyldiethylamine (929 F) in 1937 [2].

Although hymoxyethyldiethylamine was too toxic for use in humans, it opened the door for the introduction of the 1st generation H_1-antihistamines into the clinic. These included antergan in 1942 [3], followed by diphenhydramine in 1945 [4] and chlorpheniramine, brompheniramine and promethazine later the same decade [5]. It should be remembered, however, that these first generation H_1-antihistamines derive from the same chemical stem as cholinergic muscarinic antagonists. Also, early tranquilizers, anti-psychotics, antihypertensive and local anaesthetics agents were also developed from this stem. It is hardly surprising that 1st generation H_1-antihistamines have poor receptor selectivity and often interact with receptors of other biologically active amines causing anti-muscarinic, anti-α-adrenergic and anti-serotonin effects [6].

11.2 The Histamine H_1-Receptor

The histamine H_1-receptor is a member of the superfamily of G-protein coupled receptors (GPCRs). Physically they are composed of seven transmembrane domains coupling the exterior domains to the intracellular activating mechanism (Fig. 11.1a). In the way that they work, GPCRs may be viewed as 'cellular switches' that exist as an equilibrium between the inactive or 'off' state and the active or 'on' state [7]. To stimulate the receptor, histamine (red arrow) cross links domains III and V to stabilize the receptor in its active conformation or 'on' position [8] (Fig. 11.1b) this is a transient event with histamine being rapidly removed. H_1-antihistamines, which are not structurally related to histamine, do not antagonize the binding of histamine but bind to different sites on the receptor to produce the opposite effect. For example, cetirizine cross links sites on transmembrane domains IV and VI to stabilize the receptor in the inactive state and swing the equilibrium to the 'off' position [9] (Fig. 11.1c). Binding times for H_1-antihistamines vary from 25 s for diphenhydramine to 60 and 73 min for fexofenadine and bilastine, respectively [10]. Thus, H_1-antihistamines are not receptor antagonists but are inverse agonists in that they produce the opposite effect on the receptor to histamine [7]. Consequently, the preferred term to define these drugs is 'H_1-antihistamines' rather than 'histamine antagonists'.

Fig. 11.1 (**a**) Diagram of a histamine H_1-receptor in a membrane showing the 7 transmembrane domains. Histamine stimulates the receptor following its penetration into the central core of the receptor. (**b**) a surface view of an activated receptor with histamine linking domains III and V, and (**c**) a surface view of an inactive receptor with cetirizine linking domains IV and VI

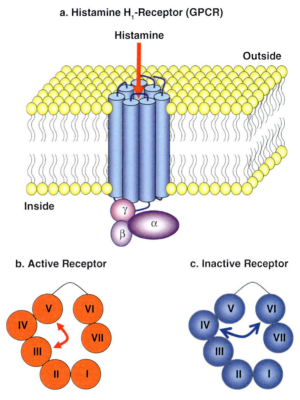

Church MK, Church DS. Pharmacology of Antihistamines. In: Urticaria. Ed Godse, K. Indian Association of Dermatologists, Venereologistsand Leprologists: Mumbai. 2012: 94–99.

11.3 H₁-Antihistamines and the Central Nervous System

Perhaps the greatest drawback of first generation H_1-antihistamines is their ability to cross blood–brain barrier and interfere with histaminergic transmission. Histamine is an important neuromediator in the human brain which contains approximately 64,000 histamine-producing neurones, emanating from the tuberomamillary nucleus [11]. Stimulation of H_1-receptors in the CNS increases arousal in the circadian sleep/wake cycle, reinforces learning and memory, and has roles in fluid balance, suppression of feeding, control of body temperature, control of cardiovascular system and mediation of stress-triggered release of ACTH and β-endorphin from the pituitary gland [12]. It is not surprising then that 1st generation H_1-antihistamines, such as chlorpheniramine, diphenhydramine, hydroxyzine and ketotifen, which, even when given at licensed doses, occupy more than 50% of brain H_1-receptors interfere with all of these processes (Fig. 11.2).

Physiologically, the release of histamine during the day causes arousal, whereas its decreased production at night results in a passive reduction of the arousal

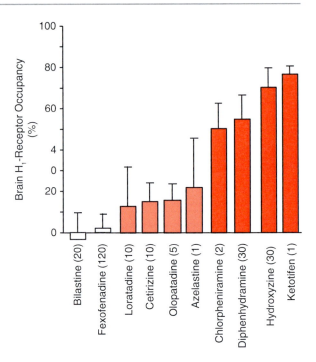

Fig. 11.2 Brain receptor occupancy of H_1-antihistamines. The doses of the drugs used are in parentheses. This diagram is based on data from references [13, 14]

response. When taken during the day, 1st generation H_1-antihistamines, even in the manufacturers' recommended doses, frequently cause daytime somnolence, sedation, drowsiness, fatigue and impaired concentration and memory [15, 16]. When taken at night, 1st generation H_1-antihistamines increase the latency to the onset of rapid eye movement (REM) sleep and reduce the duration of REM sleep (Fig. 11.3) [17, 18, 20]. The residual effects of poor sleep, including impairment of attention, vigilance, working memory and sensory-motor performance, are still present the next morning [17, 21]. This is especially problematical with drugs with a long half-life, such as chlorpheniramine (21–27 h) hydroxyzine (20–25 h) and promethazine (16–19 h). The detrimental CNS effects of 1st generation H_1-antihistamines on learning and examination performance in children and on the impairment of the ability of adults to work, drive and fly aircraft have been reviewed in detail in a recent review [6]. However, it is pertinent to emphasize the effects in children. It is well established that allergic rhinitis reduces learning ability in children and is associated with poor examination performance in teenagers. This situation is exacerbated by first-generation, H_1-antihistamines [22–24]. In an analysis of 1834 teenage students in the UK taking national examinations, those with untreated allergic rhinitis were 40% more likely to drop one or more grades compared with healthy teenagers. However, if they took a first-generation H_1 this figure increased to 70% [25].

A major advance in antihistamine development occurred in the 1980s with the introduction of second generation H_1-antihistamines, including loratadine,

11 Antihistamines

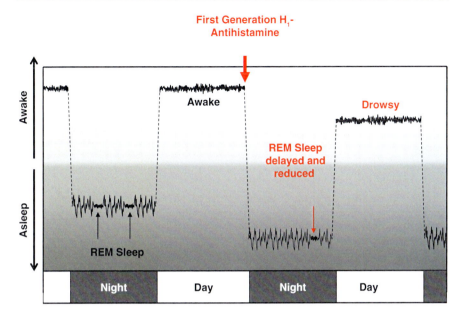

Fig. 11.3 A theoretical diagram of the sleep/wake cycle and the effects of a first-generation H_1-antihistamine leading to somnolence during the day and abnormal sleep at night. This diagram is based on data from references [17–19] and reproduced from reference [6]

desloratadine, cetirizine, levocetirizine, ebastine, azelastine and olopatadine, which have high H_1-receptor selectivity, no anti-cholinergic effects, low brain permeability and longer durations of action [26]. Unlike first generation drugs, second generation H_1-antihistamines are amphiphilic in that hydrophilic groups have been introduced into the molecule so that they are always positively or negatively charged and, therefore, have a greatly reduced passage across the blood–brain barrier occupying less than 20% of brain H_1-receptors (Fig. 11.4) [13, 28]. Although second generation H_1-antihistamines have a much reduced brain penetration, they may only be referred to as 'minimally sedating' rather than 'non-sedating'. For example, in a study of patients' perspective of effectiveness and side effects of H_1-antihistamine updosing in chronic spontaneous urticaria, more than 20% of patients reported sedation is a side effect of SGAHs [29].

More recently, studies have suggested hydrophilicity alone is not sufficient to keep drugs from entering the brain but that an active efflux transporter in the blood–brain barrier may be involved. The most extensively studied of the active efflux proteins is P-glycoprotein (P-gp), which is known to efflux a wide variety of structurally dissimilar drugs (Fig. 11.4) [30, 31]. *In vitro* studies of P-gp-mediated efflux from caco-2 cells have shown cetirizine, desloratadine and hydroxyzine to have weak but significant efflux ratios while that of fexofenadine was much greater [32]. More recently, similar studies have shown bilastine also has a high efflux ratio [33].

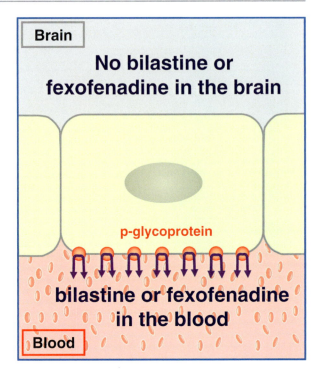

Fig. 11.4 Theoretical diagram of the p-glycoprotein membrane pump preventing bilastine from crossing the blood–brain barrier. This diagram is based on data from reference [27]

The failure of bilastine and fexofenadine to enter the brain and occupy histamine H_1-receptors has been confirmed using positron emission tomography [34]. It is also important to note that total H_1-receptor occupancy (H1RO) in the brain for bilastine and fexofenadine was less than zero. Thus, these two drugs appear to be truly 'non-sedating' H_1-antihistamines and the most likely reason for their lack of brain penetration is that they are actively pumped out of the blood–brain barrier by P-gp (Fig. 11.4) [30, 35–37].

11.4　H_1-Antihistamines and Cardiotoxicity

The introduction of the second generation H_1-antihistamines in the late 1970s and 1980s brought new and unexpected problems, with an increasing number of reports showing an association between the consumption of astemizole and terfenadine and cardiotoxicity. Both of these are essentially pro-drugs that are metabolized by the cytochrome P450 enzyme, CYP3A4, to their active antihistaminic form. However, it was soon realized that if this metabolism was blocked by the concomitant use of inhibitors of CYP3A4, such as ketoconazole, itraconazole and macrolide antibiotics, or by grapefruit juice, which causes post-translational down-regulation of CYP3A4, then this could cause the prolongation of the QT interval, leading to the appearance of polymorphic ventricular arrhythmias, syncope and even cardiac arrest in susceptible individuals [7]. The main mechanism underlying this acquired

QT syndrome and a potentially fatal torsade de pointes arrhythmia is the inhibition of the potassium channel encoded by hERG (the human ether-a-go-go-related gene).

Astemizole and terfenadine are no longer approved for use by regulatory agencies in most countries. However, some 1st generation H_1-antihistamines, such as promethazine [38], brompheniramine [39] and chlorpheniramine [40], may also be associated with a prolonged QTc and cardiac arrhythmias when taken in large doses or overdoses. Today, the concentration of a drug required to produce a half-maximal block of the hERG potassium current (IC_{50}) is used as a surrogate marker for pro-arrhythmic properties of compounds and is the primary test for cardiac safety of drugs [41]. No clinically significant cardiac effects have been reported for the second generation H_1-antihistamines fexofenadine, the metabolite of terfenadine, desloratadine, loratadine, cetirizine, levocetirizine, azelastine, ebastine, mizolastine, rupatadine and bilastine [35, 42–46].

11.5 H_1-Antihistamines in Urticaria

Most types urticaria, including chronic spontaneous urticaria (CSU) and the majority of inducible urticarias, are mediated primarily by mast cell-derived histamine [47] which reaches very high concentrations due to the poor diffusibility of substances in the dermis [48, 49]. Urticaria is characterized by short-lived wheals ranging from a few millimetres to several centimetres in diameter which are accompanied by severe itching which is usually worse in the evening or night-time [50].

The latest EAACI/GA²LEN/EDF/WAO guidelines for the management of urticaria [51] recommend that the first line treatment for urticaria should be second generation, non-sedating H_1-antihistamines. Furthermore, the guidelines state 'We recommend aiming at complete symptom control in urticaria, considering as much as possible the safety and the quality of life of each individual patient'. Because, standard licensed doses of H_1-antihistamines are often ineffective in completely relieving symptoms in many patients [29] the guidelines state 'We suggest updosing second generation H_1-antihistamines up to fourfold in patients with chronic urticaria unresponsive to second generation H_1-antihistamines onefold' (Fig. 11.5) [51]. Thus, it is clear that the attributes that dermatologists seek when choosing an H_1-antihistamine are a rapid onset of action, good efficacy, a long duration of action and freedom from unwanted effects. While some of these attributes may be predicted from pre-clinical and pharmacokinetic studies, it is only in the clinical environment that they may be definitively established [52].

11.5.1   Speed of Onset of Action and Duration of Action

The speed of onset of action of a drug is often equated to the rate of its oral absorption and its duration of action by its plasma concentration. However, this is not strictly correct as a time for a drug to diffuse into the extravascular space to produce a maximal clinical effect. In adults, the maximal inhibition of the flare response is

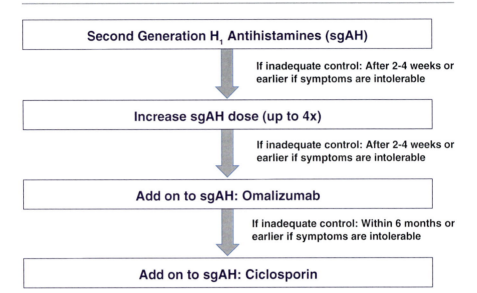

Fig. 11.5 Recommended treatment algorithm for urticaria from the EAACI/GA²LEN/EDF/WAO guideline for the definition, classification, diagnosis and management of urticaria. (*Adapted from Zuberbier T, Aberer W, Asero R, Abdul Latiff AH, Baker D, Ballmer-Weber B, et al. The EAACI/GA(2)LEN/EDF/WAO guideline for the definition, classification, diagnosis and management of urticaria. Allergy 2018;73(7):1393–1414*)

usually ~4 h for levocetirizine, fexofenadine and desloratadine [53–55] but may be longer for drugs, such as loratadine and ebastine, which require metabolism to produce their active moiety [55]. In contrast, a recent wheal and flare study has suggested that bilastine may have a more rapid onset of action because of its facilitated uptake from the duodenum [56].

The duration of action of antihistamines is also much longer than would be predicted from knowledge of their plasma concentration and for most is in the vicinity of 24 h [56, 57]. This is presumably to 'trapping' of the drug by its strong and long lasting binding to histamine H_1-receptors [9]. This may be especially so for bilastine which has an especially long residency time on the H1-receptor [10]. Because it is actively secreted into the intestine and urine by P-glycoprotein [58], the duration of action of fexofenadine is shorter, around $8^1/_2$ h [59] indicating that may be best given twice daily. In contrast, bilastine, which is also a substrate for p-glycoprotein, In contrast, bilastine has a duration of action of around 24 h. The reason for this difference is that bilastine is also a substrate for OATP1A, an intestinal pump that facilitates its uptake into the bloodstream [27, 56]. Even so, the guidelines suggest that second generation H_1-antihistamines should be taken regularly for the treatment of patients with chronic urticaria in order to obtain maximum efficacy [51].

11.5.2 Efficacy

A question that is asked repeatedly is how is the dose of an antihistamine determined. The answer is that it is a balance between the effectiveness and the unwanted or side effects of a drug. For first generation H_1-antihistamines, it is the degree somnolence that they cause limits the amount of drug that may be given. Hence drugs have relative weak efficacy. With most second generation H_1-antihistamines, their ability to penetrate the CNS to cause sedation is again a limiting factor. Drugs such as cetirizine and desloratadine may be minimally sedating at licensed doses, but updosing may cause sedation in susceptible patients. Possible exceptions to this rule are fexofenadine and bilastine which, because they are p-glycoprotein substrates and do not penetrate the CNS, may be updosed without fear of somnolence [35, 56, 60].

11.5.3 Clinical Usage

For the treatment of chronic urticaria, the guidelines are [51] that treatment should start with a standard single dose second generation H_1-antihistamine. If adequate control is not achieved after 2–4 weeks, or earlier if symptoms are intolerable, then the dose should be doubled. If adequate control is still not achieved after a further 2–4 weeks, or earlier if symptoms are intolerable, then the dose should be increased to four times the initial dose. The guidelines also recommend updosing with a single antihistamine rather than using different H_1-antihistamines at the same time. If somnolence is a problem, then either fexofenadine or bilastine should be considered.

For children, many clinicians use first generation, sedating H_1-antihistamines as their first choice assuming that the safety profile of these drugs is better known than that of the newer second generation H_1-antihistamines. However, the guidelines make a strong recommendation to discourage the use of first generation antihistamines in infants and children for the reasons stated above. Thus, in children the same first line treatment and updosing (weight and age adjusted) are recommended as in adults. It should be realized, however, that young children have more body water, as a percentage, than adults. Also, their renal function is fully developed. In contrast, liver enzymes mature more slowly reaching maximum at around 10 years of age. Consequently, in young children, only water-soluble drugs that are excreted renally, such as cetirizine, levocetirizine, fexofenadine and bilastine, should be used.

In elderly patients, again first generation antihistamines should not be used, particularly those with dementia as cumulative use of first generation antihistamines with anti-cholinergic activity is associated with an increased risk for dementia in such patients [61, 62].

11.6 Conclusions

In conclusion, the use of first generation H_1-antihistamines should be discouraged in clinical practice today for two main reasons. First, they are less effective than second generation H_1-antihistamines. Second, they have unwanted side effects and the potential for causing severe toxic reactions that are not shared by second generation H_1-antihistamines.

With regard to second generation H_1-antihistamines, there are many efficacious and safe drugs on the market for the treatment of allergic disease. Of the three drugs highlighted in this review, levocetirizine, fexofenadine and bilastine are the most potent in humans *in vivo*. However, levocetirizine may cause somnolence in susceptible individuals while fexofenadine has a relatively short duration of action and may be required to be given twice daily for all round daily protection. While desloratadine is less potent, it has the advantages of rarely causing somnolence and having a long duration of action. Of current drugs, bilastine is perhaps the most effective drug and does rarely causes somnolence.

References

1. Bovet D. Introduction to antihistamine agents and antergan derivative. Ann N Y Acad Sci. 1950;50(9):1089–126.
2. Staub AM. Action de la thymoxyethyldiethylamine (929F) et des ethers phenoliques sur le choc anaphylactique. Compt Rend Soc Biol. 1937;125:818–21.
3. Halpern BN. Les antihistaminiques de synthese. Essais de chemotherapie des etats allergiques. Arch Int Pharmacodyn Ther. 1942;681:339–408.
4. Loew ER, MacMillan R, Kaiser ME. The anti-histamine properties of benadryl, beta-dimethylaminoethyl benzhydryl ether hydrochloride. J Pharmacol Exp Ther. 1946;86:229–38.
5. Emanuel MB. Histamine and the antiallergic antihistamines: a history of their discoveries. Clin Exp Allergy. 1999;29(Suppl 3):1–11.
6. Church MK, Maurer M, Simons FE, Bindslev-Jensen C, van Cauwenberge P, Bousquet J, et al. Risk of first-generation H(1)-antihistamines: a GA(2)LEN position paper. Allergy. 2010;65(4):459–66.
7. Leurs R, Church MK, Taglialatela M. H1-antihistamines: inverse agonism, anti-inflammatory actions and cardiac effects. Clin Exp Allergy. 2002;32(4):489–98.
8. Wieland K, Laak AM, Smit MJ, Kuhne R, Timmerman H, Leurs R. Mutational analysis of the antagonist-binding site of the histamine H(1) receptor. J Biol Chem. 1999;274(42):29994–30000.
9. Gillard M, Van Der Perren C, Moguilevsky N, Massingham R, Chatelain P. Binding characteristics of cetirizine and levocetirizine to human H(1) histamine receptors: contribution of Lys(191) and Thr(194). Mol Pharmacol. 2002;61(2):391–9.
10. Bosma R, van den Bor J, Vischer HF, Labeaga L, Leurs R. The long duration of action of the second generation antihistamine bilastine coincides with its long residence time at the histamine H1 receptor. Eur J Pharmacol. 2018;838:107–11.
11. Haas H, Panula P. The role of histamine and the tuberomamillary nucleus in the nervous system. Nat Rev Neurosci. 2003;4(2):121–30.
12. Brown RE, Stevens DR, Haas HL. The physiology of brain histamine. Prog Neurobiol. 2001;63(6):637–72.
13. Yanai K, Zhang D, Tashiro M, Yoshikawa T, Naganuma F, Harada R, et al. Positron emission tomography evaluation of sedative properties of antihistamines. Expert Opin Drug Saf. 2011;10(4):613–22.

14. Farré M, et al. Brain histamine H1-receptor occupancy of bilastine, a new second-generation antihistamine, measured by positron emission tomography. XXVI Congreso de la SEFC (17–18 Oct, 2013, Cádiz-Spain). 2013.
15. Simons FE. Advances in H1-antihistamines. N Engl J Med. 2004;351(21):2203–17.
16. Juniper EF, Stahl E, Doty RL, Simons FE, Allen DB, Howarth PH. Clinical outcomes and adverse effect monitoring in allergic rhinitis. J Allergy Clin Immunol. 2005;115(3 Suppl 1):S390–413.
17. Boyle J, Eriksson M, Stanley N, Fujita T, Kumagi Y. Allergy medication in Japanese volunteers: treatment effect of single doses on nocturnal sleep architecture and next day residual effects. Curr Med Res Opin. 2006;22(7):1343–51.
18. Rojas-Zamorano JA, Esqueda-Leon E, Jimenez-Anguiano A, Cintra-McGlone L, Mendoza Melendez MA, Velazquez Moctezuma J. The H1 histamine receptor blocker, chlorpheniramine, completely prevents the increase in REM sleep induced by immobilization stress in rats. Pharmacol Biochem Behav. 2009;91(3):291–4.
19. Monti JM. Involvement of histamine in the control of the waking state. Life Sci. 1993;53(17):1331–8.
20. Adam K, Oswald I. The hypnotic effects of an antihistamine: promethazine. Br J Clin Pharmacol. 1986;22(6):715–7.
21. Kay GG, Berman B, Mockoviak SH, Morris CE, Reeves D, Starbuck V, et al. Initial and steady-state effects of diphenhydramine and loratadine on sedation, cognition, mood, and psychomotor performance. Arch Intern Med. 1997;157(20):2350–6.
22. Vuurman EF, van Veggel LM, Uiterwijk MM, Leutner D, O'Hanlon JF. Seasonal allergic rhinitis and antihistamine effects on children's learning. Ann Allergy. 1993;71(2):121–6.
23. Vuurman EF, van Veggel LM, Sanders RL, Muntjewerff ND, O'Hanlon JF. Effects of semprex-D and diphenhydramine on learning in young adults with seasonal allergic rhinitis. Ann Allergy Asthma Immunol. 1996;76(3):247–52.
24. Scadding G. Optimal management of nasal congestion caused by allergic rhinitis in children: safety and efficacy of medical treatments. Paediatr Drugs. 2008;10(3):151–62.
25. Walker S, Khan-Wasti S, Fletcher M, Cullinan P, Harris J, Sheikh A. Seasonal allergic rhinitis is associated with a detrimental effect on examination performance in United Kingdom teenagers: case-control study. J Allergy Clin Immunol. 2007;120(2):381–7.
26. Holgate ST, Canonica GW, Simons FE, Taglialatela M, Tharp M, Timmerman H, et al. Consensus Group on New-Generation Antihistamines (CONGA): present status and recommendations. Clin Exp Allergy. 2003;33(9):1305–24.
27. Lucero ML, Gonzalo A, Ganza A, Leal N, Soengas I, Ioja E, et al. Interactions of bilastine, a new oral H(1) antihistamine, with human transporter systems. Drug Chem Toxicol. 2012;35(Suppl 1):8–17.
28. Hiraoka K, Tashiro M, Grobosch T, Maurer M, Oda K, Toyohara J, et al. Brain histamine H1 receptor occupancy measured by PET after oral administration of levocetirizine, a nonsedating antihistamine. Expert Opin Drug Saf. 2015;14(2):199–206.
29. Weller K, Ziege C, Staubach P, Brockow K, Siebenhaar F, Krause K, et al. H1-antihistamine up-dosing in chronic spontaneous urticaria: patients' perspective of effectiveness and side effects—a retrospective survey study. PLoS One. 2011;6(9):e23931.
30. Chen C, Hanson E, Watson JW, Lee JS. P-glycoprotein limits the brain penetration of nonsedating but not sedating H1-antagonists. Drug Metab Dispos. 2003;31(3):312–8.
31. Seelig A, Landwojtowicz E. Structure-activity relationship of P-glycoprotein substrates and modifiers. Eur J Pharm Sci. 2000;12(1):31–40.
32. Crowe A, Wright C. The impact of P-glycoprotein mediated efflux on absorption of 11 sedating and less-sedating antihistamines using Caco-2 monolayers. Xenobiotica. 2012;42(6):538–49.
33. Burton PS, Crean C, Kagey M, Neilsen JW. Permeability characteristics of bilastine, a potent and selective H1 receptor antagonist, in caco-2 cells. AAPS J. 2007;9(Suppl 2):2910.
34. Farre M, Perez-Mana C, Papaseit E, Menoyo E, Perez M, Martin S, et al. Bilastine vs. hydroxyzine: occupation of brain histamine H1-receptors evaluated by positron emission tomography in healthy volunteers. Br J Clin Pharmacol. 2014;78(5):970–80.

35. Church MK. Safety and efficacy of bilastine: a new H(1)-antihistamine for the treatment of allergic rhinoconjunctivitis and urticaria. Expert Opin Drug Saf. 2011;10(5):779–93.
36. Schinkel AH. P-glycoprotein, a gatekeeper in the blood-brain barrier. Adv Drug Deliv Rev. 1999;36(2–3):179–94.
37. Montoro J, Mullol J, Davila I, Ferrer M, Sastre J, Bartra J, et al. Bilastine and the central nervous system. J Investig Allergol Clin Immunol. 2011;21(Suppl 3):9–15.
38. Jo SH, Hong HK, Chong SH, Lee HS, Choe H. H(1) antihistamine drug promethazine directly blocks hERG K(+) channel. Pharmacol Res. 2009;60(5):429–37.
39. Park SJ, Kim KS, Kim EJ. Blockade of HERG K+ channel by an antihistamine drug brompheniramine requires the channel binding within the S6 residue Y652 and F656. J Appl Toxicol. 2008;28(2):104–11.
40. Hong HK, Jo SH. Block of HERG k channel by classic histamine h(1) receptor antagonist chlorpheniramine. Korean J Physiol Pharmacol. 2009;13(3):215–20.
41. Polak S, Wisniowska B, Brandys J. Collation, assessment and analysis of literature in vitro data on hERG receptor blocking potency for subsequent modeling of drugs' cardiotoxic properties. J Appl Toxicol. 2009;29(3):183–206.
42. Ten Eick AP, Blumer JL, Reed MD. Safety of antihistamines in children. Drug Saf. 2001;24(2):119–47.
43. DuBuske LM. Second-generation antihistamines: the risk of ventricular arrhythmias. Clin Ther. 1999;21(2):281–95.
44. Simons FE, Prenner BM, Finn A Jr, Desloratadine Study Group. Efficacy and safety of desloratadine in the treatment of perennial allergic rhinitis. J Allergy Clin Immunol. 2003;111(3):617–22.
45. Hulhoven R, Rosillon D, Letiexhe M, Meeus MA, Daoust A, Stockis A. Levocetirizine does not prolong the QT/QTc interval in healthy subjects: results from a thorough QT study. Eur J Clin Pharmacol. 2007;63(11):1011–7.
46. Izquierdo I, Merlos M, Garcia-Rafanell J. Rupatadine: a new selective histamine H1 receptor and platelet-activating factor (PAF) antagonist. A review of pharmacological profile and clinical management of allergic rhinitis. Drugs Today (Barc). 2003;39(6):451–68.
47. Church MK, Kolkhir P, Metz M, Maurer M. The role and relevance of mast cells in urticaria. Immunol Rev. 2018;282(1):232–47.
48. Petersen LJ, Church MK, Skov PS. Histamine is released in the wheal but not the flare following challenge of human skin in vivo: a microdialysis study. Clin Exp Allergy. 1997;27(3):284–95.
49. Church MK, Bewley AP, Clough GF, Burrows LJ, Ferdinand SI, Petersen LJ. Studies into the mechanisms of dermal inflammation using cutaneous microdialysis. Int Arch Allergy Immunol. 1997;113(1–3):131–3.
50. Maurer M, Weller K, Bindslev-Jensen C, Gimenez-Arnau A, Bousquet PJ, Bousquet J, et al. Unmet clinical needs in chronic spontaneous urticaria. A GA(2)LEN task force report. Allergy. 2011;66(3):317–30.
51. Zuberbier T, Aberer W, Asero R, Abdul Latiff AH, Baker D, Ballmer-Weber B, et al. The EAACI/GA(2)LEN/EDF/WAO guideline for the definition, classification, diagnosis and management of urticaria. Allergy. 2018;73(7):1393–414.
52. Church MK, Maurer M. H(1)-antihistamines and urticaria: how can we predict the best drug for our patient? Clin Exp Allergy. 2012;42(10):1423–9.
53. Grant JA, Riethuisen JM, Moulaert B, DeVos C. A double-blind, randomized, single-dose, crossover comparison of levocetirizine with ebastine, fexofenadine, loratadine, mizolastine, and placebo: suppression of histamine-induced wheal-and-flare response during 24 hours in healthy male subjects. Ann Allergy Asthma Immunol. 2002;88(2):190–7.
54. Denham KJ, Boutsiouki P, Clough GF, Church MK. Comparison of the effects of desloratadine and levocetirizine on histamine-induced wheal, flare and itch in human skin. Inflamm Res. 2003;52(10):424–7.
55. Purohit A, Melac M, Pauli G, Frossard N. Comparative activity of cetirizine and desloratadine on histamine-induced wheal-and-flare responses during 24 hours. Ann Allergy Asthma Immunol. 2004;92(6):635–40.

56. Church MK, Labeaga L. Bilastine: a new H1-antihistamine with an optimal profile for updosing in urticaria. J Eur Acad Dermatol Venereol. 2017.
57. Purohit A, Melac M, Pauli G, Frossard N. Twenty-four-hour activity and consistency of activity of levocetirizine and desloratadine in the skin. Br J Clin Pharmacol. 2003;56(4):388–94.
58. Miura M, Uno T. Clinical pharmacokinetics of fexofenadine enantiomers. Expert Opin Drug Metab Toxicol. 2010;6(1):69–74.
59. Purohit A, Duvernelle C, Melac M, Pauli G, Frossard N. Twenty-four hours of activity of cetirizine and fexofenadine in the skin. Ann Allergy Asthma Immunol. 2001;86(4):387–92.
60. Krause K, Spohr A, Zuberbier T, Church MK, Maurer M. Up-dosing with bilastine results in improved effectiveness in cold contact urticaria. Allergy. 2013;68(7):921–8.
61. Gray SL, Anderson ML, Dublin S, Hanlon JT, Hubbard R, Walker R, et al. Cumulative use of strong anticholinergics and incident dementia: a prospective cohort study. JAMA Intern Med. 2015;175(3):401–7.
62. Tannenbaum C, Paquette A, Hilmer S, Holroyd-Leduc J, Carnahan R. A systematic review of amnestic and non-amnestic mild cognitive impairment induced by anticholinergic, antihistamine, GABAergic and opioid drugs. Drugs Aging. 2012;29(8):639–58.

Omalizumab in the Treatment of Urticaria

12

Torsten Zuberbier, Tamara Dörr, Clive Grattan, and Marcus Maurer

Core Messages
- Omalizumab, a humanized mouse monoclonal antibody against IgE has been approved for the treatment of urticaria in 2012.
- Having strong evidence on both, efficacy and safety, it is recommended as add-on to antihistamines as third-line treatment option.
- The approved dose of 300 mg subcutaneously every 4 weeks achieves complete control of disease in >40% of patients.
- Response predictors are high IgE at baseline while the presence of autoantibodies may delay response.
- Off-label treatment has shown good efficacy in children as well as CIndU

Omalizumab, an anti-IgE therapeutic antibody, is the first biological licensed for the pharmacotherapy of urticaria. In Europe, in-label use for CSU has been permitted since 2014 although allergologists have had previous experience with this monoclonal humanized antibody as it had been licensed for the use in therapy-resistant allergic asthma for almost a decade longer.

Currently, omalizumab has been licensed for three indications:

1. moderate to severe asthma with proven allergic reaction against a perennial aeroallergen and a reduced lung function (FEV$_1$ < 80%), frequent daily or nightly symptoms or exacerbations despite daily administration of high-dose inhaled corticosteroids (ICS).

T. Zuberbier · T. Dörr · M. Maurer
Institute for Allergology, Charité – Universitätsmedizin, Berlin, Germany

Fraunhofer Institute for Translational Medicine and Pharmacology ITMP, Allergology and Immunology, Berlin, Germany
e-mail: Torsten.Zuberbier@charite.de; tamara.doerr@charite.de; Marcus.Maurer@charite.de

C. Grattan (✉)
St John's Institute of Dermatology, Guy's Hospital, London, UK
e-mail: Clive.E.Grattan@gstt.nhs.uk

© Springer Nature Switzerland AG 2021
T. Zuberbier et al. (eds.), *Urticaria and Angioedema*,
https://doi.org/10.1007/978-3-030-84574-2_12

2. chronic spontaneous urticaria with insufficient symptom relief under standard treatment with H₁-antihistamines.
3. severe chronic rhinosinusitis with nasal polyps (CRSwNP) where the therapy with intranasal corticosteroids does not provide adequate disease control.

12.1 Bioavailability, Metabolism and Elimination

The mean bioavailability of omalizumab after subcutaneous injection is about 62%. Absorption of a single dose happens slowly, the peak serum concentrations being reached 7–8 days after injection. The pharmacokinetics of omalizumab has been shown to be linear in both, asthma and urticaria patients and trough serum concentrations increase proportionally with the dose [1].

Monoclonal antibodies are bound at their Fc receptor binding site by endothelial cells, are then internalized and degraded in the reticuloendothelial system (RES) to smaller proteins and single amino acids, which can then be used for de-novo synthesis of new proteins [2]. Being an IgG antibody, omalizumab is eliminated by the RES of endothelial cells and the liver. The elimination is dose-dependent and clearance of free omalizumab is slower than of omalizumab-IgE complexes or free IgE [3].

Because of its route of elimination, the pharmacokinetics of omalizumab is unlikely to be influenced by renal or hepatic impairment. Also, the genetic polymorphisms of cytochrome P450 enzymes as well as other medication metabolized by them do not interact with the pharmacokinetics of omalizumab.

12.2 Mechanisms of Action of Omalizumab in CSU

Mast cells are the key players in the formation of wheals and angioedema. They express an array of different receptors whose binding to their respective ligand leads to the cell's degranulation, releasing proinflammatory mediators such as histamine, proteases, prostaglandins and leukotrienes, as well as chemokines and cytokines.

Several routes of mast cell activation have been identified to be relevant in the pathogenesis of CSU. Most of them involve the immunoglobulin E (IgE) receptor FcεRI. FcεRI-dependent drivers of mast cell degranulation in CSU include IgE autoantibodies to thyroid peroxidase, interleukin 24 and other autoantigens, IgG and IgM autoantibodies to the alpha chain of FcεRI, and autoantibodies to IgE. Omalizumab is a recombinant DNA-derived humanized immunoglobulin G1κ monoclonal antibody that binds non-receptor bound human IgE [4]. In CSU, omalizumab is understood to prevent mast cell degranulation by decreasing free IgE and reducing the expression of FcεRI receptors.

12.3 Common Adverse Effects

Omalizumab has a favourable risk-benefit ratio with a distinct safety profile. In single doses of up to 4000 mg, no dose-limiting toxicities have been observed. The most commonly reported adverse effects of omalizumab in patients with urticaria include nausea, headaches, swelling of throat or sinuses, cough, joint pain and upper respiratory tract infection [2, 4].

Very rare cases of type I allergic reactions including anaphylaxis to omalizumab have been described. Although they may occur even after a long duration of treatment, the majority of anaphylactic reactions occurred within the first three months of omalizumab treatment [4].

Because of its mechanism of action, one might think that the immune response to parasite and helminth infection would be impaired by omalizumab. This, however, is not the case. Although a slight numerical increase of parasite infections has been reported, the course and duration of the infections were not altered [4].

12.4 Omalizumab in the Treatment of Chronic Spontaneous Urticaria: Clinical Trials

The first randomized controlled multicentre study to show that patients with chronic spontaneous urticaria benefit from the treatment with omalizumab was X-CUISITE [5]. In X-CUISITE, all patients had IgE autoantibodies to thyroid peroxidase, and omalizumab was dosed (75–375 mg) based on body weight and serum IgE levels. At the end of the treatment phase, 70% of patients showed complete control with no more wheals. This is the highest rate of complete responders ever observed in a randomized controlled trial with omalizumab in CSU [6]. The most probable explanation for this high rate of responders is that all patients had autoallergic CSU, which is held to respond well and rapidly to omalizumab treatment.

The proof-of-concept study X-CUISITE was followed by the phase II dose-ranging study MYSTIQUE (75, 300 or 600 mg fixed dose vs. placebo) [6]. MYSTIQUE confirmed the good efficacy and tolerability profile of omalizumab in CSU and was followed by three pivotal Phase III multicentre, randomized, double-blind, placebo-controlled, parallel-group studies in patients with CSU: ASTERIA I, ASTERIA II and GLACIAL [7]. In the ASTERIA studies, patients were treated with 75 mg, 150 mg, 300 mg of omalizumab or placebo every 4 weeks for 6 months (ASTERIA I) or 3 months (ASTERIA II). The GLACIAL study investigated only the 300 mg dose against placebo. All three studies showed a rapid and marked improvement of CSU symptoms: pruritus was significantly reduced in the groups treated with 150 mg or 300 mg dose of omalizumab compared to placebo, significantly more patients became symptom-free after 3 months of 300 mg omalizumab compared to placebo and significant improvements in health-related quality of life were reported for the treatment groups with 150 mg (ASTERIA II) or 300 mg (all studies).

While ASTERIA I and II assessed the efficacy and safety of omalizumab as an add-on therapy in patients who were refractory to licensed doses of H1-antihistamines, GLACIAL assessed the safety of omalizumab as add-on therapy in patients who remained refractory to up to four times the licensed dose of H1-antihistamines plus H2-antihistamines, leukotriene receptor antagonists or both [8–10]. As patients in this study showed poorly controlled CSU despite combination pharmacotherapy, this study population represents the difficult-to-control patients seen in clinical practice more accurately. Based on these studies, EMA and FDA approved omalizumab for the treatment of patients with CSU in 2014.

More recent randomized controlled clinical trials explored the long-term safety and efficacy of omalizumab treatment of patients with CSU, re-treatment efficacy in patients with relapse after stopping omalizumab and the effects of omalizumab on recurrent angioedema in patients with CSU. The X-TEND study demonstrated that omalizumab is effective and safe in patients with CSU treated for 48 weeks [11]. In the OPTIMA study, 9 of 10 patients re-treated with omalizumab after relapse post-withdrawal regained symptomatic control [9]. The X-ACT study showed, in patients with CSU and recurrent angioedema, that omalizumab treatment reduces angioedema burdened days per week threefold versus placebo, with first recurrence of angioedema after 57–63 days with omalizumab and <5 days with placebo [12]. Omalizumab also significantly reduced angioedema-specific quality of life impairment.

Several meta-analyses of the effects of omalizumab in CSU have been performed and published. They all arrive at the conclusion that the evidence provided by randomized controlled clinical trials is of high quality and supports the efficacy and safety of omalizumab in patients with CSU and for treating these patients with 300 mg every 4 weeks.

12.5 Omalizumab in the Treatment of Chronic Spontaneous Urticaria: Real-world Data

In routine clinical practice, the efficacy of omalizumab treatment, in patients with CSU, is similar to that seen in the randomized controlled trials, and often better. In one of the first real life retrospective studies performed, 83% of patients were responders, and 6 and 9 of 10 patients who achieved complete response did so within 1 week and 4 weeks, respectively [13]. In another retrospective study, with 110 CSU patients treated with omalizumab in Spain, 8 of 10 patients showed complete or significant responses [14].

Real life data also supports the efficacy of re-treatment with omalizumab in CSU patients who experience relapse after treatment discontinuation. In one study, where 25 patients with CSU or chronic inducible urticaria stopped omalizumab treatment, all experienced relapse and then received re-treatment with omalizumab. All reported a rapid and complete response within the first 4 weeks, usually during the first days of re-treatment, with no relevant side effects [15]. In another study, 20 patients re-started omalizumab treatment, and complete response was achieved in 18 of them, within 1 week to 2 months [16].

Most CSU patients treated with omalizumab show a fast response, within the first or second month of treatment. Real life studies suggest that a subpopulation of patients takes longer to respond (see Markers for response section). This is in line with the response patterns observed in controlled trials, where some patients who had not responded after 12 weeks of treatment did so after 24 weeks.

It appears to be possible to increase omalizumab dosing intervals, once patients show complete control of their CSU. On the other hand, shortening of dosing intervals or increasing the dose can benefit patients with inadequate response to standard-dosed omalizumab, and it often does. Several recent retrospective studies showed that most patients with partial response to omalizumab treatment experience substantial or complete response when switched to 450 mg/month or 600 mg/month [15]. Experts recommend using higher than standard doses of omalizumab in patients with uncontrolled symptoms throughout the treatment interval and to shorten the interval in patients who show a good response during the beginning and worsening of symptoms at the end of the interval.

Most patients with CSU have recurrent angioedema, with or without wheals. The effects of omalizumab in the latter subpopulation have not yet been investigated in controlled trials. Real life data, i.e. several case reports and case series, support the treatment of CSU with angioedema without wheals, as all reported patients ceased to develop angioedema in response to treatment [17].

The treatment of patients with chronic inducible urticaria without comorbid CSU is off label but may be very effective. A recent systematic review of more than 40 studies including several investigator-initiated randomized controlled trials showed that omalizumab treatment in patients with chronic inducible urticaria results in substantial or complete response in most patients [18]. The supporting evidence for the efficacy of omalizumab treatment of patients with chronic inducible urticaria is strongest for symptomatic dermographism, cold urticaria, solar urticaria and cholinergic urticaria.

Omalizumab is licensed for the treatment of CSU patients who are 12 years old or older. The prevalence and course of CSU in patients younger than 12 years are similar to those in older patients. As of now there are no randomized controlled trials in children under 12 years of age. Real-world data support the efficacy and safety of omalizumab in this age group but are limited. Expert opinion supports the use of omalizumab for the treatment of patients with CSU who are younger than 12 years old, but patients and their parents should understand that this is off label.

CSU, in most patients, shows spontaneous remission after several years duration. It is, therefore, important to assess patients with complete response to omalizumab treatment for the need to continue treatment. This is done by stopping the treatment, often by increasing dosing intervals by one week at a time, and monitoring patients for relapse. Experts recommend doing this after 6 to 12 months of complete response. The authors prefer the latter.

Patients with CSU who do not respond to omalizumab during the first six months of treatment should be considered for treatment with ciclosporin. Real life data and experience support combining low-dose cyclosporin with omalizumab in patients with CSU who show partial response to omalizumab [17].

A recent meta-analysis of real-world evidence on the safety of omalizumab treatment in adolescent and adult patients with CSU arrived at the conclusion that the safety profile of omalizumab in CSU is similar or superior to that found in clinical trials, where adverse event rates range from 3 to 8% versus 4% in real life [19].

12.6 Markers that Predict and Tools that Help to Monitor Treatment Responses to Omalizumab in Patients with CSU

Based on the current understanding of the pathogenesis of CSU and the mechanisms of action of omalizumab, patients with type I autoimmune (or autoallergic) CSU can be expected to show faster and better responses than those with type IIb autoimmune CSU. This is supported by the results of the X-CUISITE trial, where only patients with type I autoimmune CSU, characterized by the expression of IgE against thyroid peroxidase, were included. Patients in this trial showed very fast onset of responses and a high rate of complete responders, 70%, higher than those observed in other trials, where autoallergy was not an inclusion criterion.

In contrast, patients with type IIb autoimmune CSU, as characterized by a positive autologous serum test or a positive basophil test, show slower onset of response and lower rates of response as compared to patients who are negative for these markers. In one study with 64 patients with CSU, basophil test-positive patients had a median time to response of 29 days, as compared to only 2 days in basophil test-negative patients [19]. In another study, in 41 patients with antihistamine-refractory CSU, a negative basophil test correlated with rates of clinical response to omalizumab: of the 18 patients with a positive test, only 9 (50%) had clinical improvement with omalizumab, whereas 20 of 23 (87%) patients with a negative test were responders [20].

A low total serum IgE level is a marker of type IIb autoimmune CSU and linked to non-response to omalizumab, whereas high normal or elevated total serum IgE levels, a marker of type I autoimmune CSU, are linked to complete response. Markers of type I and IIb autoimmune CSU may, therefore, be helpful to predict treatment responses to omalizumab in patients with CSU.

Treatment responses in CSU patients should be assessed and monitored with the help of validated tools. We recommend using the Urticaria Control Test (UCT) as the primary instrument to do this. The angioedema control test (AECT), the disease activity scores UAS7 and AAS, and the disease-specific quality of life tools CU-Q2oL and AE-QoL should complement the use of UCT whenever possible and as indicated. The decision to change the treatment should be based on the results obtained with these tools using established response criteria. The UCT measures disease control, and 12 or more points indicate that the disease is well controlled, 16 points reflect complete control. The UCT can be used in CSU patients with wheals who do or do not have angioedema and patients with CIndU. The AECT is used in CSU patients with angioedema, who do or do not have wheals.

12.7 Use in Pregnancy and Breast Feeding

Omalizumab is not licensed for the use in pregnant or lactating women but may be used if it is clinically necessary [1]. Real-world data on the treatment of pregnant and breastfeeding patients with CSU are limited, but they support the notion that omalizumab is effective and safe. Based on these data and the experience with the use of omalizumab in asthma, experts recommend using omalizumab during pregnancy and breastfeeding if indicated after counselling the patient on potential risks and benefits. Although omalizumab crosses the placental barrier, clinical data showed no foetal or neonatal toxicity, and in animal studies, no reproductive toxicity has been observed.

As omalizumab is an IgG antibody, it may be present in human milk and taken orally by the breastfed neonate. IgG is quickly proteolysed in the intestines, and effects on the neonate are not to be expected, which is in line with clinical data.

12.8 Home Therapy

Omalizumab, initially, was available only as a powder for solution, which had to be prepared on-site and vortexed prior to subcutaneous injection. In 2018, the European Commission approved omalizumab self-administration by the use of prefilled syringes, allowing patients with no known history of anaphylaxis to self-inject omalizumab or be injected by a trained lay-caregiver, from the fourth dose onwards, if a physician determines that this is appropriate. This decreases the treatment burden for patients and health care systems.

12.9 Future Developments

Omalizumab is an effective and safe treatment of CSU and most patients benefit from its use. In addition, omalizumab has helped to better understand the pathogenesis of CSU especially the role of IgE and its high affinity receptor. Because of this new IgE and FcεRI-targeted treatments are under development and in clinical testing. The furthest along is ligelizumab. Like omalizumab, ligelizumab (Novartis) is a humanized IgG mAb that binds specific epitopes in the C3 region of IgE and thereby blocks its interaction with FcεRI. Compared to omalizumab, ligelizumab has a higher affinity for IgE and a lower off rate as well as higher efficacy in reducing CSU disease activity. In a recent phase II randomized controlled trial, ligelizumab showed a rapid onset of effects, dose-dependent efficacy and longer time to relapse after treatment discontinuation and a good safety profile [21]. Phase III studies with ligelizumab in adults and adolescents with CSU are ongoing.

The novel long-acting IgE Trap-Fc fusion protein GI-301 (GI Innovation) also binds circulating IgE and shows higher and more durable binding to IgE than omalizumab. GI-301 is also under development for the treatment of CSU.

12.10 Current Positioning of Omalizumab in Local and International Guidelines

Since authorities' approval of omalizumab in the therapy of chronic urticaria, it has become a valuable component of therapy-resistant urticaria internationally.

Despite minor differences, all current guidelines include omalizumab as add-on therapy in antihistamine-refractory chronic spontaneous urticaria as licensed by FDA, EMA and many national authorities such as Swissmedic. While the current guideline on definition, classification, diagnosis and management of urticaria by Zuberbier et al. [22] recommends solely omalizumab as add-on therapy to antihistamines and includes ciclosporin as a further possibility in patients being non-responding to omalizumab or having contraindications or insuperable reservations against subcutaneous injection, the US Practice Parameters guideline [23] recommends omalizumab among other immunomodulating medication (Fig. 12.1). It

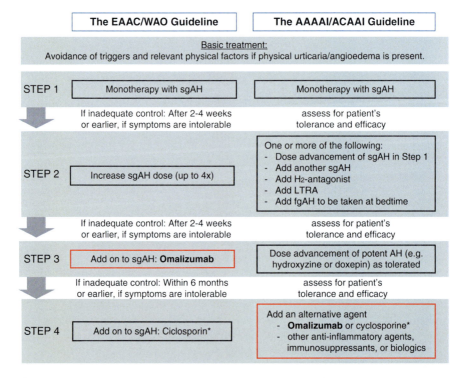

Fig. 12.1 Positioning of omalizumab in the treatment algorithms of the EAACI and the AAAAI Guidelines (Zuberbier T, Bernstein JA: A Comparison of the United States and International Perspective on Chronic Urticaria Guidelines. J Allergy Clin Immunol Pract 2018;6(4):1144–1151.)

should however be noted that the guideline by Zuberbier et al. [24] has been approved by 42 national and international societies representing 94 countries, including the UniUSA. Despite the still lacking authorization of omalizumab in the use of chronic inducible urticaria both guidelines do recommend its use also for those subtypes of chronic urticaria.

References

1. Kaplan AP, Gimenez-Arnau AM, Saini SS. Mechanisms of action that contribute to efficacy of omalizumab in chronic spontaneous urticaria. Allergy. 2017;72(4):519–33.
2. DrugBank. Omalizumab. 2020. https://www.drugbank.ca/drugs/DB00043.
3. Tabrizi MA, Tseng CM, Roskos LK. Elimination mechanisms of therapeutic monoclonal antibodies. Drug Discov Today. 2006;11(1-2):81–8.
4. EuropeanMedicinesAgency. Xolair: EPAR—Summary for the public. 2014. https://www.ema.europa.eu/en/documents/product-information/xolair-epar-product-information_en.pdf.
5. Milgrom H, Berger W, Nayak A, Gupta N, Pollard S, McAlary M, et al. Treatment of childhood asthma with anti-immunoglobulin E antibody (omalizumab). Pediatrics. 2001;108(2):E36.
6. Saini S, Rosen KE, Hsieh HJ, Wong DA, Conner E, Kaplan A, et al. A randomized, placebo-controlled, dose-ranging study of single-dose omalizumab in patients with H1-antihistamine-refractory chronic idiopathic urticaria. J Allergy Clin Immunol. 2011;128(3):567–73.e1.
7. Maurer M, Altrichter S, Bieber T, Biedermann T, Brautigam M, Seyfried S, et al. Efficacy and safety of omalizumab in patients with chronic urticaria who exhibit IgE against thyroperoxidase. J Allergy Clin Immunol. 2011;128(1):202–9.e5.
8. Saini SS, Bindslev-Jensen C, Maurer M, Grob JJ, Bulbul Baskan E, Bradley MS, et al. Efficacy and safety of omalizumab in patients with chronic idiopathic/spontaneous urticaria who remain symptomatic on H1 antihistamines: a randomized, placebo-controlled study. J Invest Dermatol. 2015;135(3):925.
9. Kaplan A, Ledford D, Ashby M, Canvin J, Zazzali JL, Conner E, et al. Omalizumab in patients with symptomatic chronic idiopathic/spontaneous urticaria despite standard combination therapy. J Allergy Clin Immunol. 2013;132(1):101–9.
10. Maurer M, Rosen K, Hsieh HJ, Saini S, Grattan C, Gimenez-Arnau A, et al. Omalizumab for the treatment of chronic idiopathic or spontaneous urticaria. N Engl J Med. 2013;368(10):924–35.
11. Maurer M, Kaplan A, Rosén K, Holden M, Iqbal A, Trzaskoma BL, et al. The XTEND-CIU study: long-term use of omalizumab in chronic idiopathic urticaria. J Allergy Clin Immunol. 2018;141(3):1138–9.
12. Sussman G, Hebert J, Gulliver W, Lynde C, Yang WH, Papp K, et al. Omalizumab re-treatment and step-up in patients with chronic spontaneous urticaria: OPTIMA trial. J Allergy Clin Immunol Pract. 2020;8(7):2372–8.e5.
13. Staubach P, Metz M, Chapman-Rothe N, Sieder C, Brautigam M, Canvin J, et al. Effect of omalizumab on angioedema in H1-antihistamine-resistant chronic spontaneous urticaria patients: results from X-ACT, a randomized controlled trial. Allergy. 2016;71(8):1135–44.
14. Metz M, Ohanyan T, Church MK, Maurer M. Omalizumab is an effective and rapidly acting therapy in difficult-to-treat chronic urticaria: a retrospective clinical analysis. J Dermatol Sci. 2014;73(1):57–62.
15. Labrador-Horrillo M, Valero A, Velasco M, Jauregui I, Sastre J, Bartra J, et al. Efficacy of omalizumab in chronic spontaneous urticaria refractory to conventional therapy: analysis of 110 patients in real-life practice. Expert Opin Biol Ther. 2013;13(9):1225–8.
16. Metz M, Ohanyan T, Church MK, Maurer M. Retreatment with omalizumab results in rapid remission in chronic spontaneous and inducible urticaria. JAMA Dermatol. 2014;150(3):288–90.

17. Turk M, Carneiro-Leao L, Kolkhir P, Bonnekoh H, Buttgereit T, Maurer M. How to treat patients with chronic spontaneous urticaria with omalizumab: questions and answers. J Allergy Clin Immunol Pract. 2020;8(1):113–24.
18. Maurer M, Metz M, Brehler R, Hillen U, Jakob T, Mahler V, et al. Omalizumab treatment in patients with chronic inducible urticaria: a systematic review of published evidence. J Allergy Clin Immunol. 2018;141(2):638–49.
19. Tharp MD, Bernstein JA, Kavati A, Ortiz B, MacDonald K, Denhaerynck K, et al. Benefits and harms of omalizumab treatment in adolescent and adult patients with chronic idiopathic (spontaneous) urticaria: a meta-analysis of "real-world" evidence. JAMA Dermatol. 2019;155(1):29–38.
20. Gericke J, Metz M, Ohanyan T, Weller K, Altrichter S, Skov PS, et al. Serum autoreactivity predicts time to response to omalizumab therapy in chronic spontaneous urticaria. J Allergy Clin Immunol. 2017;139(3):1059–61.e1.
21. Palacios T, Stillman L, Borish L, Lawrence M. Lack of basophil CD203c-upregulating activity as an immunological marker to predict response to treatment with omalizumab in patients with symptomatic chronic urticaria. J Allergy Clin Immunol Pract. 2016;4(3):529–30.
22. Maurer M, Gimenez-Arnau AM, Sussman G, Metz M, Baker DR, Bauer A, et al. Ligelizumab for chronic spontaneous urticaria. N Engl J Med. 2019;381(14):1321–32.
23. Zuberbier T, Aberer W, Asero R, Abdul Latiff AH, Baker D, Ballmer-Weber B, et al. The EAACI/GA(2)LEN/EDF/WAO guideline for the definition, classification, diagnosis and management of urticaria. Allergy. 2018;73(7):1393–414.
24. Bernstein JA, Lang DM, Khan DA, Craig T, Dreyfus D, Hsieh F, et al. The diagnosis and management of acute and chronic urticaria: 2014 update. J Allergy Clin Immunol. 2014;133(5):1270–7.

Other Interventions for Chronic Urticaria

13

Clive Grattan, Torsten Zuberbier, and Marcus Maurer

Core Messages
- In patients not responding to or having contraindications against the treatment options recommended in the guidelines, several other treatment options with low-quality evidence can be tried.
- Pharmacological interventions include oral corticosteroids, H2 antihistamines, anti-leukotrienes, immunosuppressives and the sulphone anti-inflammatories.
- Non-pharmacological interventions include diet, phototherapy and psychological assessment.

H1 antihistamines and omalizumab are currently the only licensed drugs for the treatment of chronic spontaneous urticaria. This leaves a therapeutic void for chronic urticaria patients who do not respond adequately to antihistamines or for whom omalizumab is either not available or not effective. Historically, many interventions have been used to treat urticaria off licence, most of which are still available and can be valuable for the right patients in the right circumstances. Some drugs are more likely to be effective for specific subtypes or situations and are known as 'targeted' treatments. The evidence base for many of these treatments is based on small studies, case reports, anecdotal reports or clinical experience. Particular care is required when recommending these drugs. Physicians need to be aware of potential side effects, contraindications or interaction with other medications.

Most of these interventions are summarized in Table 9 of the 2018 EAACI/GA²LEN/EDF/WAO guidelines [1]. This chapter aims to summarize the evidence

---

C. Grattan (✉)
St John's Institute of Dermatology, Guy's Hospital, London, UK
e-mail: Clive.E.Grattan@gstt.nhs.uk

T. Zuberbier · M. Maurer
Institute for Allergology, Charité – Universitätsmedizin, Berlin, Germany

Fraunhofer Institute for Translational Medicine and Pharmacology ITMP, Allergology and Immunology, Berlin, Germany
e-mail: Torsten.Zuberbier@charite.de; Marcus.Maurer@charite.de

© Springer Nature Switzerland AG 2021
T. Zuberbier et al. (eds.), *Urticaria and Angioedema*,
https://doi.org/10.1007/978-3-030-84574-2_13

and practical guidance for using unlicensed drugs and non-drug interventions, i.e. diets, phototherapy, psychotherapy and desensitization, that continue to be valuable in the real world for management of some patients with chronic urticaria in special circumstances. All low-evidence interventions should be used in conjunction with a second generation antihistamine concurrently. They should be considered when antihistamines, omalizumab and ciclosporin, alone or in combination are not available or tolerated.

13.1 Low-Evidence Pharmacological Interventions in Chronic Urticaria

13.1.1 Anti-inflammatory Sulphones

13.1.1.1 Dapsone

Dapsone is an old-fashioned sulphonamide anti-bacterial drug, which has useful properties on inflammation and is still quite widely used in Dermatology for different conditions, including chronic urticaria. It is also used as a treatment of leprosy.

Evidence for Dapsone in Urticaria

Even though dapsone is widely used for difficult urticaria there have been relatively few publications [2–4]. A study comparing a double dose of antihistamine (desloratadine) with or without dapsone 50 mg daily in CSU showed no difference in the overall disease activity when the two groups were compared at 3 months, but a few of the patients treated with dapsone remained in complete remission 3 months after finishing it (while still on the antihistamine) [5]. A chart review suggested that patients with delayed pressure urticaria responded better to dapsone than those with delayed pressure and spontaneous urticaria [6]. Another chart review in 62 CSU patients recorded a complete response in 29 (47%), with a mean time to improvement of 1.1 months and mean time to complete response of 5.2 months. Ten patients remained clear after stopping with a follow-up of 0.3–10.0 months [7]. A modest improvement was found in a placebo-controlled cross-over trial over 6 weeks. Of the 22 patients treated with dapsone, 3 showed complete resolution of hives and itch, while 31% and 41% had ≥50% resolution of hives and itch, respectively [8].

Dose and Length of Treatment

The usual starting dose is 75–100 mg of dapsone a day. This can be increased up to 150 mg daily if there are no significant side effects.

Interactions with Other Medicines

Dapsone should not usually be taken with other sulphonamides, e.g. sulphasalazine or a medicine for gout called probenecid. Concentrations in the blood increase if taken with an antibiotic called trimethoprim. It may possibly reduce the contraceptive effect of combined oral contraceptives.

13 Other Interventions for Chronic Urticaria

Checks During Treatment
Screening blood tests for anaemia, liver function and glucose-6-phosphate dehydrogenase should be done before starting dapsone. A blood count and liver function tests should be repeated a week after starting treatment, a month later and then every 3 months on treatment.

Contraindications to Treatment
Dapsone should not be taken if there is a history of reacting to sulphonamides.

Possible Side Effects of Treatment
The commonest unwanted effect is anaemia. This is more likely to be a problem at higher doses. Mild anaemia is usually unimportant, but more severe anaemia may result in becoming out of breath and feeling tired. Bluish discolouration of the lips may be apparent at high doses of dapsone due to an increase in methaemoglobin with reduced oxygen carriage and possible shortness of breath. There is a small risk of paraesthesia with long-term use although this is rare. Headache and gastrointestinal side effects may occur. A few people feel unwell 3–6 weeks after starting dapsone with fever, rash and enlarged lymph glands (dapsone hypersensitivity syndrome). The drug should be stopped immediately if this happens.

Summary
Dapsone is a useful treatment for some patterns of difficult chronic urticaria, including delayed pressure urticaria and CSU not responding to antihistamines, but the published evidence for using it is not strong. It should be taken in addition to an antihistamine. It may allow steroids to be stopped or taken at a lower dose. It is usually well tolerated but anaemia is a risk that must be checked for with blood tests before and during treatment.

13.1.1.2 Sulphasalazine
Is a long acting sulphonamide, called sulphapyridine, coupled to a derivative of salicylic acid called 5-aminosalicylic acid. It is usually used for inflammatory bowel disease, such as ulcerative colitis or Crohn's disease.

Evidence for Sulphasalazine in Urticaria
There have been reports of using sulphasalazine for severe CSU that was steroid-dependent in some patients [9, 10] and others with delayed pressure urticaria [11]. Twenty-six patients with CSU (83.9%) showed an improvement in symptoms within the first 3 months, with 51.6% of patients becoming asymptomatic within the first 6 months of starting sulphasalazine in a retrospective record review. Eleven patients (35.4%) achieved complete relief of symptoms after tapering off sulphasalazine therapy although two patients had to stop treatment because of side effects [12].

Dose and Length of Treatment
The effective dose varies between individuals. A usual starting dose might be 500 mg twice daily, increasing by 500 mg daily at intervals of 2 weeks to a maximum regular dose of 4 g (eight tablets) daily.

Possible Side Effects of Treatment
Quite a wide range of possible side effects have been described including anaemia, rashes (which may be severe), loss of appetite, dizziness and reduced sperm counts. Treatment should be stopped immediately if there is any suspicion of a serious blood disorder. This may present with bruising, infections or anaemia. Sore throat, fever, malaise or unexpected illness should be reported since these symptoms may result from side effects of the drug. Overall, about 75% of unwanted effects show themselves within 3 months of starting treatment. The urine may be coloured orange and some soft contact lenses may be stained.

Interactions with Other Medicines
Sulphasalazine should not be taken with methotrexate or azathioprine.

Checks During Treatment
Bone marrow, kidney and liver function should be checked with a blood test before starting treatment and then monthly for the first 3 months. Checks can be less frequent after this: once every 3 months should be sufficient while treatment continues, provided there are no problems. Glucose-6-phosphate dehydrogenase should also be checked before making a decision to start sulphasalazine.

Reasons for Avoiding It
Sulphasalazine should be avoided if there is a previous history of adverse reactions to sulphonamides or aspirin. It should only be used during pregnancy and breast feeding if there is no alternative.

Summary
Sulphasalazine may be useful for CSU and delayed pressure urticaria but does carry some risks of unwanted effects that may be serious and needs to be monitored.

13.1.2 Tranexamic Acid

Tranexamic acid exerts its antifibrinolytic activity by inhibiting plasmin, which breaks down clots. It is mainly used to treat women with heavy periods.

13.1.2.1 Evidence for Tranexamic Acid in Urticaria
Although a trial of tranexamic acid for chronic urticaria patients seemed to show no benefit [13], clinical experience indicates that the treatment may be effective for a few patients with unexplained ('idiopathic') nonhistaminergic angioedema,

especially those without wheals [13, 14]. Its use has been endorsed in recent guidelines on urticaria [15].

13.1.2.2 Dose and Length of Treatment

The dose of tranexamic acid for angioedema varies between patients. Daily doses range from 0.5 to 4.5 g daily with most patients finding the right balance at 1½–3 g a day. There is no limit to the length of time tranexamic acid can be taken.

13.1.2.3 Possible Side Effects of Treatment

The most likely side effects are nausea, vomiting and diarrhoea at large doses. Treatment should be stopped if changes in colour vision develop or a thrombosis occurs.

13.1.2.4 Interactions with Other Medicines

Tranexamic acid should not be taken at the same time as other medicines that promote clotting, such as epsilon aminocaproic acid.

13.1.2.5 Checks During Treatment

No checks are necessary when tranexamic acid is taken for less than 3 months. Blood testing for liver function and regular eye checks are recommended by the manufacturer for patients on long-term treatment of hereditary angioedema.

13.1.2.6 Contraindications to Treatment

The medicine should not be taken if there is a history of thromboembolic disease and should be used with caution in patients receiving oral contraceptives or on a background of ischaemic heart disease.

13.1.2.7 Summary

Tranexamic acid may be useful for some patients with unexplained recurrent angioedema who have not responded to usual treatments with antihistamines and short courses of steroid tablets. The treatment should not be taken by patients who have had thrombosis and should be stopped immediately if thrombosis or changes in colour vision develop.

13.1.3 Montelukast

Montelukast is a cysteinyl leukotriene (LTD4, E4, C4) inhibitor. It binds with high affinity and selectivity to the CysLT1 receptor. Symptoms of urticaria are mainly due to histamine release from mast cells in the skin. Failure to respond to an antihistamine may be due to other mediators of inflammation, including leukotrienes generated at the time of histamine release. The development of cysteinyl leukotriene receptor antagonists for asthma (also known as antileukotrienes) has provided an opportunity to try these medicines for chronic urticaria that does not respond well to antihistamine treatment alone. Montelukast is now the only antileukotriene available in Europe. By contrast, zileuton is an orally active inhibitor of 5-lipoxygenase that inhibits leukotriene (LTB4, LTC4, LTD4 and LTE4) formation that is only available in the USA. There are no studies of zileuton in chronic urticaria but, in theory, it might be effective. Antileukotrienes, when used, should be given with an antihistamine.

13.1.3.1 Evidence for Using Montelukast in Urticaria

Encouraging results have been seen in patients with aspirin-sensitive urticaria treated [16], delayed pressure urticaria [17] and CSU with predominant angioedema [18, 19], but CSU patients without angioedema may also benefit [20–22]. There have been anecdotal reports of patients with autoreactive CSU [23] and cold urticaria [24] improving, but this needs to be confirmed with well-designed clinical studies.

13.1.3.2 Dose and Length of Treatment

The daily adult dose of montelukast is 10 mg. It is usually taken at bedtime. The medicine may start to have a useful effect within a week, but the benefit seems to increase for up to 6 weeks [20]. There is probably no advantage in going beyond this if it has not worked by then. There is no time limit to treatment, but it is always good practice to try stopping medicines periodically to see if they are still needed.

13.1.3.3 Possible Side Effects of Treatment

Bowel symptoms, fever, headache, nausea, vomiting and increased upper respiratory tract infections may occur but there are no predictable unwanted effects from taking montelukast and it is usually well tolerated. A range of other possible side effects has been reported including anxiety, depression, dizziness, dry mouth, muscle and joint complaints and sleep disorders including dream abnormalities and nightmares (especially in children) so it is best not to increase the dose above 10 mg a day in adults and the approved dose in children. Urticaria has been reported as a side effect.

13.1.3.4 Interactions with Other Medicines and Reasons for Avoiding It

There are no important interactions with other medicines. It should not be used in pregnancy or during breastfeeding unless essential. A very rare condition of the lungs, called Churg-Strauss syndrome, may be more likely to develop in asthmatics.

13.1.3.5 Checks During Treatment

No regular checks are recommended by the manufacturer.

13.1.3.6 Summary

Montelukast blocks leukotrienes, which may contribute to the development of signs and symptoms of urticaria in some patients. It appears to work best for aspirin-sensitive chronic urticaria. It may be helpful for some patients with CSU including those with angioedema, delayed pressure urticaria. A single daily dose appears to be safe and well tolerated. It can be taken as long as it helps (with an antihistamine). It will probably not work if it has not done so within 6 weeks.

13.1.4 H2 Antihistamines

Several H2 antihistamines are available. Ranitidine was the most widely used in the context of treating chronic urticaria but is currently not available in the EU and the US because an impurity (NDMA) has been identified that may have pro-carcinogenic properties in humans pending further investigation. Cimetidine was little used until the withdrawal of ranitidine since it may interfere with hepatic metabolism of other drugs (including some H1 antihistamines) and has anti-androgenic effects, including gynaecomastia but famotidine remains available without these risks. Skin testing with H1 and H2 analogues in healthy volunteers showed that H2 receptors in skin cause vasodilatation (erythema) and whealing but not flare [25]. Blockade of H1 and H2 receptors with chlorphenamine and cimetidine, respectively, resulted in significant histamine skin test weal suppression that was non-significantly greater with combined treatment [26].

13.1.4.1 Evidence for Using H2 Antihistamines in Urticaria

Total symptom score was significantly less with cimetidine and chlorphenamine than placebo and chlorphenamine in patients with chronic idiopathic urticaria (syn. CSU) not responding to chlorphenamine alone at 4 and 8 weeks [27]. A similar outcome was found with hydroxyzine and cimetidine [28]. In a study of symptomatic dermographism, the addition of ranitidine to cetirizine raised the threshold for a whealing response, but it did not improve symptoms overall [29]. A Cochrane review of H2 antihistamines in urticaria concluded that it did not allow confident decision-making about the use of H2-receptor antagonists for urticaria. Although some of the studies reported a measure of relief of symptoms of urticaria and rather minimal clinical improvement in some of the participants, the evidence was regarded as weak and unreliable [30]. A subsequent small randomized double-blind placebo-controlled study of patients with CSU found no benefit from adding ranitidine to cetirizine but was underpowered [31]. Clinical experience, nevertheless, suggests that combining H2 antihistamines with a second generation H1 antihistamine may be beneficial in some patients with chronic urticaria, despite the lack of confirmatory large placebo-controlled trials. There are no publications on the use of famotidine in chronic urticaria.

13.1.5 Immunosuppressives

Immunosuppressives have been used successfully as an adjunct to antihistamines for severe CSU since the demonstration of functional histamine releasing autoantibodies in some patients in the late 1980s giving rise to the concept of autoimmune urticaria. Ciclosporin has been the most widely used and studied.

13.1.5.1 Ciclosporin

Ciclosporin was isolated originally from a fungus (Hypocladium inflatum gams). It is a powerful immunosuppressive, inhibiting T cell activation by blocking lymphokines including interleukin-2. It also inhibits histamine release from basophils. This may be one of the reasons it can be useful for severe urticaria even when autoantibodies cannot be demonstrated. It is included in the 2018 EAACI/GA2LENWAO/EDF guideline treatment algorithm for chronic urticaria as a fourth line intervention in patients who fail omalizumab [1].

Evidence for Using Ciclosporin in Urticaria

Studies of ciclosporin in severe CSU [32–34] have shown that about 2/3 of patients clear on treatment but the condition often relapses on stopping. In a recent systematic review of 18 studies including 2 randomized controlled trials, the overall response rate to treatment with ciclosporin (2–5 mg/kg) at 4, 8 and 12 weeks was 54%, 66% and 73%, respectively [35]. About 25% of patients who cleared after treatment with ciclosporin at 4 mg/kg body weight for 4–8 weeks were still clear on an antihistamine 5 months later [34]. Some patients with symptomatic dermographism also benefit [36]. Another systematic review of the literature indicated that a positive baseline autologous serum skin test, basophil histamine release assay or basophil activation test, elevated baseline plasma D-dimer levels and low total IgE predict a good response to treatment [37].

Dose and Length of Treatment

There is still discussion about the best dose of ciclosporin and how long it should be taken. 38 Starting at 4 mg/kg body weight/day for 4 weeks, reducing to 3 mg/kg/day for 6 weeks and then 2 mg/kg/day for a final 6 weeks works for many patients. Lower doses taken for 5 months may also be effective [38]. More than one course of ciclosporin may be given although it is probably better to look at other therapies if this proves necessary. Long-term treatment with immunosuppressive therapies for over a year should only be undertaken when there is no reasonable alternative because there are potential concerns about encouraging infections, lymphomas and skin cancers. A review of the safety and effectiveness of ciclosporin taken at low doses for up to 10 years in one centre was favourable [39].

Possible Side Effects of Treatment

Among patients treated with <2 mg/kg, 2–<4 mg/kg and 4–5 mg/kg of ciclosprin, 6%, 23% and 57% experienced one or more adverse event, respectively [35]. The main risks are hypertension, renal impairment and predisposition to infections. Hyperkalaemia and increased lipids may occur. Some side effects of ciclosporin are more unpleasant than dangerous. They include slight tremor, burning sensations of the hands and feet, and swelling of the gums, nausea, muscle weakness, missed periods and increased facial hair growth, which settle on stopping treatment. The effectiveness and safety of some immunizations may be reduced and live vaccines should not be given for 3 months after stopping treatment.

13 Other Interventions for Chronic Urticaria

Checks Before and During Treatment

The most important checks are on renal function, which may go down and blood pressure, which may go up. It is usual to check kidney function with two separate blood tests before starting treatment, every fortnight for the first month and then monthly. Blood pressure should be checked at the same time. Liver function should be checked on blood tests before, and every month on treatment because mild reversible inflammation may occur. Viral hepatitis and HIV infection should be excluded when there is clinical suspicion before starting treatment.

It is important to decide who will make these checks and who will be responsible for acting on any abnormal results. It is common practice to have 'shared care' agreements between primary care practitioners and hospitals, or hospital departments with each other. These should be worked out before treatment is started. Women of childbearing age should have a pregnancy test before starting and ensure adequate contraception throughout treatment and for 2 weeks after finishing. Breastfeeding should be avoided.

Interactions with Other Medicines

Some medicines may increase the level of ciclosporin in the blood including some antibiotics, painkillers (e.g. aspirin, ibuprofen), a treatment for gout (allopurinol) and some blood pressure treatments (e.g. nifedipine, diltiazem). Grapefruit juice can also do this. Other drugs reduce the levels of ciclosporin, such as some anticonvulsants (e.g. phenytoin, carbamazepine). It is recommended that St John's wort should not be taken at the same time. There may be an increased risk of muscle inflammation with statins.

Cautions and Contraindications

The main reasons for not using ciclosporin would be reduced kidney function, uncontrolled blood pressure, active serious infections and previous cancers.

Summary

Ciclosporin is a useful treatment for many patients with severe and disabling chronic urticaria. A decision to start it must only be taken after trying other medicines, including antihistamines, and arrangements for careful monitoring must be in place.

13.1.5.2 Methotrexate

Is used in low doses as an immunosuppressive drug for a number of conditions including psoriasis and rheumatoid arthritis. It has also been found to help patients with severe chronic urticaria, especially when they would otherwise have to take regular steroids to control their symptoms or they are unable to tolerate other immunosuppressive therapies, such as ciclosporin. Methotrexate is a derivative of folic acid, known as an antifolate, which interferes with dihydrofolate reductase and the production of DNA in actively dividing cells.

Evidence for Using Methotrexate in Urticaria
There have only been a few reports of methotrexate being used successfully for chronic urticaria [40–43]. One controlled studies comparing it against placebo for 3 months five showed no benefit but the duration of treatment was probably too short since methotrexate is usually administered long term. Clinical experience, however, has shown that it may be valuable for selected urticaria patients who do not respond to antihistamine treatment, including those who would otherwise need steroids.

Dose and Length of Treatment
A small test dose of methotrexate is usually given to check it is suitable before beginning regular treatment at a higher dose. It is essential to take the medicine only once a week rather than daily to minimize the risk of myelosuppression. The benefit is not immediate. It may take 4–6 weeks to begin working. There is no definite limit on the length of time methotrexate can be taken, provided that there are no complications. It is common practice to recommend that Methotrexate is taken on Mondays and Folic acid on Fridays as a useful 'aide memoire' or folic acid on each day that is not the methotrexate day.

Possible Side effects of Treatment
Sore throats, bad mouth ulcers or unusual bruising may be a sign of reduced bone marrow function, mandating an urgent blood count. Pneumonitis may occur occasionally with prolonged treatment, especially in the rheumatoid disease population. Methotrexate should be stopped if a persistent dry cough or unexplained breathlessness develops until the possibility of pneumonitis due to the drug has been investigated. Alcohol can be more damaging to the liver than usual when on methotrexate. It should be avoided completely if possible during treatment. Nausea may be a problem for a day or two after taking methotrexate in some people but can often be reduced by taking an anti-sickness medicine beforehand, such as prochlorperazine, dividing the dose over 36 h or administering the treatment subcutaneously.

Checks Before and During Treatment
Blood must be checked for bone marrow, kidney and liver function before starting methotrexate. Viral hepatitis and HIV infection should be excluded. It is good practice to have a baseline chest X-ray. Blood counts and liver function tests must be checked weekly for the first month, fortnightly for a month and then monthly as long as the treatment continues. It is important to decide who will make these checks and who will be responsible for acting on any abnormal results. Women of childbearing age must check that they are not pregnant with a pregnancy test before starting and ensure adequate contraception throughout treatment. Pregnancy and fathering children should be avoided for 6 months after finishing. Breastfeeding should be avoided during treatment. Keeping a personal booklet for methotrexate monitoring is recommended.

Interactions with Other Medicines
There are several types of medicine that should be taken with care or avoided:

1. Aspirin and other non-steroidal anti-inflammatory drugs (e.g. ibuprofen, diclofenac): these may reduce elimination of methotrexate by the kidneys and increase the levels of methotrexate in the body.
2. Antibacterials: some antibiotics can increase the risks of methotrexate affecting myelopoiesis. Examples of this include trimethoprim, co-trimoxazole and penicillins.
3. Others: some medicines taken for inflammatory bowel disease (e.g. sulphasalazine), malaria (e.g. pyrimethamine), gout (e.g. probenecid) and epilepsy (e.g. phenytoin).

Cautions and Contraindications
Methotrexate should not normally be used if there is an underlying blood disorder, reduced kidney function, persistent liver inflammation, peptic ulceration or ulcerative colitis.

Summary
Methotrexate is a potentially useful treatment for some patients with disabling chronic urticaria who have not responded to guideline treatments and would otherwise need steroids to control it. Its use must be monitored closely with regular blood tests and some medicines should not be taken at the same time. Symptoms of infection, including bad sore throats, may be important and usually mean that the blood should be checked and methotrexate discontinued temporarily.

13.1.5.3 Mycophenolate Mofetil
Is an immune suppressing drug used primarily for the prevention of organ transplant rejection. It is also used for some severe skin diseases, including blistering disorders. It works by reducing the formation of lymphocytes that are involved in autoimmune conditions.

Evidence for Using Mycophenolate in Urticaria
There have only been two studies published to date. Nine patients with evidence of autoimmune CSU who had not been controlled on antihistamines and courses of steroids were treated with mycophenolate for 12 weeks [44]. Four cleared completely and five improved. The improvement was still present 6 months later. A later study involving chart review looked at the results of a step-up followed by a step-down approach to using mycophenolate for CSU. The average time to achieve disease control was 14 weeks at doses of mycophenolate ranging from 1 to 6 g daily [45]. As is the case for other low level evidence interventions, mycophenolate should only be used in selected patients when other treatments, including antihistamines, omalizumab and ciclosporin, alone or in combination, have failed or have not been well tolerated.

Dose and Length of Treatment
The starting dose is usually 1g of mycophenolate twice a day, but it may be necessary to increase this up to 1.5 g twice daily (maximum). The initial course of treatment should be for 3 months but longer periods may be appropriate for some patients.

Possible Side effects of Treatment
Mycophenolate is generally safe and well tolerated when used in short courses for urticaria. A number of important side effects have been reported in patients taking it in combination with other immunosuppressives to prevent transplant rejection, including infections (including pneumonia, cold sores, thrush and shingles), gastrointestinal symptoms (including abdominal pain, diarrhoea and nausea) anxiety, tremor and headache. The effectiveness of some vaccines may be reduced and live vaccines should not be given for 3 months after stopping treatment.

Interactions with Other Medicines
There are relatively few interactions with other medicines. The blood levels of mycophenolate may be affected by other immune suppressing drugs given at the same time, but this mainly applies to transplant patients. Other drugs that may affect the levels of mycophenolate include cholestyramine and rifampicin. Oral contraceptives are not affected.

Checks During Treatment
A full blood count should be checked weekly for the first month, fortnightly for the next 2 months and then monthly. Blood must be tested for liver function once every month.

Contraindications to Treatment
Mycophenolate must be avoided during pregnancy since it can cause birth defects. Women of child-bearing age should be on effective contraception throughout treatment. It should also be avoided during breast feeding. It should be stopped if severe infections, such as pneumonia or chickenpox develop. Immune suppressing drugs, such as mycophenolate, should not be used if there is a past history of cancer.

Summary
There is only limited evidence that mycophenolate can improve the symptoms of patients with severe CSU. It has a number of important risks when it is used with other immune suppressing treatments in transplant patients, but appears to be safe and well tolerated in chronic urticaria.

13.1.5.4 Azathioprine

Azathioprine is an immune suppressing drug that has been used for serious immune skin conditions for many years including blistering disorders and atopic eczema. Azathioprine is an imidazole derivative of 6-mercaptopurine (6-MP). It is rapidly broken down *in vivo* into 6-MP. 6-MP readily crosses cell membranes and is converted intracellularly into a number of purine thioanalogues. It reduces the number and function of T and B-cells.

Evidence for Using Azathioprine in Urticaria
Azathioprine has been used occasionally for patients with difficult chronic urticaria who would otherwise need systemic steroids. Steroids were withdrawn in two patients with chronic urticaria after treatment with azathioprine [46]. It was found to be as effective as ciclosporin for CSU in a recent randomized comparison [47].

Dose and Length of Treatment
The daily dose is based on body weight. Treatment usually starts at 2 mg/kg body weight per day but may need to go up or down a little from this. The tablets are taken two or three times a day. It is common practice to start them with steroids for the first 3 weeks and then continue without steroids for 3–6 months, but azathioprine can be used in other ways. The benefits of azathioprine seem to continue for months after stopping treatment in many patients with eczema, and the same may be true for urticaria.

Possible Side Effects of Treatment
The most important side effects are bone marrow suppression and liver inflammation. Malaise, aching, fevers or vomiting may occur rarely in the first week or two of treatment. Azathioprine must be stopped immediately if unexplained bruising, bleeding or serious infections develop. The effectiveness of some vaccines may be reduced and live vaccines should not be given for 3 months after stopping treatment. Total sunblocks should be worn in strong sunlight as a precaution to minimize any risk of skin cancers developing later in life.

Interactions with Other Medicines
Azathioprine should not be taken at the same time as other medicines that suppress the immune system unless essential, and the treatment must be monitored closely. Concomitant therapy with ACE-inhibitors, trimethoprim/sulphamethoxazole, cimetidine or indomethacin increases the risk of myelosuppression.

Checks During Treatment
Thiopurine methyltransferase (TPMT) should be checked before starting treatment and blood must be monitored regularly for bone marrow and liver function. The general rule is that blood tests should be done weekly for the first month, fortnightly for a month and then monthly.

Contraindications to Treatment
In common with all immune-suppressing drugs, azathioprine should be avoided if cancer has been treated in the past, including melanoma. It should also be avoided in pregnancy unless essential and in patients who have had previous bad reactions to it. It should not be used in patients who have had HIV or hepatitis B or C infection without careful assessment.

Summary

Azathioprine may be used occasionally for very severe CSU that has not responded to antihistamine treatment and would otherwise need regular steroids to control it. The treatment must be monitored carefully with blood tests and is usually given for 3–6 months.

13.1.6 Miscellaneous

13.1.6.1 Doxepin

Doxepin, a tricyclic antidepressant, has been used as a treatment for urticaria since the 1980s. It has potent H1 and H2 antihistaminic properties. It also has anticholinergic and anti-serotoninergic effects. The doses of doxepin used for depression are usually much higher than those used for urticaria. There is unlikely to be any mood lifting effect when taken for urticaria although it may be helpful if depression is also a problem. Doxepin may be most valuable when taken at night if sleep is disturbed by itching or swellings.

Evidence for Using Doxepin in Urticaria

Doxepin was found to be more effective than diphenhydramine at a dose of 10 mg three times a day [48] and as effective as mequitazine at a dose of 5 mg twice daily [49]. It has not been compared against modern non-sedating antihistamines.

Dose and Length of Treatment

It is best to start at the lowest dose which is 25 mg at night with an option of working up to 75 mg daily. This can either be taken as a single dose at night or split into two or three smaller doses over the day. The highest total daily dose recommended for depression is 300 mg with a maximum single dose of 100 mg but these very high levels are probably never appropriate for urticaria. There is no time limit for which doxepin can be taken.

Possible Side Effects of Treatment

Sedation is the commonest unwanted effect. A dry mouth and blurring of vision are more likely as the dose increases. Other side effects may include constipation, difficulty in passing water, feeling light headed on standing up quickly, increased appetite, rashes and some rare changes in the blood. There may be heart complications in the elderly with pre-existing cardiac disease.

Interactions with Other Medicines

One of the disadvantages of doxepin is the high number of possible interactions with other medicines (and alcohol too). These include other antidepressants, certain strong painkillers (e.g. tramadol), some drugs for heart rhythm problems (e.g. amiodarone), drugs for epilepsy and some antihypertensives (e.g. diltiazem). A few treatments that may be used for urticaria, such as epinephrine and cimetidine, should be avoided concurrently if possible.

Cautions and Contraindications
Doxepin should not be taken after a recent heart attack or in severe liver disease. It should be used with caution in pregnancy and the elderly since it may cause confusion, unwanted falls in blood pressure on standing up, glaucoma of the eyes and difficulty passing water.

Checks During Treatment
No routine checks are required.

Summary
Doxepin has been used to treat difficult urticaria for about 30 years. It has a number of side effects, which tend to increase with the dose and interactions with other medicines, which need to be considered carefully before starting.

13.1.6.2 Epinephrine
The use of epinephrine, in chronic urticaria, is limited to the treatment of patients with cold urticaria who develop anaphylaxis or angioedema of the upper airways after cold liquids. Patients with cold urticaria, who are at risk of anaphylaxis or angioedema of the throat should carry two epinephrine autoinjectors but this is rare [50]. Although some patients with severe episodes of CSU describe a feeling of tightness or scratchiness in the throat, they can be reassured that throat closure is not a feature of the illness. By contrast, throat angioedema is a feature of anaphylaxis and may be experienced in very severe acute urticaria.

Evidence for Using Epinephrine in Histaminergic Angioedema
There are no studies of epinephrine for throat angioedema or anaphylaxis in cold urticaria, but it is known to work well.

Dose and Method of Administration
Epinephrine injections for self-administration are available on prescription in preloaded syringes that deliver a single dose. The standard adult dose is 300 μg. A 500 μg injector is also available. Junior pens are available for children weighing 15–30 kg, which deliver 150 μg. A second dose may be necessary if the swelling has not started to go down within 5 min.

An over-the-counter epinephrine 'puffer' spray for asthma may be used for angioedema of the throat but is currently only available in the USA. The aerosol should be puffed 4–5 times directly onto the swelling in the throat and not inhaled (as directed for asthma attacks) or sprayed underneath the tongue (unless it is too swollen). The same number of puffs can be repeated after 5–10 min. An epinephrine injection can still be given if the swelling worsens despite the inhaler.

Possible Side Effects of Treatment
Epinephrine can be life-saving in an emergency but may also raise blood pressure, cause anxiety and shaking and make the skin look pale. These effects wear off within an hour and usually present no problems. However, they may be risky for a

few people with poorly controlled high blood pressure, angina or those who are at risk of stroke.

Interactions with Other Medicines
Intramuscular epinephrine should ideally not be used at the same time as taking tricyclic antidepressants (e.g. amitriptyline, doxepin), beta-blockers (e.g. propranolol, atenolol) or angiotensin converting enzyme inhibitors (e.g. ramipril, captopril) but should be always be given in a life-threatening situation if other measures have failed.

Summary
Epinephrine is a valuable treatment for severe swelling of the tongue or throat and may be life-saving. It is usually given by intramuscular injection but it may be used as a puffer spray for throat or tongue angioedema. There are important potential interactions with tricyclic antidepressants and beta blockers. Patients with pre-existing angina and high blood pressure are at risk of exacerbation.

13.1.7 Steroids

13.1.7.1 Anabolic Steroids
Anabolic steroids are different to corticosteroids (e.g. prednisolone). Danazol is an example of an anabolic steroid. It is a synthetic steroid with properties of a weak androgen. It has complicated effects on sex hormone production and can be used for gynaecological conditions, including endometriosis. It also increases plasma proteins in the blood and may be used to treat hereditary angioedema where there is a deficiency of C1 inhibitor. It may work in cholinergic urticaria in a similar way, since a protease inhibitor called alpha-1-antichymotrypsin was found to be reduced.

13.1.7.2 Danazol

Evidence for Danazol in Cholinergic Urticaria
The level of alpha-1-antichymotrypsin increased with danazol treatment and wheal counts decreased over 4 weeks in a placebo-controlled study [51]. Several cases of patients with cholinergic urticaria responding to danazol have been reported [51, 52].

Details and Length of Treatment
Danazol is no longer available in many countries. Treatment can be continued for months or years if necessary at the lowest dose that controls symptoms. Danazol should be taken with an antihistamine. Although adverse effects are common in the HAE population on prolonged treatment, clinical experience shows that it is well tolerated in the short term (3–6 months) at doses between 200 and 600 mg daily in the cholinergic urticaria population and may allow re-establishment of symptom control with an antihistamine alone in some responders.

Possible Side Effects of Treatment
Up to 80% of patients treated with danazol in an HAE population can be expected to develop side effects in the long term, the most common ones being weight gain, virilization and menstrual disorders as well as headache, myalgia, depression and acne. There is also an increased risk of cardiovascular disease. Because of its androgenizing effects, it should be avoided or given at least doses in females. Pregnancy must be avoided. Abnormalities of liver function and lipoproteins may occur. Benign adenomas, rashes, muscle aches, depression, fatigue and changes in libido have been reported. It is not recommended in children or the elderly.

Checks Before and During Treatment
A full blood count, liver function tests and lipid profile should be done at baseline with repeat liver profile and cholesterol at 3 months. A blood count, liver profile and cholesterol should be repeated with every 6 months of continuous treatment. A liver ultrasound scan is advised every 2–3 years on long-term treatment.

Interactions with Other Medicines
Danazol may affect the plasma level of carbamazepine and other anticonvulsants. It can cause insulin resistance, potentiate the action of warfarin and oppose the action of anti-hypertensive agents, possibly through fluid retention. Taking statins metabolized by CYP3A4 (e.g. simvastatin) at the same time increases a risk of myopathy.

Cautions and Contraindications
Danazol must be avoided in pregnancy and breastfeeding, in patients with significantly impaired hepatic, renal or cardiac function and with active thrombosis.

Summary
Danazol can be considered in the short term for severe treatment-resistant cholinergic urticaria when high dose antihistamines are not effective. It is generally more suited to men since virilizing side effects in women may be unacceptable. Monitoring with blood tests is mandatory.

13.1.7.3 Corticosteroids (Steroids)
Oral steroids have been used for many years to treat severe urticaria that does not respond to antihistamines. They are useful acutely because they nearly always work if the dose is right. Larger doses given for longer (e.g. 20 mg prednisolone daily for a month) are immunosuppressive. The problem with steroids is the risk of unwanted effects if they are taken for many weeks or months without a break. They may also reduce the ability of the body to produce natural steroid (cortisol), which is essential for good health. Several different types of steroid tablets can be used. The usual one is prednisolone, which comes in plain, coated and soluble forms. Other oral formulations include prednisone (precursor of prednisolone), methyl prednisolone, betamethasone, dexamethasone and hydrocortisone.

Evidence for Using Corticosteroids in Chronic Urticaria

There is only one prospective study of prednisone for CSU, mainly because steroids were introduced before the era of evidence-based medicine [53]. About 50% of patients with antihistamine-unresponsive CSU responded well to prednisone starting at the relatively low dose of 25 mg for 3 days, 12.5 mg for 3 days, reducing to 6.25 mg/day over 4 days, but many relapsed despite antihistamines after stopping. There is a need for good studies to show how long they should be taken and the best dose.

Dose and Length of Treatment

Clinical experience has shown that taking prednisolone at around ½ mg per kilogram body weight (usually 25–40 mg daily in adults) for 1–3 days can be very helpful for the most severe attacks of urticaria or bad attacks of angioedema as 'rescue' treatment. There is little risk from doing so provided the courses are not repeated too often. Long courses of continuous steroids must generally be avoided although there may be special situations when this might be necessary in some people, such as delayed pressure urticaria that cannot be controlled in other ways. There are many ways of prescribing steroids but it is usually appropriate to reduce the dose slowly after being on them continuously for more than 3 weeks, especially if treatment has been taken for months.

Possible Side Effects of Treatment

Short courses of steroids can sometimes make people feel more energetic and wakeful, but this does not last for more than a few days. This is why steroids are usually taken in the morning to reduce wakefulness at night. It is common to feel lacking in energy as the dose comes down after a long course of treatment. There is a tendency to gain weight, unless care is taken to prevent this, and to lose muscle strength. The skin and bones may become weaker. Spots, increased body and facial hair growth and bruises may be more likely. Serious infections, such as chickenpox in adults, may be more harmful and measures may be necessary to give protection. Some vaccinations may not 'take' well and others may not be safe. Increased blood pressure and sugar diabetes may be promoted. Stopping steroids suddenly after a long period of time can lead to low blood pressure and faintness. They should therefore be reduced cautiously on medical advice after a long course of treatment.

Interactions with Other Medicines and Reasons for Being Careful

Steroids can usually be taken safely with other medicines except aspirin and other non-steroidal anti-inflammatory drugs (e.g. ibuprofen) because there is an increased risk of gastric bleeding. They should be used with care in diabetics and patients with stomach ulcers, high blood pressure and osteoporosis. Prolonged courses of corticosteroids increase susceptibility to infections and severity of infection. Patients who have never had chickenpox should be regarded as being at risk of severe infection.

Checks During Treatment
No checks are usually needed when steroids are taken for 10 days or less. It is good practice to check weight, urine (for sugar) and blood pressure in the clinic when steroids are taken regularly for weeks. Bone density scans (DEXA) should be done if steroids have to be taken for at least 6 months. Steroids should only be prescribed in the first trimester of pregnancy if essential because of concerns about abnormalities developing in the baby although they are generally very safe.

Summary
Oral corticosteroids may be necessary for the most difficult forms of urticaria but should only be taken for the shortest period necessary and at the least dose. Rescue prednisolone for one to three days can be taken in addition to antihistamines for severe urticaria outbreaks, including angioedema. Steroids should not be stopped suddenly after 6 weeks and the dose should be agreed with the specialist or GP.

13.1.8 Anticoagulants

There is a small literature on anticoagulants being effective in CSU, possibly relating to the observed activation of the extrinsic (tissue factor) pathway in chronic urticaria with increased D-Dimer and prothrombin fragment F1+2 formation being related to disease severity [54]. However the risks of anticoagulation are significant.

13.1.8.1 Heparin
A patient with treatment refractory CSU not responding to warfarin cleared completely with subcutaneous heparin given for an unrelated reason [55]. A small cohort of antihistamine-resistant CSU patients with elevated D-dimer improved with heparin and tranexamic acid [56].

13.1.8.2 Warfarin
There have been several case reports of CSU responding to warfarin. A small crossover study appeared to confirm this [57]. The same patient responded to two different coumarin anticoagulants including warfarin, suggesting a class benefit [58].

13.1.9 Antineutrophilic Drugs

13.1.9.1 Colchicine
Is mainly used in the context of neutrophilic urticaria, normocomplementaemic urticarial vasculitis and neutrophilic urticarial dermatoses but one retrospective review found that it might be helpful in chronic urticaria [59].

13.1.9.2 Biologicals

There is increasing enthusiasm to identify biological drugs to treat patients with chronic urticaria who do not respond to H1 antihistamines and omalizumab but only a few small studies and case reports have been published to date. The evidence is generally insufficient to justify the risks and costs of biological agents other than omalizumab for chronic urticaria at the present time.

13.1.9.3 Anakinra

Benefit has been reported in a case of cold contact urticaria with positive ice cube test and negative NLRP3 mutation [60] and in refractory delayed pressure urticaria [61]. By contrast, anakinra is the treatment of choice for Schnitzler syndrome and may be used in other autoinflammatory disorders presenting with urticarial rash.

13.1.9.4 Anti-TNFs

A case report [62] and open series suggest that etanercept [63], adalimumab [64] or infliximab [65] may be useful for treatment refractory CSU, especially cases that do not respond to omalizumab.

13.1.9.5 Rituximab

Although depletion of B-cells and reduction of functional autoantibodies are theoretically desirable as a way of providing long-term control of autoimmune urticaria rare reports of severe risk including progressive multifocal encephalopathy make this option unattractive. Case reports indicate that it may [66] or may not [67] be effective for CSU.

Treatment with the monoclonal antibodies secukinumab, mepolizumab, benralizumab, reslizumab and dupilumab has also been reported to benefit patients with chronic urticaria anecdotally.

13.1.10 Immunosuppressives (Other than Ciclosporin, Methotrexate, Azathioprine and Mycophenolate Mofetil)

Tacrolimus and cyclophosphamide have been reported in treatment refractory chronic urticaria in addition to the more commonly used immunosuppressive options. The evidence for using them is less and there does not appear to be a clear advantage. Cyclophosphamide carries additional risks of haemorrhagic cystitis, secondary tumours and infertility when given intravenously and should probably be avoided.

13.1.10.1 Tacrolimus

Two open series indicate a similar response rate to ciclosporin with complete resolution in some patients [68, 69].

13.1.10.2 Cyclophosphamide

Case reports have documented good outcomes with oral [70] and intravenous treatment [71].

13.1.11 Immunomodulators

Recognition that some patients have an autoimmune aetiology has promoted the use of immunomodulatory drugs as well as immunosuppressives to optimize safety. Reports to date have been encouraging but do not support the routine use of these products.

13.1.11.1 Hydroxychloroquine
A placebo-controlled study showed an improvement in quality of life of patients with CSU but no overall improvement in disease activity [72] but a later study showed a lower proportion of therapeutic failures [73].

13.1.11.2 Intravenous Immunoglobulins
There have been no double-blind studies to date but open studies suggest benefit [74–76]. However, the risk of infusion reactions, including aseptic meningitis, and relative shortage of IVIG in some communities mean that this option should only be used in exceptional cases.

13.1.11.3 Plasmapheresis
Was used as a proof of concept that functional autoantibodies were potentially pathogenic in a small case series [77]. Although it has been adopted successfully in clinical practice since then it is not very practical in the long term as urticaria relapses when autoantibodies recover weeks after treatment cessation.

13.1.12 Vitamin D

Reports of vitamin D deficiency correction in chronic urticaria leading to improvement in disease activity are interesting [78, 79], but a recent systematic review concluded that although high dose vitamin D supplementation for 4–12 weeks might help to decrease the disease activity in some CSU patients, well-designed randomized placebo-controlled studies are now needed to determine the cut-off levels of vitamin D for supplementation and treatment outcomes [80].

13.2 Non-drug Interventions

13.2.1 Diet

Although IgE-mediated food allergy is a rare underlying cause of chronic spontaneous urticaria (CSU), there are some patients in which pseudoallergic reactions to naturally occurring food ingredients or food additives have been observed. When in doubt, a pseudoallergen-free diet should be tried. Diet protocols containing low levels of natural as well as artificial food pseudoallergens are available and have been successfully used in different countries. Also, a low histamine diet may improve symptoms in some patients. This kind of treatment requires very cooperative and adherent patients, since it usually comprises a trial period of at least 2–3 weeks before beneficial effects are observable. Success rates may also vary considerably due to regional and cultural differences in eating and food preparation habits. However, those diets are not yet proven in well-designed double-blind placebo-controlled studies and are therefore still controversial [1].

Diets have been used for many years to manage urticaria but the benefits have been difficult to ascertain due to the lack of blinding in studies (except oral provocation) and the natural history of chronic urticaria to remit. There is an old literature on minimizing dietary salicylates and food additives (including colours, preservatives, stabilizers, anti-oxidants and flavour enhancers) that are incorporated into a low pseudoallergen diet that has been popular in Europe for over 20 years. More recently, low histamine diets have been promoted based on open studies. A systematic review of publications on diet in chronic urticaria divided diets into three main groups: low pseudoallergen, low histamine and fish avoidance, which induced complete remission in 4.8%, 11.7% and 10.6% of patients, with partial remission in 37.0%, 43.9% and 4.3%, respectively [81]. The authors concluded that there is evidence for the benefit of diets in symptomatic CSU patients only. However, the level of evidence is low for the benefit of systematic diets in CSU and double-blind controlled trials of diet are lacking.

13.2.1.1 Low Pseudoallergen Diet

Pseudoallergic food reactions are due to intolerance rather than allergy. This means that conventional skin and blood tests for specific IgE are negative. They resemble allergic reactions (hence the name) since histamine release from mast cells with leukotriene generation is believed to mediate the symptoms of urticaria. Urinary leukotriene levels reduced more in CSU patients responding to a low pseudoallergen diet than non-responders [82]. Dietary pseudoallergens are not restricted to food additives and natural salicylates. They include histamine (found in tuna, bananas, avocado, walnut and well-matured cheeses) and alcohol. They have been found in tomato extracts, white wine and herbs [83]. There are no simple diagnostic tests for dietary pseudoallergens. The best way of showing whether or not they aggravate or even cause urticaria is to go on a strict low pseudoallergen diet for 3 weeks. If the urticaria improves on the diet, it is likely that pseudoallergens in food or beverages were making it worse. It may then be possible to track down which foods should be avoided by reintroducing them at intervals of 3 days. Food intolerance usually settles when urticaria clears so it is often possible to reintroduce the offending foods later, unlike allergies which may be life-long.

Evidence for Low Pseudoallergen Diets in Urticaria

Over 70% of 64 In-patients with chronic spontaneous urticaria improved over 2 weeks on a strict low pseudoallergen diet after eating only cooked potatoes, rice and water for 3 days before admission [84]. Over 70% of them showed some improvement over the first 2 weeks of the diet as an inpatient but only 19% of the diet responders reacted to challenge capsules containing additives or salicylic acid, suggesting that other substances in food were relevant. Most of the patients were still improved or clear after 6 months, without antihistamines, and about half were back on a normal diet without problems. About 30% of outpatients responded to the same diet in another prospective open study by the same group but less than half of these did very well [85]. A study from Italy found similar results [86]. Patients responding to a pseudoallergen diet for 5 weeks who followed a step-wise incremental build-up challenge protocol found one or more groups of foods triggered a recurrence of their urticaria, often foods containing biogenic amines (such as histamine) and salicylates [87].

Details and Length of Treatment
The diet should be followed for 3 weeks before foods are reintroduced step-by-step every 3 days if there has been an improvement. There is no specific order for this but it makes sense to add favourite foods first and leave those that are more likely to be responsible for the urticaria (including alcohol) to the end. If, on the other hand, there has been no improvement on the low pseudoallergen diet, a full diet can be restarted.

Compatibility with Other Diets
A dietician should normally be consulted if the patient requires a diet for other medical reasons, such as diabetes, coeliac disease, high blood fats or weight reduction.

Summary
A low pseudoallergen diet may be helpful for some patients with chronic spontaneous urticaria. It may be tried instead of antihistamines or as well as them if they do not provide sufficient relief. Failure to improve within 3 weeks indicates that diet is not useful and that food is not the cause.

13.2.1.2 Low Histamine Diet
Histamine rich foods include fermented foods, beer or wine, scombroid fish, cheese, vinegar and pickles. Dietary histamine is metabolized mainly by diamine oxidase (DAO) in the bowel.

Evidence for a Low Histamine Diet
The weekly urticarial activity scores and plasma histamine levels were significantly lower after a 4 week low histamine diet in a small study of Korean CSU patients although plasma levels of DAO were unchanged [88]. A third of patients with moderate to severe CSU gave a history of histamine intolerance. They were challenged with oral histamine after a low histamine and pseudoallergen diet. During the diet, 46% of patients responded with reduced CSU activity (UAS7 reduction of ≥ 7). Following double-blind, placebo-controlled oral histamine provocation, 17% of patients gave a positive weal response. There appeared to be little relationship between patient history, response to diet and the weal response to oral histamine provocation. The authors concluded that histamine intolerance as a cause of CSU was rare and could not be diagnosed from the history [89].

Phototherapy and Photochemotherapy

In addition to a literature on using phototherapy to desensitize patients with solar urticaria, there is a small but increasing literature on narrow-band ultraviolet B phototherapy (NB-UVB) and psoralen with ultraviolet A (PUVA) therapy to treat CSU or symptomatic dermographism when antihistamines and other 'second line' medicines have been unsuccessful. The mechanism is unknown but may involve reduction of mast cell 'releasability'.

Evidence for Phototherapy in Urticaria

A comparison of NB-UVB with PUVA in steroid-dependent antihistamine unresponsive patients with CSU showed an improvement in average UAS7 over 90–180 days [90]. There was a significant reduction in UAS7 over 8–16 sessions in patients with CSU allocated randomly to loratadine alone or loratadine with phototherapy [91]. An open study showed clearance in just under half of CSU patients and improvement in the remainder with a median number of 31 exposures [92]. Open studies of antihistamine-unresponsive symptomatic dermographism have also show benefit [93, 94].

Dose and Length of Treatment

Ultraviolet treatments are given two or three times a week for at least 6 weeks but the specific details will depend on protocols in each centre, skin type and the response to treatment.

Interactions with Other Medicines

Some medicines, such as tetracycline antibiotics, make the skin more sensitive to ultraviolet therapy and should be avoided during treatment if possible. Antihistamines can be taken safely.

Checks During Treatment

The skin should be checked for cancers before starting treatment and any new moles or lumps that come up during it should be looked at.

Reasons for Avoiding Ultraviolet Treatment

Ultraviolet should not usually be given after previous skin cancers or radiation therapy. Having heat bumps (polymorphic light eruption) or other light-sensitive conditions, such as lupus erythematosus, would usually be a contraindication. Loss of skin colour (vitiligo) would put the skin at risk of burning very easily.

Possible Side Effects of Treatment

Burning can usually be avoided by increasing the doses carefully. There are slight concerns about the long-term effects of ultraviolet radiation encouraging skin cancers. These risks are probably very small initially but may increase after around 150 PUVA treatments and 300 NB-UVB exposures.

Summary

NB-UVB and PUVA treatments may be helpful for troublesome CSU and symptomatic dermographism but should only be tried if antihistamines have not worked well. There are some risks of burning and slight concern about possibly promoting skin cancers with high exposures to ultraviolet. A course of treatment usually involves at least 18 visits to hospital. It is not clear how long any relief from urticaria will last afterwards.

13.2.1.3 Psychological Therapies

There is increasing recognition of the psychological burden of chronic urticaria and its association with mental health disorders. A systematic review and meta-analysis of psychiatric co-morbidity in chronic urticaria patients revealed that almost one out of three CU patients have at least one underlying psychiatric disorder [95]. None of the studies reviewed clarified whether the psychiatric disorders pre-existed the CU onset or not, and no association was found between CU severity and duration and psychological functioning. The review highlights the need for a multidisciplinary therapeutic approach involving prompt recognition and management of any potential psychiatric disorder in addition to urticaria treatment. Another systematic review identified psychosocial factors as having a prevalence of 46% in CSU but their contribution to the development and exacerbation of illness symptoms was not quantifiable [96]. A recent report suggested that disease activity and stress are linked in a subpopulation of chronic spontaneous urticaria patients [97].

Evidence for Psychotherapy in Chronic Urticaria

There are few reported studies of psychological therapies for patients with CU promoting resolution of urticaria but no reports of pharmacological management of mental health disorders resulting in disease resolution. Four patients (three CSU and one idiopathic angioedema) were recruited into a brief Whole Person Treatment Approach course based on non-dualistic concepts of mind and body connectedness, and utilizing psychotherapy-derived listening skills for up to 10 h long sessions, once per week. Treatment efficacy rating, using Urticaria Activity Score and the Urticaria Severity Score, and reduction of drug usage, showed patients experienced long-term resolution of urticaria and cessation of hospitalization for angioedema and came off regular antihistamine medication [98]. Hypnosis provided relief of pruritus as measured by three self-report parameters in a small study by comparison with baseline and control session values but there was no change in the number of hives. Hypnotizable patients had fewer hives and were more symptomatic during the control session. At review 5–14 months after therapy, six patients were free of hives and an additional seven reported improvement [99].

13.2.1.4 Psychotherapy

Psychosocial situation should be evaluated in all patients with chronic urticaria not only to uncover and solve potential problems for treatment adherence but also to detect stress factors that may cause or contribute to urticaria symptoms.

13.2.1.5 Desensitization

Desensitization protocols do exist for several forms of inducible urticarias. As they consist of frequent re-exposure to the trigger for whealing, they are often met with adherence problems. Protocols exist for solar urticaria in which UV-light exposure is required, for cholinergic urticaria in which sweat-inducing activity is required, cold urticaria which require daily cold baths or showers and for heat urticaria which require the application of heat to the skin at the determined threshold. Desensitization in solar urticaria is not recommended due to any increase of risk for skin cancer development. All other desensitization protocols do require a great amount of commitment from the patient and do not acquire long-term tolerance. All desensitization treatments come with the risk of severe exacerbation of urticaria induced by trigger exposure.

References

1. Zuberbier T, Aberer W, Asero R, Abdul Latiff AH, Baker D, Ballmer-Weber B, et al. The EAACI/GA(2)LEN/EDF/WAO guideline for the definition, classification, diagnosis and management of urticaria. Allergy. 2018;73(7):1393–414.
2. Watanabe J, Shimamoto J, Kotani K. The Effects of Antibiotics for Helicobacter pylori Eradication or Dapsone on Chronic Spontaneous Urticaria: A Systematic Review and Meta-Analysis. Antibiotics (Basel). 2021;10(2):156.
3. Boehm I, Bauer R, Bieber T. Urticaria treated with dapsone. Allergy. 1999;54(7):765–6.
4. Noda S, Asano Y, Sato S. Long-term complete resolution of severe chronic idiopathic urticaria after dapsone treatment. J Dermatol. 2012;39(5):496–7.
5. Engin B, Ozdemir M. Prospective randomized non-blinded clinical trial on the use of dapsone plus antihistamine vs. antihistamine in patients with chronic idiopathic urticaria. J Eur Acad Dermatol Venereol. 2008;22(4):481–6.
6. Grundmann SA, Kiefer S, Luger TA, Brehler R. Delayed pressure urticaria - dapsone heading for first-line therapy? J Dtsch Dermatol Ges. 2011;9(11):908–12.
7. Liang SE, Hoffmann R, Peterson E, Soter NA. Use of dapsone in the treatment of chronic idiopathic and autoimmune urticaria. JAMA Dermatol. 2019;155(1):90–5.
8. Morgan M, Cooke A, Rogers L, Adams-Huet B, Khan DA. Double-blind placebo-controlled trial of dapsone in antihistamine refractory chronic idiopathic urticaria. J Allergy Clin Immunol Pract. 2014;2(5):601–6.
9. Jaffer AM. Sulfasalazine in the treatment of corticosteroid-dependent chronic idiopathic urticaria. J Allergy Clin Immunol. 1991;88(6):964–5.
10. McGirt LY, Vasagar K, Gober LM, Saini SS, Beck LA. Successful treatment of recalcitrant chronic idiopathic urticaria with sulfasalazine. Arch Dermatol. 2006;142(10):1337–42.
11. Engler RJ, Squire E, Benson P. Chronic sulfasalazine therapy in the treatment of delayed pressure urticaria and angioedema. Ann Allergy Asthma Immunol. 1995;74(2):155–9.
12. Orden RA, Timble H, Saini SS. Efficacy and safety of sulfasalazine in patients with chronic idiopathic urticaria. Ann Allergy Asthma Immunol. 2014;112(1):64–70.
13. Munch EP, Weeke B. Non-hereditary angioedema treated with tranexamic acid. A 6-month placebo controlled trial with follow-up 4 years later. Allergy. 1985;40(2):92–7.
14. Du-Thanh A, Raison-Peyron N, Drouet C, Guillot B. Efficacy of tranexamic acid in sporadic idiopathic bradykinin angioedema. Allergy. 2010;65(6):793–5.
15. Powell RJ, Leech SC, Till S, Huber PA, Nasser SM, Clark AT, et al. BSACI guideline for the management of chronic urticaria and angioedema. Clin Exp Allergy. 2015;45(3):547–65.

16. Pacor ML, Di Lorenzo G, Corrocher R. Efficacy of leukotriene receptor antagonist in chronic urticaria. A double-blind, placebo-controlled comparison of treatment with montelukast and cetirizine in patients with chronic urticaria with intolerance to food additive and/or acetylsalicylic acid. Clin Exp Allergy. 2001;31(10):1607–14.
17. Nettis E, Pannofino A, Cavallo E, Ferrannini A, Tursi A. Efficacy of montelukast, in combination with loratadine, in the treatment of delayed pressure urticaria. J Allergy Clin Immunol. 2003;112(1):212–3.
18. Nettis E, Colanardi MC, Soccio AL, Ferrannini A, Vacca A. Desloratadine in combination with montelukast suppresses the dermographometer challenge test papule, and is effective in the treatment of delayed pressure urticaria: a randomized, double-blind, placebo-controlled study. Br J Dermatol. 2006;155(6):1279–82.
19. Akenroye AT, McEwan C, Saini SS. Montelukast reduces symptom severity and frequency in patients with angioedema-predominant chronic spontaneous urticaria. J Allergy Clin Immunol Pract. 2018;6(4):1403–5.
20. Erbagci Z. The leukotriene receptor antagonist montelukast in the treatment of chronic idiopathic urticaria: a single-blind, placebo-controlled, crossover clinical study. J Allergy Clin Immunol. 2002;110(3):484–8.
21. Wan KS. Efficacy of leukotriene receptor antagonist with an anti-H1 receptor antagonist for treatment of chronic idiopathic urticaria. J Dermatolog Treat. 2009;20(4):194–7.
22. Sarkar TK, Sil A, Pal S, Ghosh C, Das NK. Effectiveness and safety of levocetirizine 10 mg versus a combination of levocetirizine 5 mg and montelukast 10 mg in chronic urticaria resistant to levocetirizine 5 mg: A double-blind, randomized, controlled trial. Indian J Dermatol Venereol Leprol. 2017;83(5):561–8.
23. Tedeschi A, Suli C, Lorini M, Airaghi L. Successful treatment of chronic urticaria. Allergy. 2000;55(11):1097–8.
24. Hani N, Hartmann K, Casper C, Peters T, Schneider LA, Hunzelmann N, et al. Improvement of cold urticaria by treatment with the leukotriene receptor antagonist montelukast. Acta Derm Venereol. 2000;80(3):229.
25. Robertson I, Greaves MW. Responses of human skin blood vessels to synthetic histamine analogues. Br J Clin Pharmacol. 1978;5:319–22.
26. Marks R, Greaves MW. Vascular reactions to histamine and compound 48/80 in human skin: suppression by a histamine H2-receptor blocking agent. Br J Clin Pharmacol. 1977;4(3):367–9.
27. Bleehen SS, Thomas SE, Greaves MW, Newton J, Kennedy CT, Hindley F, et al. Cimetidine and chlorpheniramine in the treatment of chronic idiopathic urticaria: a multi-centre randomized double-blind study. Br J Dermatol. 1987;117(1):81–8.
28. Minocha YC, Minocha KB, Sood VK, Dogra A. Evaluation of H2 receptor antagonists in chronic idiopathic urticaria. Indian J Dermatol Venereol Leprol. 1995;61(5):265–7.
29. Sharpe GR, Shuster S. In dermographic urticaria H2 receptor antagonists have a small but therapeutically irrelevant additional effect compared with H1 antagonists alone. Br J Dermatol. 1993;129(5):575–9.
30. Fedorowicz Z, van Zuuren EJ, Hu N. Histamine H2-receptor antagonists for urticaria. Cochrane Database Syst Rev. 2012;3
31. Guevara-Gutierrez E, Bonilla-Lopez S, Hernandez-Arana S, Tlacuilo-Parra A. Safety and efficacy of cetirizine versus cetirizine plus ranitidine in chronic urticaria: double-blind randomized placebo-controlled study. J Dermatolog Treat. 2015;26(6):548–50.
32. Barlow RJ, Kobza Black A, Greaves MW. Treatment of severe chronic urticaria with cyclosporin. Eur J Dermatol. 1993;3:273–5.
33. Toubi E, Blant A, Kessel A, Golan TD. Low-dose cyclosporin A in the treatment of severe chronic idiopathic urticaria. Allergy. 1997;52(3):312–6.
34. Grattan CE, O'Donnell BF, Francis DM, Niimi N, Barlow RJ, Seed PT, et al. Randomized double-blind study of cyclosporin in chronic 'idiopathic' urticaria. Br J Dermatol. 2000;143(2):365–72.

35. Kulthanan K, Chaweekulrat P, Komoltri C, Hunnangkul S, Tuchinda P, Chularojanamontri L, et al. Cyclosporine for chronic spontaneous urticaria: a meta-analysis and systematic review. J Allergy Clin Immunol Pract. 2018;6(2):586–99.
36. Toda S, Takahagi S, Mihara S, Hide M. Six cases of antihistamine-resistant dermographic urticaria treated with oral ciclosporin. Allergol Int. 2011;60(4):547–50.
37. Kulthanan K, Subchookul C, Hunnangkul S, Chularojanamontri L, Tuchinda P. Factors predicting the response to cyclosporin treatment in patients with chronic spontaneous urticaria: a systematic review. Allergy Asthma Immunol Res. 2019;11(5):736–55.
38. Boubouka CD, Charissi C, Kouimintzis D, Kalogeromitros D, Stavropoulos PG, Katsarou A. Treatment of autoimmune urticaria with low-dose cyclosporin A: a one-year follow-up. Acta Derm Venereol. 2011;91(1):50–4.
39. Kessel A, Toubi E. Cyclosporine-A in severe chronic urticaria: the option for long-term therapy. Allergy. 2010;65(11):1478–82.
40. Weiner MJ. Methotrexate in corticosteroid-resistant urticaria. Ann Intern Med. 1989;110(10):848.
41. Gach JE, Sabroe RA, Greaves MW, Black AK. Methotrexate-responsive chronic idiopathic urticaria: a report of two cases. Br J Dermatol. 2001;145(2):340–3.
42. Perez A, Woods A, Grattan CE. Methotrexate: a useful steroid-sparing agent in recalcitrant chronic urticaria. Br J Dermatol. 2010;162(1):191–4.
43. Saghi L, Solomon M, Baum S, Lyakhovitsky A, Trau H, Barzilai A. Evidence for methotrexate as a useful treatment for steroid-dependent chronic urticaria. Acta Derm Venereol. 2011;91:303–6.
44. Shahar E, Bergman R, Guttman-Yassky E, Pollack S. Treatment of severe chronic idiopathic urticaria with oral mycophenolate mofetil in patients not responding to antihistamines and/or corticosteroids. Int J Dermatol. 2006;45(10):1224–7.
45. Zimmerman AB, Berger EM, Elmariah SB, Soter NA. The use of mycophenolate mofetil for the treatment of autoimmune and chronic idiopathic urticaria: experience in 19 patients. J Am Acad Dermatol. 2012;66(5):767–70.
46. Tal Y, Toker O, Agmon-Levin N, Shalit M. Azathioprine as a therapeutic alternative for refractory chronic urticaria. Int J Dermatol. 2015;54(3):367–9.
47. Pathania YS, Bishnoi A, Parsad D, Kumar A, Kumaran MS. Comparing azathioprine with cyclosporine in the treatment of antihistamine refractory chronic spontaneous urticaria: a randomized prospective active-controlled non-inferiority study. World Allergy Organ J. 2019;12(5):100033.
48. Greene SL, Reed CE, Schroeter AL. Double-blind crossover study comparing doxepin with diphenhydramine for the treatment of chronic urticaria. J Am Acad Dermatol. 1985;12(4):669–75.
49. Harto A, Sendagorta E, Ledo A. Doxepin in the treatment of chronic urticaria. Dermatologica. 1985;170(2):90–3.
50. Yee CSK, El Khoury K, Albuhairi S, Broyles A, Schneider L, Rachid R. Acquired cold-induced urticaria in pediatric patients: a 22-year experience in a tertiary care center (1996-2017). J Allergy Clin Immunol Pract. 2019;7(3):1024–31.e3.
51. Wong E, Eftekhari N, Greaves MW, Ward AM. Beneficial effects of danazol on symptoms and laboratory changes in cholinergic urticaria. Br J Dermatol. 1987;116(4):553–6.
52. Berth-Jones J, Graham-Brown RA. Cholinergic pruritus, erythema and urticaria: a disease spectrum responding to danazol. Br J Dermatol. 1989;121(2):235–7.
53. Asero R, Tedeschi A. Usefulness of a short course of oral prednisone in antihistamine-resistant chronic urticaria: a retrospective analysis. J Investig Allergol Clin Immunol. 2010;20(5):386–90.
54. Chua SL, Gibbs S. Chronic urticaria responding to subcutaneous heparin sodium. Br J Dermatol. 2005;153(1):216–7.
55. Asero R, Tedeschi A, Coppola R, Griffini S, Paparella P, Riboldi P, et al. Activation of the tissue factor pathway of blood coagulation in patients with chronic urticaria. J Allergy Clin Immunol. 2007;119(3):705–10.

56. Asero R, Tedeschi A, Cugno M. Heparin and tranexamic acid therapy may be effective in treatment-resistant chronic urticaria with elevated d-dimer: a pilot study. Int Arch Allergy Immunol. 2010;152(4):384–9.
57. Parslew R, Pryce D, Ashworth J, Friedmann PS. Warfarin treatment of chronic idiopathic urticaria and angio-oedema. Clin Exp Allergy. 2000;30(8):1161–5.
58. Samarasinghe V, Marsland AM. Class action of oral coumarins in the treatment of a patient with chronic spontaneous urticaria and delayed-pressure urticaria. Clin Exp Dermatol. 2012;37(7):741–3.
59. Pho LN, Eliason MJ, Regruto M, Hull CM, Powell DL. Treatment of chronic urticaria with colchicine. J Drugs Dermatol. 2011;10(12):1423–8.
60. Bodar EJ, Simon A, de Visser M, van der Meer JW. Complete remission of severe idiopathic cold urticaria on interleukin-1 receptor antagonist (anakinra). Neth J Med. 2009;67(9):302–5.
61. Lenormand C, Lipsker D. Efficiency of interleukin-1 blockade in refractory delayed-pressure urticaria. Ann Intern Med. 2012;157(8):599–600.
62. Magerl M, Philipp S, Manasterski M, Friedrich M, Maurer M. Successful treatment of delayed pressure urticaria with anti-TNF-alpha. J Allergy Clin Immunol. 2007;119(3):752–4.
63. Sand FL, Thomsen SF. TNF-alpha inhibitors for chronic urticaria: experience in 20 patients. J Allergy (Cairo). 2013;2013:130905.
64. Bangsgaard N, Skov L, Zachariae C. Treatment of refractory chronic spontaneous urticaria with adalimumab. Acta Derm Venereol. 2017;97(4):524–5.
65. Wilson LH, Eliason MJ, Leiferman KM, Hull CM, Powell DL. Treatment of refractory chronic urticaria with tumor necrosis factor-alfa inhibitors. J Am Acad Dermatol. 2011;64(6):1221–2.
66. Chakravarty SD, Yee AF, Paget SA. Rituximab successfully treats refractory chronic autoimmune urticaria caused by IgE receptor autoantibodies. J Allergy Clin Immunol. 2011;128(6):1354–5.
67. Mallipeddi R, Grattan CE. Lack of response of severe steroid-dependent chronic urticaria to rituximab. Clin Exp Dermatol. 2007;32(3):333–4.
68. Kessel A, Bamberger E, Toubi E. Tacrolimus in the treatment of severe chronic idiopathic urticaria: an open-label prospective study. J Am Acad Dermatol. 2005;52(1):145–8.
69. Dorman SM Jr, Regan SB, Khan DA. Effectiveness and safety of oral tacrolimus in refractory chronic urticaria. J Allergy Clin Immunol Pract. 2019;7(6):2033–4.e1.
70. Asero R. Oral cyclophosphamide in a case of cyclosporin and steroid-resistant chronic urticaria showing autoreactivity on autologous serum skin testing. Clin Exp Dermatol. 2005;30(5):582–3.
71. Bernstein JA, Garramone SM, Lower EG. Successful treatment of autoimmune chronic idiopathic urticaria with intravenous cyclophosphamide. Ann Allergy Asthma Immunol. 2002;89(2):212–4.
72. Reeves GE, Boyle MJ, Bonfield J, Dobson P, Loewenthal M. Impact of hydroxychloroquine therapy on chronic urticaria: chronic autoimmune urticaria study and evaluation. Intern Med J. 2004;34(4):182–6.
73. Boonpiyathad T, Sangasapaviliya A. Hydroxychloroquine in the treatment of anti-histamine refractory chronic spontaneous urticaria, randomized single-blinded placebo-controlled trial and an open label comparison study. Eur Ann Allergy Clin Immunol. 2017;49(5):220–4.
74. O'Donnell BF, Barr RM, Black AK, Francis DM, Kermani F, Niimi N, et al. Intravenous immunoglobulin in autoimmune chronic urticaria. Br J Dermatol. 1998;138(1):101–6.
75. Dawn G, Urcelay M, Ah-Weng A, O'Neill SM, Douglas WS. Effect of high-dose intravenous immunoglobulin in delayed pressure urticaria. Br J Dermatol. 2003;149(4):836–40.
76. Mitzel-Kaoukhov H, Staubach P, Muller-Brenne T. Effect of high-dose intravenous immunoglobulin treatment in therapy-resistant chronic spontaneous urticaria. Ann Allergy Asthma Immunol. 2010;104(3):253–8.
77. Grattan CE, Francis DM, Slater NG, Barlow RJ, Greaves MW. Plasmapheresis for severe, unremitting, chronic urticaria. Lancet. 1992;339(8801):1078–80.
78. Sindher SB, Jariwala S, Gilbert J, Rosenstreich D. Resolution of chronic urticaria coincident with vitamin D supplementation. Ann Allergy Asthma Immunol. 2012;109(5):359–60.

79. Rasool R, Masoodi KZ, Shera IA, Yosuf Q, Bhat IA, Qasim I, et al. Chronic urticaria merits serum vitamin D evaluation and supplementation; a randomized case control study. World Allergy Organ J. 2015;8(1):15.
80. Tuchinda P, Kulthanan K, Chularojanamontri L, Arunkajohnsak S, Sriussadaporn S. Relationship between vitamin D and chronic spontaneous urticaria: a systematic review. Clin Transl Allergy. 2018;8:51.
81. Cornillier H, Giraudeau B, Samimi M, Munck S, Hacard F, Jonville-Bera AP, et al. Effect of diet in chronic spontaneous urticaria: a systematic review. Acta Derm Venereol. 2019;99(2):127–32.
82. Akoglu G, Atakan N, Cakir B, Kalayci O, Hayran M. Effects of low pseudoallergen diet on urticarial activity and leukotriene levels in chronic urticaria. Arch Dermatol Res. 2012;304(4):257–62.
83. Zuberbier T, Pfrommer C, Specht K, Vieths S, Bastl-Borrmann R, Worm M, et al. Aromatic components of food as novel eliciting factors of pseudoallergic reactions in chronic urticaria. J Allergy Clin Immunol. 2002;109(2):343–8.
84. Zuberbier T, Chantraine-Hess S, Hartmann K, Czarnetzki BM. Pseudoallergen-free diet in the treatment of chronic urticaria. A prospective study. Acta Derm Venereol. 1995;75(6):484–7.
85. Magerl M, Pisarevskaja D, Scheufele R, Zuberbier T, Maurer M. Effects of a pseudoallergen-free diet on chronic spontaneous urticaria: a prospective trial. Allergy. 2010;65(1):78–83.
86. Pigatto PD, Valsecchi RH. Chronic urticaria: a mystery. Allergy. 2000;55(3):306–8.
87. Bunselmeyer B, Laubach HJ, Schiller M, Stanke M, Luger TA, Brehler R. Incremental build-up food challenge--a new diagnostic approach to evaluate pseudoallergic reactions in chronic urticaria: a pilot study: stepwise food challenge in chronic urticaria. Clin Exp Allergy. 2009;39(1):116–26.
88. Son JH, Chung BY, Kim HO, Park CW. A histamine-free diet is helpful for treatment of adult patients with chronic spontaneous urticaria. Ann Dermatol. 2018;30(2):164–72.
89. Siebenhaar F, Melde A, Magerl M, Zuberbier T, Church MK, Maurer M. Histamine intolerance in patients with chronic spontaneous urticaria. J Eur Acad Dermatol Venereol. 2016;30(10):1774–7.
90. Bishnoi A, Parsad D, Vinay K, Kumaran MS. Phototherapy using narrowband ultraviolet B and psoralen plus ultraviolet A is beneficial in steroid-dependent antihistamine-refractory chronic urticaria: a randomized, prospective observer-blinded comparative study. Br J Dermatol. 2017;176(1):62–70.
91. Sheikh G, Latif I, Lone KS, Hassan I, Jabeen Y, Keen A. Role of adjuvant narrow band ultraviolet B phototherapy in the treatment of chronic urticaria. Indian J Dermatol. 2019;64(3):250.
92. Aydogan K, Karadogan SK, Tunali S, Saricaoglu H. Narrowband ultraviolet B (311 nm, TL01) phototherapy in chronic ordinary urticaria. Int J Dermatol. 2012;51(1):98–103.
93. Borzova E, Rutherford A, Konstantinou GN, Leslie KS, Grattan CE. Narrowband ultraviolet B phototherapy is beneficial in antihistamine-resistant symptomatic dermographism: a pilot study. J Am Acad Dermatol. 2008;59(5):752–7.
94. Heelan K, Murphy M. Symptomatic dermatographism treated with narrowband UVB phototherapy. J Dermatolog Treat. 2015;26(4):365–6.
95. Konstantinou GN, Konstantinou GN. Psychiatric comorbidity in chronic urticaria patients: a systematic review and meta-analysis. Clin Transl Allergy. 2019;9:42.
96. Ben-Shoshan M, Blinderman I, Raz A. Psychosocial factors and chronic spontaneous urticaria: a systematic review. Allergy. 2013;68(2):131–41.
97. Schut C, Magerl M, Hawro T, Kupfer J, Rose M, Gieler U, et al. Disease activity and stress are linked in a subpopulation of chronic spontaneous urticaria patients. Allergy. 2020;75(1):224–6.
98. Lindsay K, Goulding J, Solomon M, Broom B. Treating chronic spontaneous urticaria using a brief 'whole person' treatment approach: a proof-of-concept study. Clin Transl Allergy. 2015;5:40.
99. Shertzer CL, Lookingbill DP. Effects of relaxation therapy and hypnotizability in chronic urticaria. Arch Dermatol. 1987;123(7):913–6.

Urticaria in Pediatrics and During Pregnancy and Lactation: Highlights on Epidemiology, Diagnosis, and Management

Moshe Ben-Shoshan and Petra Staubach

Abbreviations

BAT	Basophil activation test
CAPS	Cryopyrin-associated periodic syndrome
CRP	C-reactive protein
CSU	Chronic spontaneous urticaria
CU	Chronic urticaria
PU	Physical urticaria
SSLR	Serum sickness-like reaction
UAS	Urticaria Activity Score

14.1 Introduction

Chronic urticaria (CU) in children as in adults is characterized by the presence of itchy wheals, angioedema, or both daily or almost daily for at least 6 weeks. Most cases of urticaria in the pediatric age group are acute [1–4]. CU is sub-classified as spontaneous (occurring without a known trigger) or inducible. There are also cases of spontaneous and inducible forms that co-exist. The chronic subtypes occur continuously but also recurrently, often in association with infections. In this chapter we will touch briefly on the clinical presentation, diagnosis, and management of

M. Ben-Shoshan
Division of Allergy Immunology and Dermatology, Montreal Children's Hospital, Montreal, QC, Canada
e-mail: moshe.ben-shoshan@mcgill.ca

P. Staubach (✉)
Department of Dermatology, University Medical Center, Mainz, Germany
e-mail: petra.staubach@unimedizin-mainz.de

acute urticaria in children. However, our primary goal is to highlight key findings regarding the epidemiology, diagnosis, and management approach of pediatric CU. In addition, we will summarize the data regarding the management of CU in pregnancy and lactation.

14.1.1 Acute Urticaria in Children

Only few studies discuss causes of isolated pediatric urticaria. The main known cause of acute urticaria in children is viral infections, mainly of the upper respiratory tract [5, 6]. Other less common causes include food [5] and drug hypersensitivity [7]. The diagnosis of allergic reactions involving hives is established through corroboration of a suggestive clinical history consistent with an immediate hypersensitivity reaction occurring shortly (usually within one hour after exposure) and the use of confirmatory skin tests, specific IgE levels and, potentially, provocation challenges. It is important to establish the presence of allergic triggers of urticaria with confirmatory tests to avoid mislabeling of patients as allergic. It is also important to assess the presence of atopic co-morbidities such as eczema and asthma given that these could affect the clinical presentation.

Second generation antihistamines are the main treatment for non-anaphylactic episodes of acute urticaria. The main antihistamines recommended include cetirizine (1 year: 0.25 mg/kg twice daily, 2–5 years: 2.5 mg twice daily, 6–11 years: 5 mg twice daily, 12–17 years: 10 mg once daily) [8], levocetirizine (2–5 years: 1.25 mg twice daily, 6–17 years: 5 mg once daily) [9], fexofenadine (30 mg twice daily for children 6–12 years) [10], desloratadine (1.25 mg daily and 2.5 mg daily for children 1–5 years and 6–11 years, respectively) [11], loratadine (5 mg daily for children 2–11 years, body weight up to 30 kg, 10 mg daily above 30 kg) [12], and rupatadine (2.5 mg once a day up to 25 kg and 5 mg a day for children who weight more than 25 kg) [13].

14.1.1.1 Differential Diagnosis of Acute Urticaria in Children

1. Anaphylaxis: more than 80% of patients presenting with anaphylaxis are reported to have hives [14, 15]. Prompt epinephrine administration is indicated in all cases presenting with urticaria as part of anaphylaxis (defined as involvement of at least 2 organ systems/hypotension in response to a known allergen) [16, 17].
2. Serum sickness-like reaction (SSLR) is defined when large erythematous, urticarial plaques with dusky to ecchymotic centers, often associated with hand and foot swelling, develop 7–21 days after medication exposure. In addition to the characteristics and cutaneous manifestations, patients with SSLR are reported to have fever, malaise, lymphadenopathy, abdominal pain, nausea, vomiting, diarrhea, myalgias, headaches, and a self-limited symmetric arthritis [18]. The prognosis of SSLR is excellent with symptoms resolution usually within 2 weeks after withdrawal of the offending agent. Systemic glucocorticoids are often used for more severe cases [19].

Fig. 14.1 Urticaria multiforme and hand swelling in an 18 months old boy

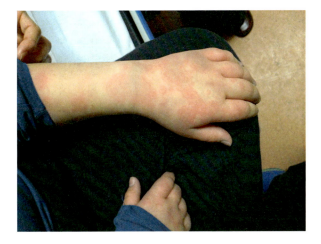

3. Viral infections can be associated rarely with a similar rash called "urticaria multiforme" that resembles acute urticaria (Fig. 14.1) [20]. However, in cases of urticaria multiforme versus SSLR, rash presents faster (1–3 days following an acute viral illness). Similar to SSLR this is a self-limited condition with favorable long-term prognoses. A hemorrhagic morphology within urticarial lesions is commonly seen in children [21].

14.1.2 CU in Children

14.1.2.1 Burden
Recent studies suggest that the one-year diagnosed prevalence of CU (including CSU and inducible forms) in pediatric patients is 1.38% (95% CI, 0.94–1.86) and that spontaneous CU (CSU) affects 0.75% (95% CI, 0.44–1.08) of children [22]. The prevalence of CSU was reported to be higher (1.2%) in selected pediatric populations (e.g., children with systemic lupus erythematosus) [23]. The majority of pediatric CU cases are reported to be spontaneous (55.9% of cases) [24]. It was published that the prevalence of CU is higher in boys than in girls among children under the age of 10 years although it was significantly higher in females than in males among adolescents and adults older than 15 years [25].

14.1.2.2 Clinical Presentation
Urticaria is characterized by the presence of pruritic, well-circumscribed, raised wheals ranging from several millimeters, sometimes merging to from lesions that are several centimeters or larger in size (Fig. 14.2a and b). The wheals can be pale to brightly erythematous in color, often with surrounding erythema. The onset of symptoms for urticaria or angioedema is rapid, usually occurring over minutes. Unlike acute urticaria, in CU individual lesions may last 24 h before they resolve spontaneously [26, 27].

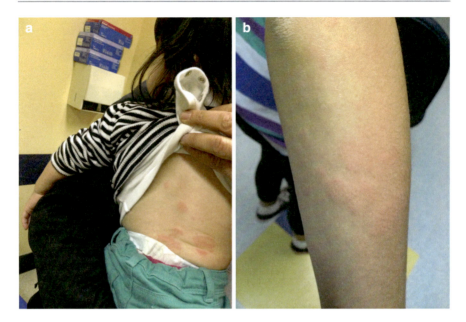

Fig. 14.2 (**a** and **b**) CU in 2 year old and 12 year old girls

Urticaria can occur with angioedema, which is localized non-pitting edema of the subcutaneous or interstitial tissue that may be painful and warm and in average not lasting more than 48 h. There are only a small number of publications available regarding the association between urticaria and angioedema in children. Mast cell-associated angioedema was reported in 6–14% of children with CU [22]. In a study in adolescents it was reported that they were less likely to have experienced angioedema compared to adults (23.1% and 44.8%, respectively) [28].

14.1.2.3 Classification

Although most CU cases in childhood are reported to be spontaneous, it is important to rule out rare forms that may require different treatment. Given that co-existence of spontaneous and inducible forms is not rare and given that patients often report only one form, it is crucial to query patients on all subtypes of urticaria.

Rare forms of CU subtypes include the following:

1. Inducible urticarias:
    (a) Physical urticaria. Physical urticaria (PU) occurs when the CU is associated with a specific physical stimulus [e.g., cold contact urticaria, solar urticaria, delayed pressure urticaria, heat contact urticaria, dermographic urticaria (Fig. 14.3), or vibratory angioedema] [29]. It is reported that PU can affect 22% of children presenting with CU and that among all cases of PU a quarter will also have CSU [30]. The most common cause of PU (38% of all cases) is dermographic urticaria [31].

Fig. 14.3 Dermatographism

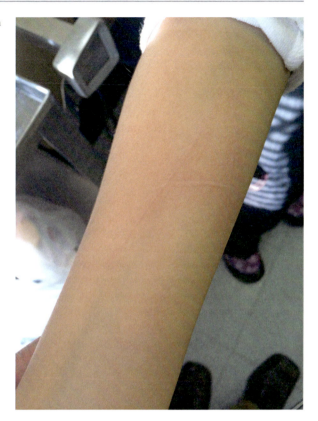

It is reported that in countries with lower temperatures during winter, cold induced PU accounts for 16% of pediatric PU cases [30]. Up to 67% cases of PU were reported to have associated angioedema [31] and only 11.6% of children become free of urticaria at one-year post-onset and 38.4% at 5 years post-onset [31]. Establishing the diagnosis of PU is based on physical provocation tests as previously published [27, 32] (Fig. 14.4).

In general, second generation H1 antihistamines should be given daily (including up-dosing as in adults, weight-adjusted) but avoidance of the physical trigger and the use of second generation H1 antihistamines to control symptoms before anticipated exposure may be sufficient in some patients. Recently successful treatment with subcutaneous omalizumab injections off-label has been reported for children with severe PU, including cold induced PU [33] and delayed pressure urticaria [34] that often respond poorly to antihistamines [35].

There are case reports on cold urticaria associated with systemic symptoms and potential fatality (e.g., when swimming in cold water), [36] and hence prescription of an epinephrine auto-injector for children presenting with cold induced PU could be considered for those deemed at risk, especially in cases presenting with a history of systemic reactions [37]. The diag-

Fig. 14.4 Cold induced urticaria : hands of a 4-year-old child

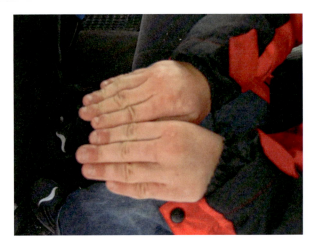

nosis is established when wheals reproduce after contact for 5 min with an ice cube (in a thin plastic bag) placed on the volar aspect of the arm. More accurate provocation testing could be conducted with the aid of computer-aided thermoelectric Peltier device (Temptest®) [29].

  (b) Cholinergic urticaria. Cholinergic urticaria affects 2.2–6.5% of children diagnosed with inducible CU, but it is likely that this is an underestimate as many cases are not reported. [30, 38] It is characterized by the development of pinpoint-sized wheals and severe itch that last 20–30 min and are associated with conditions of elevated core body temperature (e.g., as exercise and hot showers). Among children, cholinergic urticaria is most common in teenagers [35] and especially in atopics [39]. The diagnosis is established when lesions occur reproducibly with exercise and with passive warming and rest, such as might occur in a steam bath or hot pool [29]. Decreasing the degree of exercise and temperature exposure is obviously challenging in small children as well as in teenagers who engage in sports regularly. Second generation H1 antihistamines are first-line treatment, but are often not effective. Recent reports in adults suggest that off-label use of omalizumab may lead to complete control of cholinergic urticaria although symptoms recur once treatment is discontinued [40]. No similar reports in children have been published so far.

2. Other Causes of CU
  (a) Non-steroidal anti-inflammatory drugs (NSAIDs) associated urticaria. It has been recognized that almost a quarter of children and adolescents with CSU are hypersensitive to aspirin (acetylsalicylic acid), and can experience symptom aggravation when exposed to aspirin and other NSAIDs [41]. This clinical picture is known as aspirin-exacerbated cutaneous disease. It is proposed that these conditions are related to the inhibition of cyclooxygenase-1 leading to a decreased synthesis of prostaglandin E2 and an increased cysteinyl leukotriene production in the skin and subcutaneous tissues. Urticaria in these cases is managed through the use of second generation antihistamines,

avoidance of non-selective cyclooxygenase 1 (COX-1) inhibitors, and the use of alternative NSAIDs that do not inhibit COX-1 inhibitory activity for the relief of pain inflammation and fever, i.e., paracetamol (use of COX-2 inhibitors is discouraged for children younger than 16 years) [42]. Refractory cases are reported to improve with omalizumab [43]. In addition studies suggest that drug reactions to NSAIDs and beta-lactams are higher among patients (12 years and older) with CSU than in subjects without urticaria ((13% vs 0.7%) and that drug challenge tests should be offered early during medical evaluation to avoid unnecessary restrictions [44]. Given that parents often report chronic recurrent urticaria in children in the context of infections, it is crucial to assess use of NSAIDs such as ibuprofen in these cases.

(b) Parasite infections. It was reported that up to 10% of CU cases in children in endemic areas may be related to intestinal parasite infections [45], mainly strongyloidiasis and blastocystosis (established through serology for strongyloidiasis and stool tests for blastocystis hominis) [46]. Although studies report clear benefit for treatment of strongyloidiasis [47], there is still debate regarding the need to treat blastocystis hominis that is considered an opportunistic organism, associated with nonspecific symptoms [48]. Assessment for parasites should be considered in children with recent travel to tropical countries (within one year of symptoms), with gastrointestinal symptoms (e.g., abdominal pain) [49], high eosinophil count or those living in regions considered endemic for parasites (e.g., Northern Territory in Australia) [50].

14.1.2.4 Differential Diagnosis of CU

(a) Autoinflammatory diseases: Cryopyrin-associated periodic syndrome (CAPS) is a rare (1 per million persons) but important to diagnose in order to provide correct treatment. CAPS is associated with single heterozygous germline or somatic gain-of-function gene mutations in *NLRP3* (NLR Family Pyrin Domain Containing 3) gene. Cryopyrin nucleates an NLRP3 inflammasome, and the overactivation of this gene results in increased interleukin-1 (IL-1) secretion. IL-1 plays the key role in the induction of inflammation in CAPS [51]. Recently proposed diagnostic criteria include raised inflammatory markers (C-reactive protein/serum amyloid A) plus ≥2 of 6 CAPS-typical symptoms: urticaria-like rash, cold-triggered episodes, sensorineural hearing loss, musculoskeletal symptoms, chronic aseptic meningitis and skeletal abnormalities [52]. CAPS include three autoinflammatory conditions, ranging in severity from mild (familial cold autoinflammatory syndrome: FCAS), moderate (Muckle-Wells syndrome: MWS) and severe (neonatal onset multi-system inflammatory disorder: NOMID). Common presenting features included urticaria (100%), periodic fever (78%), arthralgia (72%), and sensorineural hearing loss (61%). In cases of MWS the majority will have a family member similarly affected compared. The laboratory inflammation index such as leukocyte counts, platelet counts, erythrocyte sedimentation rate (ESR), C-reactive protein (CRP), serum amyloid A (SAA), and fibrinogen (FIB) increased significantly at initial stage and during the attack, but decreased after the attack or under therapy [53].

The recommended treatment in these cases is with anti-interleukin -1 therapy [54]. Typically those urticarial symptoms are therapy-resistant to H1 antihistamines. Other autoinflammatory IL1-dependent diseases like adult still syndrome, Mevalonate Kinase Deficiency Syndrome or Tumor Necrosis Factor Receptor-associated Periodic Syndrome or systemic-onset juvenile idiopathic arthritis could present with urticarial rashes but will likely also include recurrent fever episodes, fatigue, bone pain, and/or non-response to H1 antihistamines as well as the already mentioned abnormal lab results.

(b) Urticaria associated with vasculitis. Urticaria vasculitis is a clinical–pathological variant of leukocytoclastic vasculitis that affects postcapillary venules. The prevalence is unknown and the incidence varies between 2 and 20%. Most cases occur in women in their middle ages. Pediatric urticaria vasculitis is usually preceded by an upper respiratory tract infection. The skin lesions usually present as pruritic hives that can vary in size and typically persist for more than 24 h, with a mean duration of 3–4 days. They often spread transforming themselves in extensive plaques. Pain, burning, and tenderness may occur. Skin lesions usually appear in anatomical areas of pressure and may have purpuric elements and angioedema occurs in up to 42% cases [55]. The diagnosis is confirmed by the histopathological findings that are characterized by swelling and necrosis of endothelial cells, a perivascular inflammatory infiltrate mainly neutrophilic, extravasation of red blood cells, perivascular leukocytoclasia, and interstitial fibrinoid deposit. Direct immunofluorescence can be found in 70–80% of cases with a linear or granular deposit of immunoglobulins, complement (C3), and/or fibrinogen in the vascular endothelium and/or in the basement membrane [55, 56]. Although rare in children, urticaria vasculitis may be the first manifestation of juvenile systemic lupus erythematosus [57]. Hence, rigorous follow-up in children and adolescents with CU is required, and investigation should be performed to rule out a collagen disease in cases who develop other characteristic symptoms, such as arthritis or autoimmune hematologic abnormalities.

(c) Mastocytosis. Mastocytosis refers to a group of myeloproliferative disorders characterized by excessive proliferation and accumulation of mast cells in tissues. It affects 1 in 10,000 inhabitants [58]. Cutaneous mastocytosis (CM) is limited to the skin while systemic mastocytosis (SM) develops in extracutaneous organs, with or without skin involvement. Childhood onset mastocytosis is assumed to be mostly cutaneous and transient while in adults the condition commonly progresses to a systemic form [59–61]. CM is diagnosed through collaborating clinical findings with laboratory tests (mainly elevated baseline tryptase levels). Darier's sign is often used to diagnose CM in the clinical context. Lesional skin biopsy specimens exemplifying mast cell hyperplasia confirm the diagnosis of CM [62, 63]. Urticaria pigmentosa (UP), diffuse cutaneous mastocytosis (DCM), and mastocytoma (MS) of the skin are the three major forms of CM [60]. Typical UP lesions consist of red-brown to yellowish long lasting macules, papules, or nodules that vary in size from several millimeters to centimeters in diameter. Clinical features of DCM consist of diffuse skin infiltration and spontaneous blistering with erosions and crusts, various degrees of erythroderma, prominent dermographism, and pruritus [62]. By contrast, mastocytoma is defined by the presence of one or several brownish red plaques or nodular lesions usually 4–5 cm in diameter [59–61]. Of the three cutaneous variants, UP is the most common type and represents approximately 65% of all pediatric cases [60, 63]. Cutaneous mastocytosis is associated with gain-of-function *KIT* mutations in approximately 60–80% of cases. Children with typical cutaneous lesions usually do not require a bone marrow biopsy if hepatosplenomegaly, lymphadenopathy, or peripheral-blood abnormalities are absent [64]. Patients with all forms of mastocytosis are at increased risk of hymenoptera sting anaphylaxis, food, drug induced anaphylaxis, and perioperative anaphylaxis [65, 66].

Behavioral intervention includes avoidance of triggers such as heat, cold, pressure, exercise, sunlight, and strong emotions. Epinephrine autoinjectors (for possible anaphylaxis) is often prescribed [67]. Various medications are used for cutaneous and systemic mastocytosis including antihistamines, steroids, phototherapy, biologics, combination therapy, and allo-hematopoietic stem cell transplantation [63].

(d) Angioedema occurring without wheals. Angioedema is a rare condition which manifests as sudden localized, non-pitting swelling of certain body parts including skin and mucous membranes. Although we will discuss briefly causes and management of angioedema in children, full discussion of the pathogenesis and management of this condition are beyond the scope of this chapter. Angioedema can occur in isolation, accompanied by urticaria, or as a feature of anaphylaxis in mast cell-mediated disorders or bradykinin mediated disorders. Angioedema can also occur in other conditions with unknown mechanisms, such as infections, rare disorders, or idiopathic angioedema [68]. In certain forms the main mediators are histamine, whereas in other forms the main mediator is bradykinin. Bradykinin mediated angioedema can be caused by C1-inhibitor deficiency/impaired function [due to mutations in the C1-inhibitor (SERPING1) gene], mutations in coagulation factor XII, plasminogen gene [69], or angiopoietin-1 gene [70]. Bradykinin mediated angioedema due to angiotensin-converting enzyme inhibitors is unlikely to occur in the pediatric age group.

Several treatments are licensed for hereditary C1-INH deficiency [71]. For acute attacks different types of C1 inhibitors are available including Berinert : (intravenous 20 U/kg body weight), cinryze (1000 U, intravenous, irrespective of the body weight), and Ruconest [recombinant C1-INHs : 50 U/kg (maximum dose of 4200 U in patients with body weight >84 kg, maximum of two doses within of 24 h)]. Other options for acute attacks in children include the bradykinin receptor blocker icatibant, and the plasma kallikrein inhibitor ecallantide [72, 73]. The dosing recommendation for icatibant is 30 mg, subcutaneous (prefilled syringe), with a maximum of three doses within 24 h [72]. For ecallantide the dosing recommendation is three times 10 mg given subcutaneously, with a maximum of two doses within 24 h [72]. The only treatment option for long-term prophylaxis in children is the plasma derived C1-inhibitor.

Prophylactic treatments with attenuated androgen and antifibrinolytics are reported in the literature [74]. However, androgen therapy is less recommended in children due to the potential side effects including pituitary suppression and virilization [75, 76]. Data on the efficacy of tranexamic acid is limited and hence its use is debatable [72, 73].

Isolated angioedema mediated by histamine and responding to H1 antihistamines is considered a form of CU and its differentiation from bradykinin mediated forms may be challenging. It is important to query caregivers of children presenting with isolated angioedema on family history of angioedema, presence of abdominal pain and/laryngospasm, and use of medications to rule out bradykinin mediated hereditary forms that require different management.

14.1.2.5 The Natural History of Pediatric CU

Chronic urticaria in adults is considered a self-limited disease, yet it resolves spontaneously within 5 years in only 30–55% of adult patients [77–80]. Data on the natural history of CU and its subtypes in children are scarce. In a recent Canadian study it was reported that the mean age at disease onset was 6.7 ± 4.7 years (range: 0–17 years). Similar to adult studies, the resolution rate was low, 10.3 per 100 patients-years. The most common type of CU was CSU (78%). A quarter of patients had concomitant angioedema symptoms [30].

In previous studies in adults, it was reported that resolution is less likely in females, cases of long duration of the disorder at the initial examination, cases with angioedema, and physical urticarias [81]. Factors affecting disease resolution in children included CD63 upregulation on basophil measured by the basophil activation test (BAT) and absence of peripheral-blood basophils. Those two parameters were previously biologically linked—basopenia was observed mainly in the autoimmune subset of CSU and hypothesized to be a result of recruitment of circulating basophils into the skin during disease activity [82]. Similar findings were reported in a study conducted on adults with CU, where 56.5% of autoimmune CU cases resolved after 1.2 years (only 15 patients) compared to 34.5% of idiopathic forms in 1 year [83, 84].

14.1.2.6 CU—Diagnostic Approach

CU is not considered an allergic condition even though histamine release from cutaneous mast cells is a primary pathogenic event. Routine extensive blood work or skin tests are not indicated. A complete blood count and sedimentation rate/C-reactive protein (CRP) levels are often the only tests ordered [85, 86]. To monitor diseases activity it is recommended to record daily wheal numbers and pruritus severity using a standardized urticaria activity score (UAS) [27].

There is controversy regarding the effect of systematic diets (including pseudoallergen-free diet, low-histamine diet, and diet without fish products) in CU. Given that at this point systematic double-blind controlled trials of diet are lacking [87] and given that recent studies suggest that unnecessary elimination diets may increase the risk of IgE mediated food allergies [88, 89], we do not recommend the use of systematic diets to manage children with CU.

14.1.2.7 Pathogenesis

Studies support auto-immunity as the main mechanisms contributing to the development of CSU. There are two main autoimmune pathways that play a role in the pathogenesis of CSU: Type I involves IgE autoantibodies against self-antigens and type IIb involves IgG antibodies against the constant region of IgE or the IgE receptor [90, 91]. Both types will lead mast cell degranulation and CSU. In adults it is reported that type I mechanisms account for the majority of CSU cases mainly IgE autoantibodies directed interleukin- 24 (IL-24) [92]. There are no studies up to this point assessing the presence of type I autoantibodies in children. Up to 40% of adults and children with CSU are considered to have a type IIb autoimmune basis for their disease [93]. Patients can be screened for the presence of autoantibodies either *in vivo* with the use of the autologous serum skin test or *in vitro* with the basophil histamine release assay or the BAT measuring CD63 or CD203 upregulation on healthy donor basophils incubated with heterologous serum from the patient [94, 95]. Practical challenges in conducting the autologous skin test favor the *in vitro* methods for the assessment of functional autoantibodies. More recently it was reported that in children with CSU the BAT reveals high CD63 expression on basophils and that high levels (>1.8% of basophils) or absence of basophils on complete blood counts were associated with earlier disease resolution [30, 96]. However, currently the use of BAT is limited to research and is not offered in clinical practice routinely.

14.1.2.8 Drug Management of CSU in Childhood

There are three major drug management strategies used for the treatment of CSU in children: [97]

1. Second generation H1 antihistamines
2. Omalizumab (anti-IgE)
3. Ciclosporin

Second generation H1 antihistamines, compared with their first generation counterparts, have demonstrated improved peripheral H1-receptor selectivity and decreased lipophilicity (which minimizes CNS adverse effects). Numerous randomized controlled trials in adults indicate high efficacy and safety for levocetirizine [98], rupatadine [13], desloratadine [13], and bilastine [99] for the treatment of CSU. There are limited studies on antihistamine response in pediatrics. Although there are no studies reporting the percentage of children failing to respond to standard dose, two studies reported that 13–35% will fail treatment with high doses (double dose) [100, 101].

Agents currently authorized for use in children aged 2–11 years include cetirizine, desloratadine (1 year of age), levocetirizine, loratadine, and rupatadine [102]. Bilastine, is highly selective for the H1 histamine receptor, has a rapid onset and prolonged duration of action, does not interact with the cytochrome P450 system but so far its efficacy and safety were established only in adults with CSU [103]. In a head to head study comparing rupatadine and desloratadine, rupatadine had been shown to be superior regarding control of itchiness. However, a trial comparing levocetirizine and rupatadine reported more significant ($P < 0.001$) improvement in the levocetirizine group although symptoms improved in both groups [104]. There were no studies comparing levocetirizine and bilastine or rupatadine and bilastine in children.

According to current European, Canadian, and WHO guidelines, the dose of second generation H1 antihistamines should be increased up to four times for a trial if the standard dose is not effective [3, 32, 105]. Few studies in adults demonstrated that CU adult patients receiving up to 4 times the dose have better control of symptoms [106] and do not experience more side effects [107]. However, the efficacy of these dose escalations was not established in children although they are suggested to be applicable in children based on extrapolated data from rhinitis studies [108].

Studies suggest that in teenagers and adults, cetirizine use may promote somnolence and decreased motivation to perform activities during the workday compared with loratadine even at recommended doses [109, 110]. Thus, we recommend using other second generation antihistamines at higher than normal doses (e.g., desloratadine, rupatadine, or bilastine (in children 12 years old and above).

In a systematic review on pediatric CSU management [97] it was reported that four randomized controlled trials demonstrated high efficacy and safety for the use of omalizumab involving adults and teenagers in doses of 150–300 mg subcutaneously once a month for 6 months [111–114]. However, only a minority of the study population were teenagers and no children below 12 years were included. More limited studies mainly case reports support the efficacy and safety of omalizumab [34, 43, 115] and ciclosporin (3–4 mg/kg/day) [100, 101, 116] in severe cases of CSU in teenagers as well as in younger children. There was one case report demonstrating the benefit of rituximab [117].

There are also substantial knowledge gaps regarding the optimal dose and duration of antihistamines and biologics in children and large scale RCT are required to establish their appropriate use in children. Future studies are required to establish the safety of high dose second generation H1 antihistamines and to define the optimal dose and duration of treatment in the pediatric CSU with omalizumab. Although ciclosporin had been reported to be effective in limited sample size studies in children [100, 101, 116], potential toxicity that can occur in more than half of patients treated with moderate doses (4–5 mg/kg/day) and the need to monitor renal function and blood levels [118] is a significant limitation to the use of ciclosporin in children with CU for a short period of 3–4 months.

Given the poor adherence to current guidelines [119] and reports on frequent use of steroids in patients with CU [120], educational programs contributing to implementation of current guidelines and discouraging the use of long-term use of steroids are required, except as rescue treatment for acute severe flares [121]. This is especially important in young children given reports of behavioral abnormalities [122], adrenal suppression [123], and avascular necrosis [124].

14.1.3 CU in Pregnancy and Lactation

During pregnancy there are substantial endocrine and immunological changes. Changes in the hormonal state and the shift toward anti-inflammation are postulated to affect mast cells. Indeed, altered sex hormone serum levels have been described in subgroups of CSU patients. However, predicting the clinical consequences of these effects is challenging [125]. There are reports on CU flares during pregnancy in some cases as well as improvement in others [125]. Further pruritic urticarial papules and plaques of pregnancy (PUPPP) and other pregnancy-related dermatoses associated with pruritus should be considered as differential diagnosis if wheals and itch newly occur in pregnancy, especially during the third trimester.

For cases of clear CU the international guidelines state clearly, potential treatments. In general, systemic treatment should be avoided, if possible, in pregnant or lactating women. There are data available for the use of loratadine and cetirizine during pregnancy. Loratadine had previously been proposed as a possible factor for the increased incidence of hypospadias in infants born to mothers who had taken loratadine during pregnancy [126]. However, recent studies have ruled out this possibility and suggest that this agent does not represent a major teratogenic. However, loratadine is still considered as a category B drug by FDA [127].

Fexofenadine and desloratadine have been classified as pregnancy category C. Animal studies reveal reduction in pup weight and survival associated with fexofenadine treatment during pregnancy. There are no human data on fexofenadine and desloratadine and hence they are not categorized as safe during pregnancy. All H_1 antihistamines are excreted in breast milk. Old first generation antihistamines should no longer be used in pregnancy and lactating women due to higher risk of sedation [127].

Omalizumab has been recently assigned a pregnancy category B by the FDA [128], based mainly on data from the Xolair pregnancy registry (Expect) [129]. There are a few reports on omalizumab use during pregnancy without apparent toxicity for the offspring and achieving disease control during pregnancy [130–132]. Thus, omalizumab can be considered as a safe and successful therapeutic alternative, after careful consideration of risk-benefit profile in pregnant women with uncontrolled CU. No information is available on the clinical use of omalizumab during breastfeeding. Given that omalizumab is a large protein molecule, the amount in milk is likely to be very low. Further, absorption in the breast fed infant is unlikely because it is probably destroyed in the infant's gastrointestinal tract. However, given lack of data, omalizumab should be used with caution during breastfeeding, especially while nursing a newborn or preterm infants [133]. There are no studies on the effects of ciclosporin as treatment for CU in pregnant or breastfeeding women. However, there are limited reports on its effects mainly in the context of treating pregnant women with inflammatory bowel diseases and transplantation. In general there are more concerns raised regarding the use of ciclosporin during pregnancy [134, 135], although in a meta-analysis it was concluded that ciclosporin does not appear to be a major human teratogen and it is recommended during pregnancy in some autoimmune diseases [136]. More research is needed to establish the safe use of ciclosporin during pregnancy.

Ciclosporin concentration in milk is variable. With typical maternal ciclosporin blood levels, a completely breastfed infant would usually receive no more than about 2% of the mother's weight-adjusted dosage or pediatric transplantation maintenance dosage. However, it was reported that in 2 infants ciclosporin levels were measurable. Some reviewers believe breastfeeding should be discouraged during ciclosporin use, but these opinions appear to be based on limited, early data [137] while European experts, the National Transplantation Pregnancy Registry and other experts consider ciclosporin to be probably safe to use for inflammatory bowel disease during breastfeeding [138, 139]. Breastfed infants should be monitored if this drug is used during lactation, possibly including measurement of serum levels to rule out toxicity if there is a concern [140]. Although short-term use of steroids is sometimes necessary, betamethasone should be avoided given reports on teratogenicity in animal studies and its classification as category C by the FDA [141, 142].

In conclusion, recommendation for up-dosing second generation H1 antihistamines, use of omalizumab or ciclosporin for the treatment of CU during pregnancy and lactation should be discussed with patients and decision may vary from case to case given the sparse data available. Clearly large scale RCT are required to establish recommendations for the drug management of CU in pregnancy and lactation.

References

1. Gaig P, Olona M, Munoz LD, Caballero MT, Dominguez FJ, Echechipia S, et al. Epidemiology of urticaria in Spain. J Investig Allergol Clin Immunol. 2004;14(3):214–20.
2. Greaves MW. Chronic urticaria. N Engl J Med. 1995;332(26):1767–72.
3. Sussman G, Hebert J, Gulliver W, Lynde C, Waserman S, Kanani A, et al. Insights and advances in chronic urticaria: a Canadian perspective. Allergy Asthma Clin Immunol. 2015;11(1):7.
4. Maurer M, Weller K, Bindslev-Jensen C, Gimenez-Arnau A, Bousquet P, Bousquet J, et al. Unmet clinical needs in chronic spontaneous urticaria. A GA(2) LEN task force report. Allergy. 2011;66(3):317–30.
5. Konstantinou GN, Papadopoulos NG, Tavladaki T, Tsekoura T, Tsilimigaki A, Grattan CE. Childhood acute urticaria in northern and southern Europe shows a similar epidemiological pattern and significant meteorological influences. Pediatr Allergy Immunol. 2011;22(1 Pt 1):36–42.
6. Liu TH, Lin YR, Yang KC, Tsai YG, Fu YC, Wu TK, et al. Significant factors associated with severity and outcome of an initial episode of acute urticaria in children. Pediatr Allergy Immunol. 2010;21(7):1043–51.
7. Sackesen C, Sekerel BE, Orhan F, Kocabas CN, Tuncer A, Adalioglu G. The etiology of different forms of urticaria in childhood. Pediatr Dermatol. 2004;21(2):102–8.
8. Simons FE. Prevention of acute urticaria in young children with atopic dermatitis. J Allergy Clin Immunol. 2001;107(4):703–6.
9. Simons FE. H1-antihistamine treatment in young atopic children: effect on urticaria. Ann Allergy Asthma Immunol. 2007;99(3):261–6.
10. Hampel FC, Kittner B, van Bavel JH. Safety and tolerability of fexofenadine hydrochloride, 15 and 30 mg, twice daily in children aged 6 months to 2 years with allergic rhinitis. Ann Allergy Asthma Immunol. 2007;99(6):549–54.

11. Bloom M, Staudinger H, Herron J. Safety of desloratadine syrup in children. Curr Med Res Opin. 2004;20(12):1959–65.
12. Salmun LM, Herron JM, Banfield C, Padhi D, Lorber R, Affrime MB. The pharmacokinetics, electrocardiographic effects, and tolerability of loratadine syrup in children aged 2 to 5 years. Clin Ther. 2000;22(5):613–21.
13. Potter P, Mitha E, Barkai L, Mezei G, Santamaria E, Izquierdo I, et al. Rupatadine is effective in the treatment of chronic spontaneous urticaria in children aged 2-11 years. Pediatr Allergy Immunol. 2016;27(1):55–61.
14. Chan JCK, Peters RL, Koplin JJ, Dharmage SC, Gurrin LC, Wake M, et al. Food challenge and community-reported reaction profiles in food-allergic children aged 1 and 4 years: a population-based study. J Allergy Clin Immunol Pract. 2017;5(2):398–409.
15. Fernandes RA, Regateiro F, Pereira C, Faria E, Pita J, Todo-Bom A, et al. Anaphylaxis in a food allergy outpatient department: one-year review. Eur Ann Allergy Clin Immunol. 2018;50(2):81–8.
16. Simons FE, Ardusso LR, Bilo MB, El-Gamal YM, Ledford DK, Ring J, et al. World Allergy Organization anaphylaxis guidelines: summary. J Allergy Clin Immunol. 2011;127(3):587–93.
17. Sampson HA, Munoz-Furlong A, Campbell RL, Adkinson NF Jr, Bock SA, Branum A, et al. Second symposium on the definition and management of anaphylaxis: summary report—second National Institute of Allergy and Infectious Disease/Food Allergy and Anaphylaxis Network symposium. Ann Emerg Med. 2006;47(4):373–80.
18. Mathur AN, Mathes EF. Urticaria mimickers in children. Dermatol Ther. 2013;26(6):467–75.
19. Chiong FJ, Loewenthal M, Boyle M, Attia J. Serum sickness-like reaction after influenza vaccination. BMJ Case Rep. 2015;2015:bcr2015211917.
20. Starnes L, Patel T, Skinner RB. Urticaria multiforme—a case report. Pediatr Dermatol. 2011;28(4):436–8.
21. Mortureux P, Leaute-Labreze C, Legrain-Lifermann V, Lamireau T, Sarlangue J, Taieb A. Acute urticaria in infancy and early childhood: a prospective study. Arch Dermatol. 1998;134(3):319–23.
22. Balp MM, Weller K, Carboni V, Chirilov A, Papavassilis C, Severin T, et al. Prevalence and clinical characteristics of chronic spontaneous urticaria in pediatric patients. Pediatr Allergy Immunol. 2018;29(6):630–6.
23. Ferriani MP, Silva MF, Pereira RM, Terreri MT, Saad MC, Bonfa E, et al. Chronic spontaneous urticaria: a survey of 852 cases of childhood-onset systemic lupus erythematosus. Int Arch Allergy Immunol. 2015;167(3):186–92.
24. Caffarelli C, Cuomo B, Cardinale F, Barberi S, Dascola CP, Agostinis F, et al. Aetiological factors associated with chronic urticaria in children: a systematic review. Acta Derm Venereol. 2013;93(3):268–72.
25. Lee N, Lee JD, Lee HY, Kang DR, Ye YM. Epidemiology of chronic urticaria in korea using the Korean Health Insurance Database, 2010-2014. Allergy Asthma Immunol Res. 2017;9(5):438–45.
26. Schaefer P. Acute and chronic urticaria: evaluation and treatment. Am Fam Physician. 2017;95(11):717–24.
27. Powell RJ, Du Toit GL, Siddique N, Leech SC, Dixon TA, Clark AT, et al. BSACI guidelines for the management of chronic urticaria and angio-oedema. Clin Exp Allergy. 2007;37(5):631–50.
28. Goldstein S, Gabriel S, Kianifard F, Ortiz B, Skoner DP. Clinical features of adolescents with chronic idiopathic or spontaneous urticaria: review of omalizumab clinical trials. Ann Allergy Asthma Immunol. 2017;118(4):500–4.
29. Trevisonno J, Balram B, Netchiporouk E, Ben-Shoshan M. Physical urticaria: review on classification, triggers and management with special focus on prevalence including a meta-analysis. Postgrad Med. 2015;127(6):565–70.
30. Netchiporouk E, Sasseville D, Moreau L, Habel Y, Rahme E, Ben-Shoshan M. Evaluating comorbidities, natural history, and predictors of early resolution in a cohort of children with chronic urticaria. JAMA Dermatol. 2017;153(12):1236–42.

31. Khakoo G, Sofianou-Katsoulis A, Perkin MR, Lack G. Clinical features and natural history of physical urticaria in children. Pediatr Allergy Immunol. 2008;19(4):363–6.
32. Magerl M, Altrichter S, Borzova E, Gimenez-Arnau A, Grattan CE, Lawlor F, et al. The definition, diagnostic testing, and management of chronic inducible urticarias—The EAACI/GA(2) LEN/EDF/UNEV consensus recommendations 2016 update and revision. Allergy. 2016;71(6):780–802.
33. Alba Marin JC, Martorell AA, Satorre VP, Gastaldo SE. Treatment of severe cold-induced urticaria in a child with omalizumab. J Investig Allergol Clin Immunol. 2015;25(4):303–4.
34. Netchiporouk E, Nguyen CH, Thuraisingham T, Jafarian F, Maurer M, Ben-Shoshan M. Management of pediatric chronic spontaneous and physical urticaria patients with omalizumab: case series. Pediatr Allergy Immunol. 2015;26(6):585–8.
35. Greaves MW. Chronic urticaria in childhood. Allergy. 2000;55(4):309–20.
36. Alangari AA, Twarog FJ, Shih MC, Schneider LC. Clinical features and anaphylaxis in children with cold urticaria. Pediatrics. 2004;113(4):e313–7.
37. Hochstadter EF, Ben-Shoshan M. Cold-induced urticaria: challenges in diagnosis and management. BMJ Case Rep. 2013;2013.
38. Azkur D, Civelek E, Toyran M, Msrlolu ED, Erkoolu M, Kaya A, et al. Clinical and etiologic evaluation of the children with chronic urticaria. Allergy Asthma Proc. 2016;37(6):450–7.
39. Altrichter S, Koch K, Church MK, Maurer M. Atopic predisposition in cholinergic urticaria patients and its implications. J Eur Acad Dermatol Venereol. 2016;30(12):2060–5.
40. Metz M, Ohanyan T, Church MK, Maurer M. Retreatment with omalizumab results in rapid remission in chronic spontaneous and inducible urticaria. JAMA Dermatol. 2014;150(3):288–90.
41. Cavkaytar O, Arik YE, Buyuktiryaki B, Sekerel BE, Sackesen C, Soyer OU. Challenge-proven aspirin hypersensitivity in children with chronic spontaneous urticaria. Allergy. 2015;70(2):153–60.
42. Sanchez-Borges M, Caballero-Fonseca F, Capriles-Hulett A, Gonzalez-Aveledo L. Aspirin-exacerbated cutaneous disease (AECD) is a distinct subphenotype of chronic spontaneous urticaria. J Eur Acad Dermatol Venereol. 2015;29(4):698–701.
43. Porcaro F, Di MA, Cutrera R. Omalizumab in patient with aspirin exacerbated respiratory disease and chronic idiopathic urticaria. Pediatr Pulmonol. 2017;52(5):E26–8.
44. Sanchez JJ, Sanchez A, Cardona R. Prevalence of drugs as triggers of exacerbations in chronic urticaria. J Investig Allergol Clin Immunol. 2019;29(2):112–7.
45. Arik YE, Karaatmaca B, Sackesen C, Sahiner UM, Cavkaytar O, Sekerel BE, et al. Parasitic infections in children with chronic spontaneous urticaria. Int Arch Allergy Immunol. 2016;171(2):130–5.
46. Kolkhir P, Balakirski G, Merk HF, Olisova O, Maurer M. Chronic spontaneous urticaria and internal parasites—a systematic review. Allergy. 2016;71(3):308–22.
47. Mehta RK, Shah N, Scott DG, Grattan CE, Barker TH. Case 4. Chronic urticaria due to strongyloidiasis. Clin Exp Dermatol. 2002;27(1):84–5.
48. Stenzel DJ, Boreham PF. Blastocystis hominis revisited. Clin Microbiol Rev. 1996;9(4):563–84.
49. Laodim P, Intapan PM, Sawanyawisuth K, Laummaunwai P, Maleewong W. A hospital-based study of epidemiological and clinical data on blastocystis hominis infection. Foodborne Pathog Dis. 2012;9(12):1077–82.
50. Fisher D, McCarry F, Currie B. Strongyloidiasis in the Northern Territory. Under-recognised and under-treated? Med J Aust. 1993;159(2):88–90.
51. Kuemmerle-Deschner JB. CAPS—pathogenesis, presentation and treatment of an autoinflammatory disease. Semin Immunopathol. 2015;37(4):377–85.
52. Kuemmerle-Deschner JB, Ozen S, Tyrrell PN, Kone-Paut I, Goldbach-Mansky R, Lachmann H, et al. Diagnostic criteria for cryopyrin-associated periodic syndrome (CAPS). Ann Rheum Dis. 2017;76(6):942–7.

53. Li C, Tan X, Zhang J, Li S, Mo W, Han T, et al. Gene mutations and clinical phenotypes in 15 Chinese children with cryopyrin-associated periodic syndrome (CAPS). Sci China Life Sci. 2017;60(12):1436–44.
54. Mehr S, Allen R, Boros C, Adib N, Kakakios A, Turner PJ, et al. Cryopyrin-associated periodic syndrome in Australian children and adults: epidemiological, clinical and treatment characteristics. J Paediatr Child Health. 2016;52(9):889–95.
55. Imbernon-Moya A, Vargas-Laguna E, Burgos F, Fernandez-Cogolludo E, Aguilar-Martinez A, Gallego-Valdes MA. Urticaria vasculitis in a child: a case report and literature review. Clin Case Rep. 2017;5(8):1255–7.
56. Kaur S, Thami GP. Urticarial vasculitis in infancy. Indian J Dermatol Venereol Leprol. 2003;69(3):223–4.
57. Spadoni M, Jacob C, Aikawa N, Jesus A, Fomin A, Silva C. Chronic autoimmune urticaria as the first manifestation of juvenile systemic lupus erythematosus. Lupus. 2011;20(7):763–6.
58. Brockow K. Epidemiology, prognosis, and risk factors in mastocytosis. Immunol Allergy Clin North Am. 2014;34(2):283–95.
59. Tamay Z, Ozceker D. Current approach to cutaneous mastocytosis in childhood. Turk Pediatri Ars. 2016;51(3):123–7.
60. Ben-Amitai D, Metzker A, Cohen HA. Pediatric cutaneous mastocytosis: a review of 180 patients. Isr Med Assoc J. 2005;7(5):320–2.
61. Horny HP, Sotlar K, Valent P. Mastocytosis: state of the art. Pathobiology. 2007;74(2):121–32.
62. Lange M, Nedoszytko B, Gorska A, Zawrocki A, Sobjanek M, Kozlowski D. Mastocytosis in children and adults: clinical disease heterogeneity. Arch Med Sci. 2012;8(3):533–41.
63. Le M, Miedzybrodzki B, Olynych T, Chapdelaine H, Ben-Shoshan M. Natural history and treatment of cutaneous and systemic mastocytosis. Postgrad Med. 2017;129(8):896–901.
64. Theoharides TC, Valent P, Akin C. Mast cells, mastocytosis, and related disorders. N Engl J Med. 2015;373(2):163–72.
65. Sokol KC, Ghazi A, Kelly BC, Grant JA. Omalizumab as a desensitizing agent and treatment in mastocytosis: a review of the literature and case report. J Allergy Clin Immunol Pract. 2014;2(3):266–70.
66. Kaplan AP, Gimenez-Arnau AM, Saini SS. Mechanisms of action that contribute to efficacy of omalizumab in chronic spontaneous urticaria. Allergy. 2017;72(4):519–33.
67. Pettigrew HD, Teuber SS, Kong JS, Gershwin ME. Contemporary challenges in mastocytosis. Clin Rev Allergy Immunol. 2010;38(2-3):125–34.
68. Nedelea I, Deleanu D. Isolated angioedema: an overview of clinical features and etiology. Exp Ther Med. 2019;17(2):1068–72.
69. Belbezier A, Hardy G, Marlu R, Defendi F, Dumestre PC, Boccon-Gibod I, et al. Plasminogen gene mutation with normal C1 inhibitor hereditary angioedema: three additional French families. Allergy. 2018;73(11):2237–9.
70. Bafunno V, Firinu D, D'Apolito M, Cordisco G, Loffredo S, Leccese A, et al. Mutation of the angiopoietin-1 gene (ANGPT1) associates with a new type of hereditary angioedema. J Allergy Clin Immunol. 2018;141(3):1009–17.
71. Pattanaik D, Lieberman JA. Pediatric angioedema. Curr Allergy Asthma Rep. 2017;17(9):60.
72. Wahn V, Aberer W, Eberl W, Fasshauer M, Kuhne T, Kurnik K, et al. Hereditary angioedema (HAE) in children and adolescents—a consensus on therapeutic strategies. Eur J Pediatr. 2012;171(9):1339–48.
73. Farkas H, Kohalmi KV. Icatibant for the treatment of hereditary angioedema with C1-inhibitor deficiency in adolescents and in children aged over 2 years. Expert Rev Clin Immunol. 2018;14(6):447–60.
74. Cicardi M, Suffritti C, Perego F, Caccia S. Novelties in the diagnosis and treatment of angioedema. J Investig Allergol Clin Immunol. 2016;26(4):212–21.
75. Rosen FS, Austen KF. Androgen therapy in hereditary angioneurotic edema. N Engl J Med. 1976;295(26):1476–7.
76. Farkas H, Harmat G, Gyeney L, Fust G, Varga L. Danazol therapy for hereditary angio-oedema in children. Lancet. 1999;354(9183):1031–2.

77. Kozel MM, Sabroe RA. Chronic urticaria: aetiology, management and current and future treatment options. Drugs. 2004;64(22):2515–36.
78. O'Donnell BF, Lawlor F, Simpson J, Morgan M, Greaves MW. The impact of chronic urticaria on the quality of life. Br J Dermatol. 1997;136(2):197–201.
79. Sahiner UM, Civelek E, Tuncer A, Yavuz ST, Karabulut E, Sackesen C, et al. Chronic urticaria: etiology and natural course in children. Int Arch Allergy Immunol. 2011;156(2):224–30.
80. van der Valk PG, Moret G, Kiemeney LA. The natural history of chronic urticaria and angioedema in patients visiting a tertiary referral centre. Br J Dermatol. 2002;146(1):110–3.
81. Gregoriou S, Rigopoulos D, Katsambas A, Katsarou A, Papaioannou D, Gkouvi A, et al. Etiologic aspects and prognostic factors of patients with chronic urticaria: nonrandomized, prospective, descriptive study. J Cutan Med Surg. 2009;13(4):198–203.
82. Kolkhir P, Andre F, Church MK, Maurer M, Metz M. Potential blood biomarkers in chronic spontaneous urticaria. Clin Exp Allergy. 2017;47(1):19–36.
83. Kulthanan K, Jiamton S, Thumpimukvatana N, Pinkaew S. Chronic idiopathic urticaria: prevalence and clinical course. J Dermatol. 2007;34(5):294–301.
84. Nuzzo V, Tauchmanova L, Colasanti P, Zuccoli A, Colao A. Idiopathic chronic urticaria and thyroid autoimmunity: experience of a single center. Dermatoendocrinol. 2011;3(4):255–8.
85. Schaefer P. Urticaria: evaluation and treatment. Am Fam Physician. 2011;83(9):1078–84.
86. Chen J, Zhou DH, Nisbet AJ, Xu MJ, Huang SY, Li MW, et al. Advances in molecular identification, taxonomy, genetic variation and diagnosis of Toxocara spp. Infect Genet Evol. 2012;12(7):1344–8.
87. Cornillier H, Giraudeau B, Samimi M, Munck S, Hacard F, Jonville-Bera AP, et al. Effect of diet in chronic spontaneous urticaria: a systematic review. Acta Derm Venereol. 2019;99(2):127–32.
88. Du TG, Roberts G, Sayre PH, Bahnson HT, Radulovic S, Santos AF, et al. Randomized trial of peanut consumption in infants at risk for peanut allergy. N Engl J Med. 2015;372(9):803–13.
89. Flinterman AE, Knulst AC, Meijer Y, Bruijnzeel-Koomen CA, Pasmans SG. Acute allergic reactions in children with AEDS after prolonged cow's milk elimination diets. Allergy. 2006;61(3):370–4.
90. Gruber BL, Baeza ML, Marchese MJ, Agnello V, Kaplan AP. Prevalence and functional role of anti-IgE autoantibodies in urticarial syndromes. J Invest Dermatol. 1988;90(2):213–7.
91. Kaplan AP, Greaves M. Pathogenesis of chronic urticaria. Clin Exp Allergy. 2009;39(6):777–87.
92. Schmetzer O, Lakin E, Topal FA, Preusse P, Freier D, Church MK, et al. IL-24 is a common and specific autoantigen of IgE in patients with chronic spontaneous urticaria. J Allergy Clin Immunol. 2018;142(3):876–82.
93. Grattan C. Autoimmune chronic spontaneous urticaria. J Allergy Clin Immunol. 2017;139(6):1772–1781.e1.
94. Grattan CE, Wallington TB, Warin RP, Kennedy CT, Bradfield JW. A serological mediator in chronic idiopathic urticaria—a clinical, immunological and histological evaluation. Br J Dermatol. 1986;114(5):583–90.
95. Altrich ML, Halsey JF, Altman LC. Comparison of the in vivo autologous skin test with in vitro diagnostic tests for diagnosis of chronic autoimmune urticaria. Allergy Asthma Proc. 2009;30(1):28–34.
96. Netchiporouk E, Moreau L, Rahme E, Maurer M, Lejtenyi D, Ben-Shoshan M. Positive CD63 basophil activation tests are common in children with chronic spontaneous urticaria and linked to high disease activity. Int Arch Allergy Immunol. 2016;171(2):81–8.
97. Ben-Shoshan M, Grattan CE. Management of pediatric urticaria with review of the literature on chronic spontaneous urticaria in children. J Allergy Clin Immunol Pract. 2018;6(4):1152–61.
98. Hampel F, Ratner P, Haeusler JM. Safety and tolerability of levocetirizine dihydrochloride in infants and children with allergic rhinitis or chronic urticaria. Allergy Asthma Proc. 2010;31(4):290–5.
99. Novak Z, Yanez A, Kiss I, Kuna P, Tortajada-Girbes M, Valiente R. Safety and tolerability of bilastine 10 mg administered for 12 weeks in children with allergic diseases. Pediatr Allergy Immunol. 2016;27(5):493–8.

100. Doshi DR, Weinberger MM. Experience with cyclosporine in children with chronic idiopathic urticaria. Pediatr Dermatol. 2009;26(4):409–13.
101. Neverman L, Weinberger M. Treatment of chronic urticaria in children with antihistamines and cyclosporine. J Allergy Clin Immunol Pract. 2014;2(4):434–8.
102. Fitzsimons R, van der Poel LA, Thornhill W, Du TG, Shah N, Brough HA. Antihistamine use in children. Arch Dis Child Educ Pract Ed. 2015;100(3):122–31.
103. Wang XY, Lim-Jurado M, Prepageran N, Tantilipikorn P, Wang DY. Treatment of allergic rhinitis and urticaria: a review of the newest antihistamine drug bilastine. Ther Clin Risk Manag. 2016;12:585–97.
104. Johnson M, Kwatra G, Badyal DK, Thomas EA. Levocetirizine and rupatadine in chronic idiopathic urticaria. Int J Dermatol. 2015;54(10):1199–204.
105. Zuberbier T, Asero R, Bindslev-Jensen C, Walter CG, Church MK, Gimenez-Arnau A, et al. EAACI/GA(2)LEN/EDF/WAO guideline: definition, classification and diagnosis of urticaria. Allergy. 2009;64(10):1417–26.
106. Staevska M, Popov TA, Kralimarkova T, Lazarova C, Kraeva S, Popova D, et al. The effectiveness of levocetirizine and desloratadine in up to 4 times conventional doses in difficult-to-treat urticaria. J Allergy Clin Immunol. 2010;125(3):676–82.
107. Finn AF Jr, Kaplan AP, Fretwell R, Qu R, Long J. A double-blind, placebo-controlled trial of fexofenadine HCl in the treatment of chronic idiopathic urticaria. J Allergy Clin Immunol. 1999;104(5):1071–8.
108. Church MK, Weller K, Stock P, Maurer M. Chronic spontaneous urticaria in children: itching for insight. Pediatr Allergy Immunol. 2011;22(1 Pt 1):1–8.
109. Salmun LM, Gates D, Scharf M, Greiding L, Ramon F, Heithoff K. Loratadine versus cetirizine: assessment of somnolence and motivation during the workday. Clin Ther. 2000;22(5):573–82.
110. Howarth PH, Stern MA, Roi L, Reynolds R, Bousquet J. Double-blind, placebo-controlled study comparing the efficacy and safety of fexofenadine hydrochloride (120 and 180 mg once daily) and cetirizine in seasonal allergic rhinitis. J Allergy Clin Immunol. 1999;104(5):927–33.
111. Saini S, Rosen KE, Hsieh HJ, Wong DA, Conner E, Kaplan A, et al. A randomized, placebo-controlled, dose-ranging study of single-dose omalizumab in patients with H1-antihistamine-refractory chronic idiopathic urticaria. J Allergy Clin Immunol. 2011;128(3):567–73.
112. Saini SS, Bindslev-Jensen C, Maurer M, Grob JJ, Bulbul BE, Bradley MS, et al. Efficacy and safety of omalizumab in patients with chronic idiopathic/spontaneous urticaria who remain symptomatic on H1 antihistamines: a randomized, placebo-controlled study. J Invest Dermatol. 2015;135(3):925.
113. Maurer M, Rosen K, Hsieh HJ, Saini S, Grattan C, Gimenez-Arnau A, et al. Omalizumab for the treatment of chronic idiopathic or spontaneous urticaria. N Engl J Med. 2013;368(10):924–35.
114. Kaplan A, Ledford D, Ashby M, Canvin J, Zazzali JL, Conner E, et al. Omalizumab in patients with symptomatic chronic idiopathic/spontaneous urticaria despite standard combination therapy. J Allergy Clin Immunol. 2013;132(1):101–9.
115. Asero R, Casalone R, Iemoli E. Extraordinary response to omalizumab in a child with severe chronic urticaria. Eur Ann Allergy Clin Immunol. 2014;46(1):41–2.
116. Giuliodori K, Ganzetti G, Campanati A, Simonetti O, Marconi B, Offidani A. A non-responsive chronic autoimmune urticaria in a 12-year-old autistic girl treated with cyclosporin. J Eur Acad Dermatol Venereol. 2009;23(5):619–20.
117. Arkwright PD. Anti-CD20 or anti-IgE therapy for severe chronic autoimmune urticaria. J Allergy Clin Immunol. 2009;123(2):510–1.
118. Kulthanan K, Chaweekulrat P, Komoltri C, Hunnangkul S, Tuchinda P, Chularojanamontri L, et al. Cyclosporine for chronic spontaneous urticaria: a meta-analysis and systematic review. J Allergy Clin Immunol Pract. 2018;6(2):586–99.
119. Weller K, Viehmann K, Brautigam M, Krause K, Siebenhaar F, Zuberbier T, et al. Management of chronic spontaneous urticaria in real life—in accordance with the guidelines? A cross-sectional physician-based survey study. J Eur Acad Dermatol Venereol. 2013;27(1):43–50.

120. Broder MS, Raimundo K, Antonova E, Chang E. Resource use and costs in an insured population of patients with chronic idiopathic/spontaneous urticaria. Am J Clin Dermatol. 2015;16(4):313–21.
121. Waljee AK, Rogers MA, Lin P, Singal AG, Stein JD, Marks RM, et al. Short term use of oral corticosteroids and related harms among adults in the United States: population based cohort study. BMJ. 2017;357:j1415.
122. Upadhyay A, Mishra OP, Prasad R, Upadhyay SK, Schaefer F. Behavioural abnormalities in children with new-onset nephrotic syndrome receiving corticosteroid therapy: results of a prospective longitudinal study. Pediatr Nephrol. 2016;31(2):233–8.
123. Harel S, Hursh BE, Chan ES, Avinashi V, Panagiotopoulos C. Adrenal suppression in children treated with oral viscous budesonide for eosinophilic esophagitis. J Pediatr Gastroenterol Nutr. 2015;61(2):190–3.
124. Salem KH, Brockert AK, Mertens R, Drescher W. Avascular necrosis after chemotherapy for haematological malignancy in childhood. Bone Joint J. 2013;95-B(12):1708–13.
125. Woidacki K, Zenclussen AC, Siebenhaar F. Mast cell-mediated and associated disorders in pregnancy: a risky game with an uncertain outcome? Front Immunol. 2014;5:231.
126. Schwarz EB, Moretti ME, Nayak S, Koren G. Risk of hypospadias in offspring of women using loratadine during pregnancy: a systematic review and meta-analysis. Drug Saf. 2008;31(9):775–88.
127. Kar S, Krishnan A, Preetha K, Mohankar A. A review of antihistamines used during pregnancy. J Pharmacol Pharmacother. 2012;3(2):105–8.
128. Highlights of prescribing information. 2015. Ref Type: Online Source.
129. Namazy J, Cabana MD, Scheuerle AE, Thorp JM Jr, Chen H, Carrigan G, et al. The Xolair Pregnancy Registry (EXPECT): the safety of omalizumab use during pregnancy. J Allergy Clin Immunol. 2015;135(2):407–12.
130. Dos Santos RV, Locks BB, de Souza JR, Maurer M. Effects of omalizumab in a patient with three types of chronic urticaria. Br J Dermatol. 2014;170(2):469–71.
131. Cuervo-Pardo L, Barcena-Blanch M, Radojicic C. Omalizumab use during pregnancy for CIU: a tertiary care experience. Eur Ann Allergy Clin Immunol. 2016;48(4):145–6.
132. Ghazanfar MN, Thomsen SF. Successful and safe treatment of chronic spontaneous urticaria with omalizumab in a woman during two consecutive pregnancies. Case Rep Med. 2015;2015:368053.
133. Omalizumab. 2018. Drugs and Lactation Database (LactMed) [Internet]. Bethesda: National Library of Medicine (US. Ref Type: Online Source
134. Gonzalez-Estrada A, Geraci SA. Allergy medications during pregnancy. Am J Med Sci. 2016;352(3):326–31.
135. Unver DN, Uysal II, Fazliogullari Z, Karabulut AK, Acar H. Investigation of developmental toxicity and teratogenicity of cyclosporine A, tacrolimus and their combinations with prednisolone. Regul Toxicol Pharmacol. 2016;77:213–22.
136. Bar OB, Hackman R, Einarson T, Koren G. Pregnancy outcome after cyclosporine therapy during pregnancy: a meta-analysis. Transplantation. 2001;71(8):1051–5.
137. Janssen NM, Genta MS. The effects of immunosuppressive and anti-inflammatory medications on fertility, pregnancy, and lactation. Arch Intern Med. 2000;160(5):610–9.
138. van der Woude CJ, Kolacek S, Dotan I, Oresland T, Vermeire S, Munkholm P, et al. European evidenced-based consensus on reproduction in inflammatory bowel disease. J Crohns Colitis. 2010;4(5):493–510.
139. Gotestam SC, Hoeltzenbein M, Tincani A, Fischer-Betz R, Elefant E, Chambers C, et al. The EULAR points to consider for use of antirheumatic drugs before pregnancy, and during pregnancy and lactation. Ann Rheum Dis. 2016;75(5):795–810.
140. Cyclosporine. 2006.
141. Derks JB, Mulder EJ, Visser GH. The effects of maternal betamethasone administration on the fetus. Br J Obstet Gynaecol. 1995;102(1):40–6.
142. Product information. Celestone (betamethasone). 2019. Schering Corporation, Kenilworth, NJ. Ref Type: Online Source.

Urticaria Therapy and Management. Looking Forward

15

Emek Kocatürk, Zuotao Zhao, and Ana M. Giménez-Arnau

Core Messages

The future of chronic urticaria depends on three major steps in the understanding of the disease. First, how shall we best manage the disease? Urticaria Reference and Excellence centers are the answer to this question; these are the centers established by GA²LEN where the excellence in care and management of chronic urticaria is based on particular criteria and assured to follow the most recent guidelines. Second, does precision medicine apply to the treatment of chronic urticaria, are there biomarkers to show disease activity and response to treatment? The answer to this question is not established currently but CRP, D-Dimer or Total IgE/IgERI were suggested as biomarkers of disease activity response to treatments. Third, what are the future drugs for the treatment of chronic urticaria? We have a wide range of future drugs that are currently being tested for the treatment of chronic urticaria such as ligelizumab, siglec-8, bruton kinase inhibitors, anti-IL-5, Syk-inhibitors, and dupilumab. Future will show how effective these drugs will be and if there will be specific endotypes of chronic urticaria that will benefit from silencing a particular pathway in the pathogenesis of the disease.

E. Kocatürk
Department of Dermatology, Koç University School of Medicine, Istanbul, Turkey

Z. Zhao
Department of Dermatology, First Hospital, Peking University, Beijing, China

A. M. Giménez-Arnau (✉)
Department of Dermatology, Hospital del Mar, IMIM, Universitat Autònoma,
Barcelona, Spain
e-mail: 22505aga@comb.cat

15.1 Looking Forward, Clinical Knowledge of Chronic Urticaria (CU)

Chronic Urticaria (CU) is a heterogeneous condition that causes significant morbidity [1, 2]. CU is characterized by the sudden appearance of wheals, angioedema, or both that persist for 6 weeks or longer [2]. Spontaneous CU (CSU) shows unpredictable symptoms, while inducible CU (CIndU) is provoked by, e.g., cold, heat, pressure, friction, or protein contact among others. Both types can be concomitantly present in the same patient. The average duration of CSU episodes is from 1 to 5 years [3, 4]. CSU is estimated to affect from 0.5 to 1% of the general population, with an annual incidence rate of 1.4% and it seems to increase [5, 6]. The exact CU prevalence and patient characteristics are still unknown in many countries. Because CSU imposes a significant economic burden and also has a substantial negative impact on patients' quality of life (QoL) there is an evident interest to identify such patients that are not medically controlled. An effective treatment as soon as the CSU or CIndU episodes start is crucial [7–9].

The EAACI/GA²LEN/EDF/WAO Urticaria Guidelines, acknowledged and accepted by the European Union of Medical Specialists (UEMS) with the participation of 48 delegates of 42 national and international societies is the most global guideline in urticaria, specially focused in chronic urticaria [2]. It is a clear and evidence based guideline nevertheless the degree of monitoring the urticaria guidelines by primary care physicians and specialists is generally still poor [10]. It is important to develop anticipated efforts in continuing medical education that can improve the critical judgment of the guidelines and their implementation in daily medical assistance.

Successful approach to CU patients would preferentially be developed in local, national, or international networks of experts. In this sense "Centers of reference and excellence in urticaria" (UCAREs) can help to improve the management of hard to treat conditions such as urticaria. The main aims of GA²LEN UCAREs are to provide excellence in urticaria management, to increase the knowledge of urticaria by research and education, and to promote the awareness of urticaria by advocacy activities. This program was created in 2016 and promotes the "never give up attitude" treating CU [11]. In the immediate future coming from a communal work some present unmet needs will have a global answer as, e.g., the dilemma of differential diagnosis, indicators of urticaria prognosis, or the management of urticaria in pregnancy/lactation or geriatrics.

Very little is known about the genetic profile of the urticaria patients who suffer CSU or CIndU. Some recent approach to the transcriptome of patients suffering a severely active CSU refractory to antihistamine treatment through the bioinformatic analysis of the whole Human Genome with Oligo Microarrays and Quantitative Real-Time Polymerase Chain Reaction (qPCR) showed an overall immunological skin involvement showing a peculiar gene profile involving lesional and non-lesional skin. The wheal overexpressed genes are involved in a variety of biological functions as epidermal differentiation, intracellular signal function, transcriptional factors, cell cycle differentiation, inflammation, or coagulation. Differentially expressed genes uniformly increase or decrease along the skin worsening until the wheal appearance [12]. Omalizumab's effect on gene expression in skin biopsies from CSU patients was shown over upregulated transcript in lesional skin (vs non-lesional and/or healthy volunteers skin) suggested increased mast cell/leukocyte infiltration (FCER1G, C3AR1, CD93, S100A8, and S100A9), increased oxidative stress, vascularization (CYR61), and skin repair events (KRT6A, KRT16) [13]. Nevertheless genotype expression and its further correlation with CSU phenotypes are still unknown.

CSU shows a heterogeneous activity, evolution, associated comorbidities, and response to treatment. The identification of clinical prognostic factors that help to predict disease course and response to standardized treatments would be very useful. Factors that have been described as worst prognostic factors in terms of CSU duration and/or CSU activity: suffer multiple CSU episodes (19.2% suffered more than one lifetime CSU), late-onset (63.6% showed >45 years once the CSU started), concomitant CIndU (20.2%), and functional serum autoreactivity [14]. CSU+CIndU patients required more frequent therapy after 5 years and higher doses of second-generation H1-antihistamines [14]. According to Curto L et al, 84.6% of patients with a baseline Urticaria Activity Score 7 (UAS7) between 16 and 42 required ciclosporin or omalizumab to achieve symptom control in contrast to 15.4% of patients with baseline UAS7 between 0 and 15 ($p = 0.0013$) [14]. Although different types of CU shared a common clinical expression, phenotypically the patients may show differences regarding triggers, activity, prognosis, and therapeutic response. The knowledge of phenotypical differences observed in CU helps to design an individual management plan improving symptoms control and quality of life, decreasing the burden of the disease.

The success of the management of CSU lies on a strategic plan. The EAACI/GA2LEN/EDF/WAO Urticaria guideline is continuously updated [2]. By consensus, a successful therapy should target the rapid and complete resolution of signs (hives and angioedema) and symptoms (itch and pain). A basic principle of efficacy and safety is desirable; it is the therapeutic goal, as the clinical experience holds that treatment should continue for extended periods of time, with adaptations according to changes in symptoms. Nowadays, the unique recommended third line treatment consists of adding omalizumab and we can define accurately a protocol of its use in daily practice. We have learned from our practice and we have data on prediction of CSU fast-slow or no response, the need to up-dose, relapse, and retreatment, use in special populations, efficacy for angioedema and CIndUs, or safety of long-term treatment [15]. Recently, several reports have suggested that certain parameters could be considered as potential disease-related biomarkers. Moreover, with the advent of such biomarkers, newer biologic agents are coming forth to revolutionize management of CSU. Based on molecular and genetic pathogenic findings several new treatments can also be proposed for CU. Ongoing new therapeutic development includes more potent anti-IgE therapy and other drugs targeting different pathogenic pathways.

15.2 Emerging Biomarkers in CU, Looking Forward

According to the National Institute of Health (NIH) Biomarkers Definitions Working Group, a biomarker is a "characteristic that is objectively measured and evaluated as an indicator of normal biological processes, pathogenic processes or pharmacological responses to a therapeutic intervention." Essential characteristics of a good biomarker are its sensitivity, specificity, and reproducibility for the identification and/ or measurement of a particular disease state [16]. In addition, the ease with which the biomarker can be collected and measured at the point of care is crucial [17]. The identification and validation of reliable biomarkers in CSU would be useful in CU to define the patient's disease status leading to a more individualized and personalized treatment and follow-up not only in everyday clinical care, but also in clinical trials.

15.2.1 Biomarkers for Disease Activity

Several markers have been investigated for their possible link to CSU activity. Inflammatory mediators such as the C-reactive protein (CRP) and interleukin (IL)-6 are increased in patients with more active CSU and are significantly lower upon spontaneous remission [18–29]. Likewise, levels of mean platelet volume (MPV), which is considered a marker of platelet reactivity, also show a positive correlation with CSU activity [30–42]. CSU is an immune-mediated chronic inflammatory disease resulting from immunological activation events following the exposure to different triggers [43]. The detection of increased levels of D-dimer and prothrombin fragment 1+2 (F1+2) in patients with more active disease demonstrates the involvement of the coagulation cascade and fibrinolysis in CSU, positioning themselves as potential biomarkers of disease activity [18–29, 34–46].

On the other hand, various abnormalities related to basophils and their functions have also been described in patients with active disease. For example, a negative correlation between blood basophil count and CSU activity suggesting that circulating basophils may be recruited from blood into urticarial skin lesions during the activity of the disease [47–50]. Increased levels of basophil CD63 or CD203c expression induced by CSU serum may also predict the highest CSU activity reflected by impairment in quality of life, higher frequency of emergency department use, and higher itch severity [51–53]. Several studies also support the notion that a positive autologous serum skin test (ASST), which is a simple in-vivo clinical test suggesting an autoimmune pathogenesis, is linked to more active CSU [54–57].

In summary, CRP, IL-6, MPV, D-dimer, and F1+2 deserve further exploration for their value as biomarkers of disease activity based on the high level of evidence (i.e., several studies from different centers showing the same association), consistency (i.e., reproducibility), feasibility, and clinical relevance. Nevertheless, other suggested biomarkers, especially those related to inflammation and coagulation, are not specific enough for urticaria. Its interpretation in CSU should be prudent.

15.2.2 Biomarkers for Response to Treatment

The establishment of personalized treatment plans remains one of the biggest challenges in CSU. In this regard, and given the emergence of new therapies in CSU, there is a growing interest to look for objective markers that reliably predict the disease prognosis and the effectiveness of a specific therapeutic intervention.

In the case of antihistamine therapy, D-dimer is the most promising biomarker. In an Italian study, patients with insufficient response to antihistamines were more likely to present elevated D-dimer levels [58]. This observation was confirmed by Kolkhir et al., who suggest that the evaluation not only of D-dimer, but also fibrinogen, CRP and erythrocyte sedimentation rate (ESR) should be considered before starting treatment with non-sedating antihistamines, since high levels of these markers may predict an unsatisfactory therapeutic response [28]. Another investigation reported that antihistamine-resistant CSU might show increased complement C5a fraction, higher disease activity; longer duration of wheals, and higher positivity of ASST [59].

Baseline levels of D-dimer have been also linked to response to ciclosporin. D-dimer levels showed a highly significant negative correlation with response to treatment and were also considered a useful tool to monitor this clinical response [60]. Another biomarker for ciclosporin responsiveness could be the basophil histamine release assay (BHRA). Thus, two independent investigations, including a double-blind placebo-controlled study, showed that patients with a positive BHRA are more likely to show a satisfactory response to ciclosporin than those with a negative BHRA [61, 62].

Regarding the undergoing treatment with omalizumab, a significant association has been shown between levels of IL-31, a major dermal pruritogen, and response to anti-IgE therapy, with lower baseline levels observed in patients showing a satisfactory clinical response [63]. Levels of total serum IgE and the high-affinity IgE receptor (FcεRI) expression on basophils are also interesting biomarkers for omalizumab responsiveness. In two recent studies Deza and coworkers reported how slow and complete non-responders CSU patients to omalizumab showed significantly lower baseline levels of basophil FcεRI expression than fast responders, suggesting that the deficient FcεRI downregulation experienced during treatment could be an explanation for the non-responder status [64, 65]. Ertas and coworkers postulate that total IgE levels and their change may also predict omalizumab responsiveness during treatment, particularly by the week 4/baseline ratio of total IgE [66]. Lastly, Palacios et al observed that the lack of basophil CD203-c upregulating activity, which is thought to reflect the presence of autoantibodies to IgE and/or FcεRI receptor, might also correlate with the clinical response to anti-IgE therapy [67]. In addition to the response to treatment, some studies investigated potential biomarkers for different categories of omalizumab response. For example, a positive BHRA and ASST have been proposed as predictors of slow therapeutic response, [68] while increased IgE levels seem to be linked to faster relapse in patients with omalizumab-discontinued CSU [69].

15.2.3 Biomarkers for Disease Course

The biomarkers discussed by their usefulness to predict the course of the disease, i.e., the time to spontaneous remission, show still a low level of evidence due to the small number of available studies. The most promising biomarker for CSU course seems to be the presence of serum anti-thyroid antibodies (ATA). Disease duration is significantly longer if ATA are detected in CSU patients [70]. Levels of vitamin D and total IgE have been also linked to disease duration. Woo et al showed that serum vitamin D levels are more likely to be critically low in CSU patients and can also be inversely related to disease duration [71, 72]. Meanwhile, Kessel et al. showed a significant association between increased total serum IgE levels and urticaria duration lasting more than 2 years [73].

Due to limited published data and different methodologies and/or study designs used, there is sometimes conflicting evidence for a particular biomarker. For example, profound basopenia has been linked to increased serum autoreactivity, greater impairment in quality of life, and poorly controlled disease in adult patients with CSU [47]. However, the same markers have been associated with a better prognosis in pediatric CSU. Children with CSU showed high scores on the basophil activation test using CD63 marker expression and absence of blood basophils being more likely to exhibit an earlier spontaneous resolution of urticaria [74]. This favorable prognosis associated with higher CD63 expression could be related to autoantibody production induced by transient viral and bacterial infections, which are quite common in children and represent well-known triggers of urticaria. Differences in etiologic and/or pathogenic factors (e.g., differences in the mechanism of autoimmunity) in both groups of patients could explain such results [75–77].

In addition to laboratory values, some clinical markers have been also linked to CSU duration. Concomitant angioedema or inducible urticaria may show longer disease duration, longer time to remission, and/or lower resolution rates [78–81]. Also, disease activity, evaluated through clinical scores, could also be related to CSU duration [57, 73, 82]. Some rare clinical features, such as arterial hypertension or hypersensitivity reactions to non-steroidal anti-inflammatory drugs, may result in a distinct CSU phenotype showing longer disease duration [83, 84].

To conclude, modern techniques allowed the identification of potential useful CSU biomarkers, such as RNA sequencing, microarrays, and proteomic or metabolomic analysis [12]. For example, by proteomics analysis, serum clusterin, a protein involved in multiple functions including modulation of the complement system, regressing angiogenesis, and cleaning bioactive cell debris, has been found to be increased in patients with a positive ASST and in those showing a satisfactory clinical response to antihistamine therapy [85]. Similarly, polymorphisms determined by Sequenom Mass Array technology on the FCER1A gene, which encodes the α-chain of the FcεRI receptor, have been linked to the therapeutic efficacy of non-sedating antihistamines and also to the risk for CSU in Chinese patients [86]. Recently, certain microRNAs were found to be significantly increased in patients with positive CU index (a functional anti-FcεRI test that supports the autoimmune basis of the disease) [87]. These microRNAs, which may be considered potential biomarkers for chronic autoimmune urticaria, target some genes that are associated with several biologic functions such as cellular movement, tissue development, regulation of leukocyte migration or inflammatory response. Although larger population sizes and multicenter studies are needed to confirm such preliminary observations, the implementation of these techniques might help in the near future to not only identify potential disease biomarkers of the disease, but also to increase our knowledge regarding the pathogenesis of CSU.

15.3 Treatments for Chronic Urticaria, Looking Forward

Treatment of chronic urticaria (CU) moved forward in the recent few years after the introduction of omalizumab into standard treatment. Treatment with omalizumab provides effective and safe symptom control in 52–90% of the patients and urticaria activity scores decrease significantly in clinical trials and real life studies [3, 88–94]. Still there is a proportion of CU patients that require more effective treatments. There are a number of clinical trials now running on for the treatment of CU (Table 15.1). Potential other molecules will also be mentioned which could be targets of treatment in the future (Fig. 15.1).

Table 15.1 Drugs under investigation for CU

Study drug	Type of the drug	Clinicaltrials.gov identifier	Phase
Ligelizumab (QGE-031)	Anti-IgE	NCT02477332	P2b
		NCT02649218	P2
		NCT03437278	P2b
		NCT03580356	P3
		NCT03580369	P3
UB-221	Anti-IgE	NCT03632291	P1
GSK2646264	Syk inhibitor	NCT02424799	P1
AK002	Siglec-8	NCT03436797	P2
Abatacept	Soluble protein[a]	NCT00886795	P1/P2
Canakinumab	Anti-IL-1	NCT01635127	P2
Rilonacept	Anti-IL-1	NCT02171416	P2
Fenebrutinib	Bruton kinase inhibitor	NCT03137069	P2
		NCT03693625	P2
Benralizumab	Anti-IL-5Rα	NCT03183024	P4
Mepolizumab	Anti-IL-5	NCT03494881	P1
Dupilumab	Anti-IL-4Rα		P2

[a]Abatacept is a fusion protein binds to CD80 and CD86 receptors on APC and blocks the interaction of CD80/CD86 receptors to CD28 and inhibiting T cell proliferation and B cell immunological response

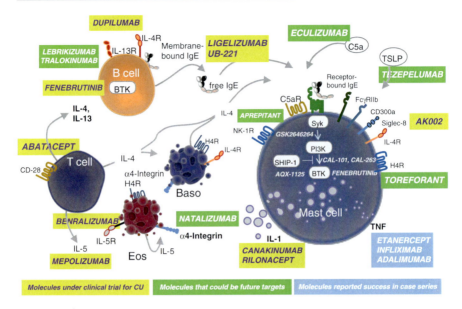

Fig. 15.1 Potential future targets of CU treatment. *Baso* basophil, *Eos* eosinophil, *H4R* histamine 4 receptor, *NK* neurokinin, *C5* complement 5, *IgE* immunoglobulin, *IL* interleukin, *LTR*, *PI3K* Phosphoinositide 3-kinase, *SHIP* Src-homology-containing inositol phosphatase 1, *Syk* spleen tyrosine kinase, *TSLP* thymic stromal lymphopoietin, *TNF* tumor necrosis factor, *BTK* Bruton kinase, *Siglec* sialic acid-binding, immunoglobulin-like lectins

15.3.1 Mast Cells/Basophils

15.3.1.1 Anti-IgEs

The most frequent cause of chronic spontaneous urticaria (CSU) is considered to be autoimmunity where two types of reactions are implicated. Type I autoimmunity is characterized by IgE to autoallergens and also termed as "autoallergy" while type-IIb autoimmunity is characterized by, e.g., IgG autoantibodies to IgE or its receptor (type 2b) and is different from cytotoxic/cytolytic hypersensitivity (type 2a) involving complement induced lysis [95, 96]. The fast responders to omalizumab are considered to have type I autoimmunity in which omalizumab rapidly binds free IgE autoantibodies and thus reduce mast cell activation, while slow responders are suggested to have type 2b autoimmunity in which the response depends on FcεRI receptor loss [95].

The growing interest on IgE as a therapeutical target promoted the production of new IgE-targeting strategies among which ligelizumab has the highest evidence and will be available soon.

Ligelizumab (QGE031)

Ligelizumab is a humanized IgG1 monoclonal antibody that binds with higher affinity to IgE than omalizumab. Like omalizumab, it inhibits the binding of free IgE to mast cells and basophils, thereby blocking the allergic reaction cascade. It shows 6 to 9-fold greater suppression of allergen-induced skin prick tests and provides greater and longer suppression of free IgE and IgE on the surface of circulating basophils [97]. The phase 2b study of ligelizumab included 382 patients with CSU (NCT02477332) and examined the efficacy and safety of ligelizumab compared to omalizumab. At the end of week 20, both ligelizumab 72 mg and 240 mg showed earlier and greater improvements in clinical responses compared to ligelizumab 24 mg, omalizumab 300 mg, and placebo [98]. Four studies are running to evaluate the efficacy and safety of ligelizumab in adolescent and adult patients with CSU (NCT03437278, NCT03580356, NCT03580369) as well as a safety extension study to evaluate the long-term safety of 240 mg subcutaneous (sc) ligelizumab given every 4 weeks for 52 weeks (NCT02649218). It seems that ligelizumab would be more effective than omalizumab in treating slow responders where type-IIb autoimmunity has been implicated.

UB-221

UB-221 is a third generation humanized anti-IgE monoclonal antibody which can neutralize IgE and can also regulate B cells through CD23, thereby blocking the production of IgE [99]. A phase I, open-label, dose-escalation study to evaluate the safety, tolerability, pharmacokinetics, and pharmacodynamics of a single dose of UB-221 as an add-on therapy in patients with CSU is now running (NCT03632291).

15.3.1.2 Other Anti-IgE Strategies

Many strategies to target IgE are on the way of production, which focus on IgE neutralization in blood, IgE-effector cell elimination, or IgE+ B cell reduction [100]. IgE-Fc3-4 mutant (IgE-R419NFc3-4), MEDI4212, recombinant single chain variable fragment (ScFv) antibody, antiFcεRI Fab conjugated celastrol loaded polymeric micelles, bispecific IgECD3 antibody, XmAb7195 constitute examples for new anti-IgE strategies [101–107]. DARPins (designed ankyrin repeat protein) are genetically engineered antibody mimetic proteins, which are small, inexpensive, rapidly acting, and can be used as oral drugs [108]. DARPins bi53_79 and E2_79 have shown to be promising inhibitors of IgE-mediated MC activation [108]. DARPins are promising candidates for the treatment of allergic diseases as well as CSU but their potential for use in humans should be confirmed [109].

15.3.1.3 Molecules that Target Intracellular Signalling Pathways in Mast Cells

The heightened releasability of mast cells and basophils in patients with urticaria might indicate potential treatment targets at this pathway [49]. Spleen tyrosine kinase (Syk) is a promoter, while Src homology 2 containing inositol phosphatases (SHIP-1 and SHIP-2) are inhibitors of histamine release and cytokine, leukotriene and prostaglandin synthesis [110]. Phosphatidylinositol 3-kinase (PI3K) is not only involved in IgE-dependent MC activation, but is also important for KIT-mediated (and other stimulatory receptor) signals [111]. Syk-inhibitors, SHIP-activators, and PI3K inhibitors can block the release of all mediator types from mast cells and might have implications in treating disorders where mast cells play a role. PI3K inhibitors CAL-101 and CAL-263 have been evaluated for allergic rhinitis [(NCT00836914) and (NCT01066611) and a SHIP-1 activator (AQX-1125) is evaluated for patients with atopic dermatitis (NCT02324972). A Syk inhibitor GSK2646264 is currently being evaluated in a cream formulation in a randomized, double blinded study to assess its safety, tolerability, pharmacodynamics, and pharmacokinetics in healthy controls and patients with cold urticaria or CSU (NCT02424799) [112]. The study was completed in November 2017 but no study results published yet.

15.3.1.4 Other Targets on Mast Cells

The surface inhibitory receptors on mast cells could also be targets of treatment for CSU and allergic disorders. The inhibitory receptors, CD300a, FcγRIIB, and Siglec-8 were shown expressed on mast cells and basophils [113]. AK002 is a humanized non-fucosylated immunoglobulin G1 (IgG1) monoclonal antibody targeting Siglec-8, a member of the CD33-related family of sialic acid-binding, immunoglobulin-like lectins (Siglecs) [114]. A Phase 2a, pilot study is now assessing the efficacy and safety of AK002 (Siglec-8) in subjects with antihistamine-resistant CU (NCT03436797). The drug will be given as monthly intravenous infusions at up to 3 mg/kg for 3 doses. All patients enrolled in the study will receive 6 monthly infusions of AK002 and will then be followed for another 8 weeks.

15.3.2 T Cells

The histopathology of CU wheals is characterized by a perivascular mixed infiltrate composed of predominantly CD4+T lymphocytes similar to allergen-mediated late-phase skin reactions, but the cytokine profile is characterized by an increase in IL-4, IL-5, and interferon-gamma, which is suggestive of a mixed Th1/Th2 response [115–117]. Interventions targeting T cells and T cell cytokines could provide benefit for the treatment of CSU.

15.3.2.1 Abatacept

Abatacept is a fusion protein, which inhibits T cell activation by blocking the specific interaction of CD80/CD86 receptors with CD28 and thereby inhibiting T cell proliferation and B cell immunological response [118]. A pilot study of the safety and efficacy of abatacept in patients with CU (NCT00886795) has been completed and 4 of the 4 participants provided a clinically detectable improvement with none of them reporting serious adverse events.

15.3.2.2 Anti-IL-4/IL-13

The inhibition of the cytokines IL-4 or IL-13 suppresses IgE synthesis. Dupilumab is a fully humanized monoclonal antibody (mAb) which blocks the effects of IL-4 and IL-13 by binding to the common α-chain of the IL-4 receptor and it decreases IgE levels by approximately 40% [119, 120]. Approved by the FDA for the treatment of moderate-to-severe atopic dermatitis in 2017 [121]. Biologicals directed against IL-4Rα receptors are AMG-317, dupilumab, and pitrakinra [122]. Anti-IL-13 mAbs are ABT-308, anrukinzumab, IMA-026, lebrikizumab, CNTO, 5825, GSK679586, QAX576, and tralokinumab [123]. Given the effectivity of these agents in lowering IgE levels and the Th1/Th2 mixed infiltrate shown in wheals, dupilumab targeting IL-4 and IL-13 is now being investigated in a phase 2 clinical trial (NCT03749135) for the treatment of CSU patients who are symptomatic despite H1-antihistamine treatment.

15.3.2.3 Anti-IL-1 Therapies

Different types of urticaria including delayed pressure urticaria and cold urticaria could benefit from IL-1 blocking therapies [124, 125]. The efficacy of canakinumab (human monoclonal antibody that specifically targets IL-1β is now being evaluated in patients with moderate-to-severe CU (URTICANA)) (NCT01635127) while rilonacept (is a soluble decoy receptor, neutralizes either IL-1α or IL-1β) is being investigated for cold contact urticaria (NCT02171416). The latter study has been completed but no results have been posted yet.

15.3.3 B Cells

15.3.3.1 Bruton's Tyrosine Kinase (BTK) Inhibitor GDC-0853

Bruton's tyrosine kinase (BTK) is critically involved in the signalling cascades of B cell antigen receptor (BCR) activation in B cells, some toll-like receptor (TLR) signalling events in B cells, myeloid cells, and dendritic cells as well as Fc receptor binding of immune complexes in myeloid cells [126]. Preclinical studies have indicated that inhibition of BTK activity might offer a potential treatment in autoimmune diseases such as rheumatoid arthritis and systemic lupus erythematosus. GDC-0853 (fenebrutinib) is a small, highly selective, orally administered inhibitor of BTK which is now being evaluated in an ongoing phase IIA, multicenter, randomized, double-blind, placebo-controlled pilot study in patients with refractory CSU (NCT03137069). A long-term safety and efficacy study of fenebrutinib is also running (NCT03693625) in which participants will receive open-label fenebrutinib at a dose of 200 milligram (mg) orally twice a day. Other BTK inhibitors for CSU are in development.

15.3.4 Eosinophils

15.3.4.1 Anti- IL-5 Pathway

The eosinophils role in CU pathophysiology, by means of triggering the tissue factor pathway of coagulation cascade and as a source of vascular endothelial growth factor, was postulated [127]. IL-5 induces the maturation, activation, and recruitment of eosinophils. Successful use of anti-IL-5 inhibitors, mepolizumab and reslizumab has been reported in two patients with CSU [128, 129]. Benralizumab binds to the α-chain of the IL-5 receptor present on both eosinophils and basophils, resulting in depletion of these key inflammatory cells through antibody-dependent cell-mediated cytotoxicity [17]. The efficacy of benralizumab is now being evaluated in a Phase 4 study in CSU patients who are refractory to treatment with H1-antihistamines (NCT03183024). The drug will be given once a month for 3 months and the estimated study completion date will be June 2018. A phase 1 study (NCT03494881) now evaluates the efficacy of 100 mg subcutaneous injections of mepolizumab at week zero, 2, 4, 6, and 8 for a total of 5 doses in CSU patients.

15.3.5 Other Targets that Might have Implications for the Future

As the role of neuroinflammation has been repeatedly reported for CSU [130, 131], therapies that target neuropeptide induced inflammation such as aprepitant, serlopitant, tradipitant, and orvepitant could be future treatment options especially for patients showing stress induced exacerbations [132]. Cellular adhesion molecules such as ICAM-1, ELAM-1, VCAM-1, and P-selectin shows an upregulation in CU and cell adhesion inhibitors such as natalizumab (monoclonal antibody against α-4-integrin) might have a role in the treatment of CSU in the future [133–135]. TSLP is an epithelial-cell-derived cytokine that drives allergic inflammatory responses by acting through the innate immune system and has been shown to be increased in lesional but not non-lesional skin of CSU patients [120, 136]. Drugs such as Tezepelumab (AMG 157) which is a humanized monoclonal antibody that binds TSLP and prevents interaction with its receptor could also be an option to treat CSU patients. C5a receptor blockade of basophils or complement depletion has been shown to reduce the histamine-releasing function of autoantibody-positive sera from CSU patients in vitro [137], this observation might open a new approach like targeting C5 with antibodies such as eculizumab [138]. The discovery of the histamine H4 receptor (H4R) provided a new drug target for the development of novel antihistamines. H4 receptors have been shown to modulate the function of mast cells and basophils, and in experimental models they show some promise in alleviating histamine-evoked itch [139–141]. An H4R antagonist, toreforant has been tested in clinical studies in patients with rheumatoid arthritis, asthma, or psoriasis and it could be a promising target for the future approach in CSU treatment [142]. TNF-α antagonists have been reported to be effective in 60% of 20 CSU patients of a retrospective case series [143], including some omalizumab non-responders, and therefore TNF-α antagonists could be an option in patients not responding to omalizumab and cyclosporine.

As the biologicals market extend, more drugs will be tested in clinical trials and a precision medicine approach will be available in CU patients which will consider the comorbidities and pathomechanisms enrolled in an individual patient.

15.4 Unmet Needs for Chronic Urticaria, Looking Forward

Looking forward in CU implies to improve some unmet needs, as it is, the early identification of such patients that are not medically controlled because the implementation of effective treatments as soon as the CSU or CIndU episodes start is crucial. With this objective a continuous effort in medical education can improve guidelines implementation in daily medical assistance. Active CU networks would help to increase CU knowledge solving global clinical and epidemiologic dilemmas. Phenotype and genotype approach started but genotype expression and its further correlation with CSU phenotypes are still unknown. The identification and validation of reliable biomarkers in CSU would be useful in CU to define the patient's disease status leading to a more individualized and personalized treatment and follow-up. This individual management plan improving symptoms control and quality of life would decrease the burden of CU. Ongoing new therapeutic developments to improve CU management are based on the principle defined by efficacy and safety with the objective to obtain as fast as possible the complete control of symptoms.

References

1. Labrador-Horrillo M, Ferrer M. Profile of omalizumab in the treatment of chronic spontaneous urticaria. Drug Des Devel Ther. 2015;9:4909–15.
2. Zuberbier T, Aberer W, Asero R, Abdul Latiff AH, Baker D, Ballmer-Weber B, Bernstein JA, Bindslev-Jensen C, Brzoza Z, Buense Bedrikow R, Canonica GW, Church MK, Craig T, Danilycheva IV, Dressler C, Ensina LF, Giménez-Arnau A, Godse K, Gonçalo M, Grattan C, Hebert J, Hide M, Kaplan A, Kapp A, Katelaris CH, Kocatürk E, Kulthanan K, Larenas-Linnemann D, Leslie TA, Magerl M, Mathelier-Fusade P, Meshkova RY, Metz M, Nast A, Nettis E, Oude-Elberink H, Rosumeck S, Saini SS, Sánchez-Borges M, Schmid-Grendelmeier P, Staubach P, Sussman G, Toubi E, Vena GA, Vestergaard C, Wedi B, Werner RN, Zhao Z, Maurer M. The EAACI/GA^{2}LEN/EDF/WAO guideline for the definition, classification, diagnosis and management of urticaria. The 2017 revision and update. Allergy. 2018;73(7):1393–414.
3. Maurer M, Rosén K, Hsieh HJ, Saini S, Grattan C, Giménez-Arnau A, et al. Omalizumab for the treatment of chronic idiopathic or spontaneous urticaria. N Engl J Med. 2013;368(10):924–35.
4. Beltrani VS. An overview of chronic urticaria. Clin Rev Allergy Immunol. 2002;23(2):147–69.
5. Bernstein JA, Lang DM, Khan DA, Craig T, Dreyfus D, Hsieh F, et al. The diagnosis and management of acute and chronic urticaria: 2014 update. J Allergy Clin Immunol. 2014;133(5):1.270–7.
6. Lapi F, Cassano N, Pegoraro V, Cataldo N, Heiman F, Cricelli I, et al. Epidemiology of chronic spontaneous urticaria: results from a nationwide, population-based study in Italy. Br J Dermatol. 2016;174(5):996–1.004.
7. Yosipovitch G, Greaves M. Chronic idiopathic urticaria: a "Cinderella" disease with a negative impact on QoL and health care costs. Arch Dermatol. 2008;144(1):102–3.
8. Ferrer M. Epidemiology, healthcare, resources, use and clinical features of different types of urticaria. Alergológica 2005. J Investig Allergol Clin Immunol. 2009;19(Suppl 2):21–6.
9. Maurer M, Abuzakouk M, Bérard F, Canonica W, Oude Elberink H, Giménez-Arnau A, et al. The burden of chronic spontaneous urticaria is substantial: real-world evidence from ASSURE-CSU. Allergy. 2017;72(12):2005–16.

10. Maurer M, Abuzakouk M, Bérard F, Canonica W, Oude Elberink H, Giménez-Arnau A, Grattan C, Hollis K, Knulst A, Lacour JP, Lynde C, Marsland A, McBride D, Nakonechna A, de Frutos JO, Proctor C, Sussman G, Sweeney C, Tian H, Weller K, Wolin D, Balp MM. The burden of chronic spontaneous urticaria is substantial: real-world evidence from ASSURE-CSU. Allergy. 2017;72(12):2005–16. https://doi.org/10.1111/all.13209. Epub 2017 Jul 10.
11. Maurer M, Metz M, Bindslev-Jensen C, Bousquet J, Canonica GW, Church MK, Godse KV, Grattan CE, Hide M, Kocatürk E, Magerl M, Makris M, Meshkova R, Saini SS, Sussman G, Toubi E, Zhao Z, Zuberbier T, Gimenez-Arnau A. Definition, aims, and implementation of GA(2) LEN Urticaria Centers of Reference and Excellence. Allergy. 2016;71(8):1210–8.
12. Giménez-Arnau A, Curto-Barredo L, Nonell L, Puigdecanet E, Yelamos J, Gimeno R, Rüberg S, Santamaria-Babi L, Pujol RM. Transcriptome analysis of severely active chronic spontaneous urticaria shows an overall immunological skin involvement. Allergy. 2017;72(11):1778–90.
13. Metz M, Torene R, Kaiser S, Beste MT, Staubach P, Bauer A, Brehler R, Gericke J, Letzkus M, Hartmann N, Erpenbeck VJ, Maurer M. Omalizumab normalizes the gene expression signature of lesional skin in patients with chronic spontaneous urticaria: a randomized, double-blind, placebo-controlled study. Allergy. 2019;74(1):141–51. https://doi.org/10.1111/all.13547. [Epub ahead of print].
14. Curto-Barredo L, Archilla LR, Vives GR, Pujol RM, Giménez-Arnau AM. Clinical features of chronic spontaneous urticaria that predict disease prognosis and refractoriness to standard treatment. Acta Derm Venereol. 2018;98(7):641–7.
15. Giménez Arnau AM, Valero Santiago A, Bartra Tomás J, Jáuregui Presa I, Labrador-Horrillo M, Miquel Miquel FJ, de Frutos JO, Sastre J, Silvestre Salvador FJ, Ferrer Puga M. Therapeutic strategy according to the differing patient response profiles to omalizumab in chronic spontaneous urticaria. J Investig Allergol Clin Immunol. 2019;29:338–48.
16. Biomarkers Definitions Working Group. Biomarkers and surrogate endpoints: preferred definitions and conceptual framework. Clin Pharmacol Ther. 2001;69:89–95.
17. Casale TB. Biologics and biomarkers for asthma, urticaria, and nasal polyposis. J Allergy Clin Immunol. 2017;139:1411–21.
18. Kasperska-Zajac A, Grzanka A, Misiolek M, Mazur B, Machura E. Pentraxin-3 as a local inflammatory marker in chronic spontaneous urticaria. Cytokine. 2015;76:566–8.
19. Grzanka A, Machura E, Mazur B, et al. Relationship between vitamin D status and the inflammatory state in patients with chronic spontaneous urticaria. J Inflamm (Lond). 2014;11:2.
20. Aleem S, Masood Q, Hassan I. Correlation of C-reactive protein levels with severity of chronic urticaria. Indian J Dermatol. 2014;59:636.
21. Rajappa M, Chandrashekar L, Sundar I, Munisamy M, Ananthanarayanan PH, Thappa DM, et al. Platelet oxidative stress and systemic inflammation in chronic spontaneous urticaria. Clin Chem Lab Med. 2013;51:1789–94.
22. Ucmak D, Akkurt M, Toprak G, Yesilova Y, Turan E, Yıldız I. Determination of dermatology life quality index, and serum C-reactive protein and plasma interleukin-6 levels in patients with chronic urticaria. Postepy Dermatol Alergol. 2013;30:146–51.
23. Kasperska-Zajac A, Grzanka A, Machura E, Misiolek M, Mazur B, Jochem J. Increased serum complement C3 and C4 concentrations and their relation to severity of chronic spontaneous urticaria and CRP concentration. J Inflamm (Lond). 2013;10:22.
24. Tedeschi A, Asero R, Lorini M, Marzano AV, Cugno M. Serum eotaxin levels in patients with chronic spontaneous urticaria. Eur Ann Allergy Clin Immunol. 2012;44:188–92.
25. Takahagi S, Mihara S, Iwamoto K, et al. Coagulation/fibrinolysis and inflammation markers are associated with disease activity in patients with chronic urticaria. Allergy. 2010;65:649–56.
26. Tedeschi A, Asero R, Lorini M, Marzano AV, Cugno M. Plasma levels of matrix metalloproteinase-9 in chronic urticaria patients correlate with disease severity and C-reactive protein but not with circulating histamine-releasing factors. Clin Exp Allergy. 2010;40:875–81.
27. Kasperska-Zajac A, Sztylc J, Machura E, Jop G. Plasma IL-6 concentration correlates with clinical disease activity and serum C-reactive protein concentration in chronic urticaria patients. Clin Exp Allergy. 2011;41:1386–91.

28. Kolkhir P, Pogorelov D, Olisova O. CRP, D-dimer, fibrinogen and ESR as predictive markers of response to standard doses of levocetirizine in patients with chronic spontaneous urticaria. Eur Ann Allergy Clin Immunol. 2017;49:189–92.
29. Rasool R, Ashiq I, Shera IA, Yousuf Q, Shah ZA. Study of serum interleukin (IL) 18 and IL-6 levels in relation with the clinical disease severity in chronic idiopathic urticaria patients of Kashmir (North India). Asia Pac Allergy. 2014;4:206–11.
30. Magen E, Mishal J, Zeldin Y, Feldman V, Kidon M, Schlesinger M, et al. Increased mean platelet volume and C-reactive protein levels in patients with chronic urticaria with a positive autologous serum skin test. Am J Med Sci. 2010;339:504–8.
31. Aleem S, Masood Q, Hassan I. Correlation of mean platelet volume levels with severity of chronic urticaria. J Dermatol Dermatol Surg. 2015;19:9–14.
32. Chandrashekar L, Rajappa M, Sundar I, et al. Platelet activation in chronic urticaria and its correlation with disease severity. Platelets. 2014;25:162–5.
33. Puxeddu I, Pratesi F, Ribatti D, Migliorini P. Mediators of inflammation and angiogenesis in chronic spontaneous urticaria: are they potential biomarkers of the disease? Mediators Inflamm. 2017;2017:4123694.
34. Cugno M, Tedeschi A, Borghi A, et al. Activation of blood coagulation in two prototypic autoimmune skin diseases: a possible link with thrombotic risk. PLoS One. 2015;10:e0129456.
35. Baek YS, Jeon J, Kim JH, Oh CH. Severity of acute and chronic urticaria correlates with D-dimer level, but not C-reactive protein or total IgE. Clin Exp Dermatol. 2014;39:795–800.
36. Asero R, Cugno M, Tedeschi A. Activation of blood coagulation in plasma from chronic urticaria patients with negative autologous plasma skin test. J Eur Acad Dermatol Venereol. 2011;25:201–5.
37. Wang D, Tang H, Shen Y, Wang F, Lin J, Xu J. Activation of the blood coagulation system in patients with chronic spontaneous urticaria. Clin Lab. 2015;61:1283–8.
38. Lu T, Jiao X, Si M, et al. The correlation of serums CCL11, CCL17, CCL26, and CCL27 and disease severity in patients with urticaria. Dis Markers. 2016;2016:1381760.
39. Farres MN, Refaat M, Melek NA, Ahmed EE, Shamseldine MG, Arafa NA. Activation of coagulation in chronic urticaria in relation to disease severity and activity. Allergol Immunopathol (Madr). 2015;43:162–7.
40. Triwongwaranat D, Kulthanan K, Chularojanamontri L, Pinkaew S. Correlation between plasma D-dimer levels and the severity of patients with chronic urticaria. Asia Pac Allergy. 2013;3:100–5.
41. Criado PR, Antinori LCL, Maruta CW, dos Reis VMS. Evaluation of D-dimer serum levels among patients with chronic urticaria, psoriasis and urticarial vasculitis. An Bras Dermatol. 2013;88:355–60.
42. Zhu H, Liang B, Li R, et al. Activation of coagulation, anti-coagulation, fibrinolysis and the complement system in patients with urticaria. Asian Pac J Allergy Immunol. 2013;31:43–50.
43. Takeda T, Sakurai Y, Takahagi S, et al. Increase of coagulation potential in chronic spontaneous urticaria. Allergy. 2011;66:428–33.
44. Asero R, Tedeschi A, Riboldi P, Griffini S, Bonanni E, Cugno M. Severe chronic urticaria is associated with elevated plasma levels of D-dimer. Allergy. 2008;63:176–80.
45. Asero R, Tedeschi A, Coppola R, et al. Activation of the tissue factor pathway of blood coagulation in patients with chronic urticaria. J Allergy Clin Immunol. 2007;119:705–10.
46. Asero R, Tedeschi A, Riboldi P, Cugno M. Plasma of patients with chronic urticaria shows signs of thrombin generation, and its intradermal injection causes wheal-and-flare reactions much more frequently than autologous serum. J Allergy Clin Immunol. 2006;117:1113–7.
47. Rauber MM, Pickert J, Holiangu L, Möbs C, Pfützner W. Functional and phenotypic analysis of basophils allows determining distinct subtypes in patients with chronic urticaria. Allergy. 2017;72:1904–11.
48. Oliver ET, Sterba PM, Saini SS. Interval shifts in basophil measures correlate with disease activity in chronic spontaneous urticaria. Allergy. 2015;70:601–3.
49. Saini SS. Basophil responsiveness in chronic urticaria. Curr Allergy Asthma Rep. 2009;9:286–90.

50. Grattan CEH, Dawn G, Gibbs S, Francis DM. Blood basophil numbers in chronic ordinary urticaria and healthy controls: diurnal variation, influence of loratadine and prednisolone and relationship to disease activity. Clin Exp Allergy. 2003;33:337–41.
51. Baker R, Vasagar K, Ohameje N, Gober L, Chen SC, Sterba PM, et al. Basophil histamine release activity and disease severity in chronic idiopathic urticaria. Ann Allergy Asthma Immunol. 2008;100:244–9.
52. Curto-Barredo L, Yelamos J, Gimeno R, Mojal S, Pujol RM, Giménez-Arnau A. Basophil activation test identifies the patients with chronic spontaneous urticaria suffering the most active disease. Immun Inflamm Dis. 2016;4:441–5.
53. Ye YM, Yang EM, Yoo HS, Shin YS, Kim SH, Park HS. Increased level of basophil CD203c expression predicts severe chronic urticaria. J Korean Med Sci. 2014;29:43–7.
54. Vohra S, Sharma NL, Mahajan VK, Shanker V. Clinicoepidemiologic features of chronic urticaria in patients having positive versus negative autologous serum skin test: a study of 100 Indian patients. Indian J Dermatol Venereol Leprol. 2011;77:156–9.
55. George M, Balachandran C, Prabhu S. Chronic idiopathic urticaria: comparison of clinical features with positive autologous serum skin test. Indian J Dermatol Venereol Leprol. 2008;74:105–8.
56. Caproni M, Volpi W, Giomi B, Cardinali C, Antiga E, Melani L, et al. Chronic idiopathic and chronic autoimmune urticaria: clinical and immunopathological features of 68 subjects. Acta Derm Venereol. 2004;84:288–90.
57. Alyasin S, Hamidi M, Karimi AA, Amiri A, Ghaffarpasand F, Ehsaei MJ. Correlation between clinical findings and results of autologous serum skin test in patients with chronic idiopathic urticaria. South Med J. 2011;104:111–5.
58. Asero R. D-dimer: a biomarker for antihistamine-resistant chronic urticaria. J Allergy Clin Immunol. 2013;132:983–6.
59. Huilan Z, Bihua L, Runxiang L, Jiayan L, Luyang L, Zhenjie L. Features of antihistamine-resistant chronic urticaria and chronic urticaria during exacerbation. Indian J Dermatol. 2015;60:323.
60. Asero R. Plasma D-dimer levels and clinical response to ciclosporin in severe chronic spontaneous urticaria. J Allergy Clin Immunol. 2015;135:1401–3.
61. Grattan CE, O'Donnell BF, Francis DM, Niimi N, Barlow RJ, Seed PT, et al. Randomized double-blind study of cyclosporin in chronic "idiopathic" urticaria. Br J Dermatol. 2000;143:365–72.
62. Iqbal K, Bhargava K, Skov PS, Falkencrone S, Grattan CE. A positive serum basophil histamine release assay is a marker for ciclosporin-responsiveness in patients with chronic spontaneous urticaria. Clin Transl Allergy. 2012;2:19.
63. Altrichter S, Hawro T, Hänel K, Czaja K, Lüscher B, Maurer M, et al. Successful omalizumab treatment in chronic spontaneous urticaria is associated with lowering of serum IL-31 levels. J Eur Acad Dermatol Venereol. 2016;30:454–5.
64. Deza G, Bertolín-Colilla M, Pujol RM, Curto-Barredo L, Soto D, García M, et al. Basophil FcεRI expression in chronic spontaneous urticaria: a potential immunological predictor of response to omalizumab therapy. Acta Derm Venereol. 2017;97:698–704.
65. Deza G, Bertolín-Colilla M, Sánchez S, Soto D, Pujol RM, Gimeno R, Giménez-Arnau AM. Basophil FcεRI expression is linked to time to omalizumab response in chronic spontaneous urticaria. J Allergy Clin Immunol. 2018;141(6):2313–6.
66. Ertas R, Ozyurt K, Atasoy M, Hawro T, Maurer M. The clinical response to omalizumab in CSU patients is linked to and predicted by IgE levels and their change. Allergy. 2018;73(3):705–12. https://doi.org/10.1111/all.13345. [Epub ahead of print].
67. Palacios T, Stillman L, Borish L, Lawrence M. Lack of basophil CD203c-upregulating activity as an immunological marker to predict response to treatment with omalizumab in patients with symptomatic chronic urticaria. J Allergy Clin Immunol Pract. 2016;4:529–30.
68. Gericke J, Metz M, Ohanyan T, Weller K, Altrichter S, Skov PS, et al. Serum autoreactivity predicts time to response to omalizumab therapy in chronic spontaneous urticaria. J Allergy Clin Immunol. 2017;139:1059–61.e1.

69. Ertas R, Ozyurt K, Ozlu E, Ulas Y, Avci A, Atasoy M, et al. Increased IgE levels are linked to faster relapse in patients with omalizumab-discontinued chronic spontaneous urticaria. J Allergy Clin Immunol. 2017;140:1749–51.
70. Gangemi S, Saitta S, Lombardo G, Patafi M, Benvenga S. Serum thyroid autoantibodies in patients with idiopathic either acute or chronic urticaria. J Endocrinol Invest. 2009;32:107–10.
71. Woo YR, Jung KE, Koo DW, Lee JS. Vitamin D as a marker for disease severity in chronic urticaria and its possible role in pathogenesis. Ann Dermatol. 2015;27:423–30.
72. Rasool R, Masoodi KZ, Shera IA, Yosuf Q, Bhat IA, Qasim I, et al. Chronic urticaria merits serum vitamin D evaluation and supplementation; a randomized case control study. World Allergy Organ J. 2015;8:15.
73. Kessel A, Helou W, Bamberger E, Sabo E, Nusem D, Panassof J, et al. Elevated serum total IgE—a potential marker for severe chronic urticaria. Int Arch Allergy Immunol. 2010;153:288–93.
74. Netchiporouk E, Sasseville D, Moreau L, Habel Y, Rahme E, Ben-Shoshan M. Evaluating comorbidities, natural history, and predictors of early resolution in a cohort of children with chronic urticaria. JAMA Dermatol. 2017;153:1236–42.
75. Maurer M, Church MK, Weller K. Chronic urticaria in children: still itching for insight. JAMA Dermatol. 2017;153:1221–2.
76. Chansakulporn S, Pongpreuksa S, Sangacharoenkit P, Pacharn P, Visitsunthorn N, Vichyanond P, et al. The natural history of chronic urticaria in childhood: a prospective study. J Am Acad Dermatol. 2014;71:663–8.
77. Sahiner UM, Civelek E, Tuncer A, Yavuz ST, Karabulut E, Sackesen C, et al. Chronic urticaria: etiology and natural course in children. Int Arch Allergy Immunol. 2011;156:224–30.
78. Champion RH, Roberts SO, Carpenter RG, Roger JH. Urticaria and angio-oedema. A review of 554 patients. Br J Dermatol. 1969;81:588–97.
79. Juhlin L. Recurrent urticaria: clinical investigation of 330 patients. Br J Dermatol. 1981;104:369–81.
80. Kozel MM, Mekkes JR, Bossuyt PM, Bos JD. Natural course of physical and chronic urticaria and angioedema in 220 patients. J Am Acad Dermatol. 2001;45:387–91.
81. Hiragun M, Hiragun T, Mihara S, Akita T, Tanaka J, Hide M. Prognosis of chronic spontaneous urticaria in 117 patients not controlled by a standard dose of antihistamine. Allergy. 2013;68:229–35.
82. Lee HC, Hong JB, Chu CY. Chronic idiopathic urticaria in Taiwan: a clinical study of demographics, aggravating factors, laboratory findings, serum autoreactivity and treatment response. J Formos Med Assoc. 2011;110:175–82.
83. Nebiolo F, Bergia R, Bommarito L, Bugiani M, Heffler E, Carosso A, et al. Effect of arterial hypertension on chronic urticaria duration. Ann Allergy Asthma Immunol. 2009;103:407–10.
84. Sánchez-Borges M, Caballero-Fonseca F, Capriles-Hulett A, González-Aveledo L. Aspirin-exacerbated cutaneous disease (AECD) is a distinct subphenotype of chronic spontaneous urticaria. J Eur Acad Dermatol Venereol. 2015;29:698–701.
85. Kim JH, Lee HY, Ban GY, Shin YS, Park HS, Ye YM. Serum clusterin as a prognostic marker of chronic spontaneous urticaria. Medicine (Baltimore). 2016;95:e3688.
86. Guo A, Zhu W, Zhang C, Wen S, Chen X, Chen M, et al. Association of FCER1A genetic polymorphisms with risk for chronic spontaneous urticaria and efficacy of nonsedating H1-antihistamines in Chinese patients. Arch Dermatol Res. 2015;307:183–90.
87. Lin CE, Kaptein JS, Sheikh J. Differential expression of microRNAs and their possible roles in patients with chronic idiopathic urticaria and active hives. Allergy Rhinol (Providence). 2017;8:67–80.
88. Kaplan A, Ledford D, Ashby M, et al. Omalizumab in patients with symptomatic chronic idiopathic/spontaneous urticaria despite standard combination therapy. J Allergy Clin Immunol. 2013;132:101–9.
89. Saini SS, Bindslev-Jensen C, Maurer M, et al. Efficacy and safety of omalizumab in patients with chronic idiopathic/spontaneous urticaria who remain symptomatic on H1-antihistamines: a randomized, placebo-controlled study. J Invest Dermatol. 2015 Mar;135(3):925.

90. Vadasz Z, Tal Y, Rotem M, et al. Omalizumab for severe chronic spontaneous urticaria: real-life experiences of 280 patients. J Allergy Clin Immunol Pract. 2017;5(6):1743–5.
91. Sussman G, Hebert J, Barron C, et al. Real-life experiences with omalizumab for the treatment of chronic urticaria. Ann Allergy Asthma Immunol. 2014;112:170–4.
92. Metz M, Ohanyan T, Church MK, Maurer M. Omalizumab is an effective and rapidly acting therapy in difficult-to-treat chronic urticaria: a retrospective clinical analysis. J Dermatol Sci. 2014 Jan;73(1):57–62. https://doi.org/10.1016/j.jdermsci.2013.08.011.
93. Ghazanfar MN, Sand C, Thomsen SF. Effectiveness and safety of omalizumab in chronic spontaneous or inducible urticaria: evaluation of 154 patients. Br J Dermatol. 2016;175(2):404–6.
94. Bernstein JA, Kavati A, Tharp MD, Ortiz B, MacDonald K, Denhaerynck K, Abraham I. Effectiveness of omalizumab in adolescent and adult patients with chronic idiopathic/spontaneous urticaria: a systematic review of 'real-world' evidence. Expert Opin Biol Ther. 2018;18(4):425–48.
95. Kolkhir P, Church MK, Weller K, Metz M, Schmetzer O, Maurer M. Autoimmune chronic spontaneous urticaria: what we know and what we do not know. J Allergy Clin Immunol. 2017;139:1772–81.
96. Grattan C. Autoimmune chronic spontaneous urticaria. J Allergy Clin Immunol. 2018;141:1165–6.
97. Arm JP, Bottoli I, Skerjanec A, et al. Pharmacokinetics, pharmacodynamics and safety of QGE031 (ligelizumab), a novel high-affinity anti-IgE antibody, in atopic subjects. Clin Exp Allergy. 2014;44(11):1371–85.
98. Maurer M, Gimenez Arnau A, Sussman G, et al. Ligelizumab achieves rapid onset of action, improved and sustained efficacy compared with omalizumab in patients with chronic spontaneous urticaria not adequately controlled by H1-antihistamines. Poster presented at 27th EADV Congress, 12–16 September 2018, Paris, France.
99. http://www.unitedbiopharma.com/UB-221.php.
100. Hu J, Chen J, Ye L, Cai Z, Sun J, Ji K. Anti-IgE therapy for IgE-mediated allergic diseases: from neutralizing IgE antibodies to eliminating IgE+ B cells. Clin Transl Allergy. 2018;8:27.
101. Navinés-Ferrer A, Serrano-Candelas E, Molina-Molina GJ, Martín M. IgE-related chronic diseases and anti-IgE-based treatments. J Immunol Res. 2016;2016:8163803. https://doi.org/10.1155/2016/8163803. Very good review on anti-IgE treatments.
102. Pennington LF, Tarchevskaya S, Brigger D, et al. Structural basis of omalizumab therapy and omalizumab-mediated IgE exchange. Nat Commun. 2016;7:11610.
103. Nyborg AC, Zacco A, Ettinger R. Development of an antibody that neutralizes soluble IgE and eliminates IgE expressing B cells. Cell Mol Immunol. 2016;13:391–400.
104. Lupinek C, Roux KH, Lafer S, Rauter I, Reginald K, Kneidinger M, et al. Trimolecular complex formation of IgE, Fc epsilon RI, and a recombinant nonanaphylactic single-chain antibody fragment with high affinity for IgE. J Immunol. 2009;182:4817–29.
105. Peng X, Wang J, Li X, Lin L, Xie G, Cui Z, et al. Targeting mast cells and basophils with anti-FcεRIα Fab-conjugated celastrol-loaded micelles suppresses allergic inflammation. J Biomed Nanotechnol. 2015;11:2286–99.
106. Kirak ORG. A novel, nonanaphylactogenic, bispecifc IgE-CD3 antibody eliminates IgE(+) B cells. J Allergy Clin Immunol. 2015;136(3):800–2.
107. Chu SY, Horton HM, Pong E, Leung IW, Chen H, Nguyen DH, et al. Reduction of total IgE by targeted coengagement of IgE B-cell receptor and Fc gamma RIIb with Fc-engineered antibody. J Allergy Clin Immunol. 2012;129:1102–15.
108. Kim B, Eggel A, Tarchevskaya SS, Vogel M, Prinz H, et al. Accelerated disassembly of IgE receptor complexes by a disruptive macromolecular inhibitor. Nature. 2012;491:613–7.
109. Kocatürk E. Role of biologics and future perspectives in the treatment of urticaria. Curr Treat Options Allergy. 2017;4:428.
110. Altman K, Chang C. Pathogenic intracellular and autoimmune mechanisms in urticaria and angioedema. Clin Rev Allergy Immunol. 2013;45:47–62.
111. Siebenhaar F, Redegeld FA, Bischoff SC, et al. Mast cells as drivers of disease and therapeutic targets. Trends Immunol. 2018 Feb;39(2):151–62.

112. https://adisinsight.springer.com/drugs/800042342.
113. Harvima IT, Levi-Schaffer F, Draber P, et al. Molecular targets on mast cells and basophils for novel therapies. J Allergy Clin Immunol. 2014;134(3):530–44.
114. https://adisinsight.springer.com/drugs/800045646.
115. Elias J, Boss E, Kaplan AP. Studies of the cellular infiltrate of chronic idiopathic urticaria: prominence of T lymphocytes, monocytes and mast cells. J Allergy Clin Immunol. 1986;78(5):914–8.
116. Caproni M, Giomi B, Volpi W, Melani L, Schincaglia E, Macchia D, Manfredi M, D'Agata A, Fabbri P. Chronic idiopathic urticaria: infiltrating cells and related cytokines in autologous serum-induced weals. Clin Immunol. 2005;114:284–92.
117. Smith CH, Kepley C, Schwartz LB, Lee TH. Mast cell number and phenotype in chronic idiopathic urticaria. J Allergy Clin Immunol. 1995;96:360–4.
118. Herrero-Beaumont G, Martínez Calatrava MJ, Castañeda S. Abatacept mechanism of action: concordance with its clinical profile. Reumatol Clin. 2012;8(2):78–83.
119. Wenzel S, Ford L, Pearlman D, et al. Dupilumab in persistent asthma with elevated eosinophil levels. N Engl J Med. 2013;368:2455–66.
120. Manka LA, Wechsler ME. New biologics for allergic diseases. Expert Rev Clin Immunol. 2018;14(4):285–96.
121. Shirley M. Dupilumab first global approval. Drugs. 2017;77:1115–21.
122. Boyman O, Kaegi C, Akdis M, et al. EAACI IG biologicals task force paper on the use of biologic agents in allergic disorders. Allergy. 2015;70(7):727–54.
123. Kocatürk E, Zuberbier T. New biologics in the treatment of urticaria. Curr Opin Allergy Clin Immunol. 2018;18(5):425–31.
124. Lenormand C, Lipsker D. Efficiency of interleukin-1 blockade in refractory delayed pressure urticaria. Ann Intern Med. 2012;157(8):599–600.
125. Bodar EJ, Simon A, de Visser M, van der Meer JW. Complete remission of severe idiopathic cold urticaria on interleukin-1 receptor antagonist (anakinra). Neth J Med. 2009;67(9):302–5.
126. Herman AE, Chinn LW, Kotwal SG, et al. Safety, pharmacokinetics, and pharmacodynamics in healthy volunteers treated with GDC-0853, a selective reversible Bruton's tyrosine kinase inhibitor. Clin Pharmacol Ther. 2018;103(6):1020–8.
127. Asero R, Cugno M, Tedeschi A. Eosinophils in chronic urticaria: supporting or leading actors? World Allergy Organ J. 2009;2(9):213–7.
128. Magerl M, Terhorst D, Metz M, Altrichter S, Zuberbier T, Maurer M, Bergmann KC. Benefit from mepolizumab treatment in a patient with chronic spontaneous urticaria. J Dtsch Dermatol Ges. 2018;16(4):477–8.
129. Maurer M, Altrichter S, Metz M, et al. Benefit from reslizumab treatment in a patient with chronic spontaneous urticaria and cold urticaria. J Eur Acad Dermatol Venereol. 2018;32(3):e112–3.
130. Metz M, Krull C, Hawro T, Saluja R, Groffik A, Stanger C, Staubach P, Maurer M. Substance P is upregulated in the serum of patients with chronic spontaneous urticaria. J Invest Dermatol. 2014;134(11):2833–6.
131. Başak PY, Vural H, Kazanoglu OO, Erturan I, Buyukbayram HI. Effects of loratadine and cetirizine on serum levels of neuropeptides in patients with chronic urticaria. Int J Dermatol. 2014;53(12):1526–30.
132. Kocatürk E, Maurer M, Metz M, Grattan C. Looking forward to new targeted treatments for chronic spontaneous urticaria. Clin Transl Allergy. 2017;7:1.
133. Haas N, Hermes B, Henz BM. Adhesion molecules and cellular infiltrate: histology of urticaria. J Investig Dermatol Symp Proc. 2001;6:137–8.
134. Zuberbier T, Schadendorf D, Haas N, et al. Enhanced P-selectin expression in chronic and dermographic urticaria. Int Arch Allergy Immunol. 1997;114:86–9.
135. Barlow RJ, Ross EL, Macdonald D, Kobza Black A, Greaves MW. Adhesion molecule expression and the inflmmatory cell infiltrate in delayed pressure urticaria. Br J Dermatol. 1994;131:341–7.

136. Kay AB, Clark P, Maurer M, Ying S. Elevations in T-helper-2-initiating cytokines (interleukin-33, interleukin-25 and thymic stromal lymphopoietin) in lesional skin from chronic spontaneous ("idiopathic") urticaria. Br J Dermatol. 2015;172:1294–302.
137. Fiebiger E, Hammerschmid F, Stingl G, Maurer D. Anti-FcεRIα autoantibodies in autoimmune-mediated disorders: identification of a structure-function relationship. J Clin Invest. 1998;101(1):243–51.
138. Horiuchi T, Tsukamoto H. Complement-targeted therapy: development of C5- and C5a-targeted inhibition. Inflammation and Regeneration. 2016;36:11.
139. Hofstra CL, Desai PJ, Thurmond RL, Fung-Leung WP. Histamine H4 receptor mediates chemotaxis and calcium mobilization of mast cells. J Pharmacol Exp Ther. 2003;305:1212–21.
140. Thurmond RL, Desai PJ, Dunford PJ, Fung-Leung WP, Hofstra CL, Jiang W, et al. A potent and selective histamine H4 receptor antagonist with antiinflammatory properties. J Pharmacol Exp Ther. 2004;309:404–13.
141. Shiraishi Y, Jia Y, Domenico J, Joetham A, Karasuyama H, Takeda K, et al. Sequential engagement of FcεRI on mast cells and basophil histamine H(4) receptor and FcεRI in allergic rhinitis. J Immunol. 2013;190:539–48.
142. Thurmond RL, Venable J, Savall B, La D, Snook S, Dunford PJ, Edwards JP. Clinical development of histamine H4 receptor antagonists. Handb Exp Pharmacol. 2017;241:301–20.
143. Sand FL, Thomsen SF. TNF-alpha inhibitors for chronic urticaria: experience in 20 patients. J Allergy (Cairo). 2013;2013:130905.

Index

A
Abatacept, 236
Acute urticaria
  aetiology, 59, 60
  clinical aspects, 58
  definition, 57
  diagnosis, 61
  EAACI anaphylaxis guideline, 57
  epidemiology, 58
  natural course, 61
  treatment, 61, 62
  upper respiratory infections, 60
Anabolic steroids, 192
Anakinra, 196
Anaphylaxis, 208
Angioedema (AE), 28, 30, 31
  bradykinin mediated AE, 135, 139, 140
    clinical description, 139, 140
    with C1Inh deficiency, 140–142
    with normal C1Inh, 142, 143
    pathophysiology, 140
  Gleich syndrome, 136
  isolated angioedema, 137
  kallikrein-kinin pathway, 135
  mast cell AE, 135, 137–139
  prevalence, 135
  pseudo angioedema, 135
  Schnitzler syndrome, 136
  in subcutaneous/submucosal tissues, 134
  vascular permeability, 134
Angioedema activity score (AAS), 35
Angioedema control test (AECT), 47, 50, 73, 172
Angio-oedemas, 65
Angiotensin converting enzyme (ACE), 16
Anisakis simplex, 34, 91
Anticoagulants
  heparin, 195
  warfarin, 195
Antihistamines, 5–6
  and cardiotoxicity, 158, 159
  and central nervous system, 155–158
  clinical usage, 161
  duration of action, 160
  efficacy, 161
  H_1-antihistamines, 153
  histamine H_1-receptor, 154
  hymoxyethyldiethylamine, 154
  laboratory methods, 153
  onset of action, 159
  in urticaria, 159
Anti-IgE-treatment, 34
Anti-inflammatory sulphones
  dapsone, 178, 179
  sulphasalazine, 179, 180
Antineutrophilic drugs
  anakinra, 196
  colchicine, 195
Aquagenic urticaria (AqU), 124, 125
Aspirin-induced urticaria, 13
Assessment of disease activity, 30
Auto-allergic CSU (aaCSU), 17
Autoimmune CSU (aiCSU), 17
Autologous serum skin test (ASST), 17, 18, 34, 72
Azathioprine, 188–190

B
Basophil activation assays, 19
Basophil activation test (BAT), 17, 34, 70, 216
Basophil histamine release assay (BHRA), 19, 70
Basophil tests (BTs), 72
Basophils, 15
B-cell activation, 15
Biological drugs, 196
Blastocystis hominis, 70, 90, 91

Bradykinin, 15
Bradykinin mediated AE (BK-AE), 135
  clinical description, 139, 140
  with C1Inh deficiency, 140–142
  with normal C1Inh, 142, 143
  pathophysiology, 140
Bruton kinase (BTK) inhibitor, 237

C

Candida albicans, 93
Causative factors, 150
CD40L expression, 15
"Centers of reference and excellence in urticaria" (UCAREs), 228
Cholinergic urticaria (CholU), 13, 120–122, 212
Cholinergic Urticaria Activity Score (CholUAS), 50
Chronic "idiopathic" urticaria (CIU), 3, 4, 29
Chronic inducible urticaria (CIndU), 40, 43, 78, 79, 228
  classification of, 110
  diagnosis of, 109
  HRQoL, 46
  nonphysical urticaria, 109
  physical urticaria, 109
  prevalence of, 109
  PROMs, 50, 51
Chronic spontaneous urticaria (CSU), 10, 109
  allergic diseases, 94, 95
  angio-oedema, 65, 66
  autoallergy and autoimmunity, 68–70
  autoimmune diseases, 88, 89
  bacterial infection, 89, 90
  B cells, 237
  biomarkers, 230–233
  cellular adhesion molecules, 238
  chronic itch, sleep impairment, and psychiatric comorbidity, 43
  classification, 67
  comorbid diseases, 78, 80–86
  comorbidities, 77, 78
  definition, 65
  diagnosis, 71–73
  eosinophils, 237
  epidemiology, 67
  etiopathogenesis, 67–71
  fungal infection, 92, 93
  genetic profile, 228
  HRQoL, 44, 45
  impairment of daily activities and work productivity, 43
  itch, sleep impairment, and psychiatric comorbidities, 42, 43
  malignant diseases, 95, 96
  management, 229
  mast cells/basophils
    anti-IgEs, 234, 235
    surface inhibitory receptors, 236
    target intracellular signalling pathways, 235
  mast cell degranulation, 68
  mental disorders, 87
  metabolic syndrome, 97, 98
  parasitic infection, 90–92
  patient-reported outcome measures, 48
  physical, social, and emotional burden, 40, 42
  PROMs, 46, 47, 49, 50
  receptor ligand interactions, 68, 69
  signs and symptoms, 65, 66
  stress, infections and food intolerance, modulators, 70, 71
  quality of life, 228
  symptoms, 228
  T cells, 236, 237
  therapy, 73, 74
  TSLP, 238
  viral infection, 92
  weals, 65, 66
Chronic urticaria (CU), 10, 219, 220
Chronic urticaria patient perspective (CUPP), 49
Chronic urticaria quality of life questionnaire (CU-Q2oL), 49
Ciclosporin, 171, 184, 185
Classification of urticaria, 30
Colchicine, 195
Cold urticaria, 13, 112–113, 212
Connective tissue mast cell, 13
Contact urticaria, 122, 123
Corticosteroids (steroids), 193–195
Cryopyrin-associated periodic syndrome (CAPS), 213
Cutaneous mastocytosis (CM), 214
Cyclophosphamide, 196
Cysteinyl leukotrienes (LT), 13

D

Danazol, 192–193
Dapsone, 178, 179
Delayed pressure urticaria (DPU), 13, 28, 114–115
Dermatographism, 211
Dermatology life quality index (DLQI), 45
Dermographic urticaria, *see* Symptomatic dermographism (SD)
Desensitisation protocols, 202

Index

Diagnosis
    ASST, 34
    baseline assessment, 31
    basophil activation tests, 34
    patient physical examination, 32
    patient's history, 32
    recommended diagnostic tests, 33
    UAS7, 34
Dientamoeba fragilis, 91
Diet
    dietary salicylates and food additives, 198
    low histamine diet, 199
    low pseudoallergen diet, 198–199
    pseudoallergen-free diet, 197
Doxepin, 190, 191

E
2018 EAACI/ GA²LEN/EDF/WAO guidelines, 177
Enterobius vermicularis, 90
Eosinophils, 14
Epinephrine, 191, 192

F
Filaria medinensis, 90
Focal bacterial infections, 89
FricTest®, 111

G
G protein–coupled receptors (GPCRs), 71
Gleich syndrome, 136

H
Hageman factor XII, 16
H_1-antihistamines, 153, 170, 177
H_2 antihistamines, 183
Health-related quality of life (HRQoL), 44–46
Heat urticaria (HeatU), 13, 118
Helicobacter pylori-gastritis, 71
Helicobacter pylori (HP) infection, 29, 70, 89
Heparin, 195
Histamine, 13
Histamine H_1-receptor, 154
Histamine H4 receptor (H4R), 238
Histamine-induced wheals, 31
Histopathology, 11–12
24-h self-evaluation scores, 31
Hydroxychloroquine, 197
Hymoxyethyldiethylamine, 154

I
IgE-mediated food allergy, 197
Immunoglobulin E, 11
Immunomodulators
    hydroxychloroquine, 197
    intravenous immunoglobulins, 197
    plasmapheresis, 197
    vitamin D, 197
Immunsuppressives, 196
    azathioprine, 188–190
    ciclosporin, 184, 185
    methotrexate, 185–187
    mycophenolate mofetil, 187, 188
Inducible urticarias, 210
Intestinal candidosis, 71
Isolated angioedema, 138, 216

K
Kallikrein-kininogen-kinin system, 15

L
Ligelizumab, 173
Low histamine diet, 199

M
Major basic protein (MBP), 18
Malassezia furfur infection, 93
Management principles
    drugs, 150
    food intolerance, 150
    lifestyle adjustments, 151
    pharmacological treatment, 151, 152
    physical stimuli, 150
    shared-decision-making concept, 149
    tolerance induction protocols, 151
Mast cell degranulation, 12, 68
Mast cell density, 12
Mastocytosis, 214
Mechanism of whealing, 12
Methotrexate, 185–187
Montelukast, 181, 182
Mycophenolate mofetil, 187–188

N
Neuropeptide-induced degranulation, 18
Neutrophilic urticaria, 12
Neutrophilic urticarial dermatoses (NUD)
    biopsies, 12

O

Occasional acute allergic urticaria, 10
Omalizumab, 17, 18, 34, 74, 177
    adverse effects, 169
    ASTERIA study, 169, 170
    bioavailability, metabolism, and elimination, 168
    EAACI and AAAAI Guidelines, 174
    GLACIAL study, 169, 170
    home therapy, 173
    indications, 167, 168
    in local and international guidelines, 174, 175
    mechanisms of action, 168
    MYSTIQUE study, 169
    in pregnancy and breast feeding, 173
    randomized controlled clinical trials, 170, 171
    real life studies, 171
    X-ACT study, 170
    X-CUISITE study, 169, 172
    X-TEND study, 170

P

Pediatric chronic urticaria (CU)
    allergic triggers, 208
    burden, 209
    causes of, 208, 212, 213
    classification, 210, 211
    clinical presentation, 209, 210
    diagnosis, 208
    diagnostic approach, 216
    differential diagnosis, 208–209, 213–216
    drug management, 217, 218
    natural history, 216
    pathogenesis, 217
    second generation antihistamines, 208
    viral infections, 208
Peripheral blood eosinophilia, 91
Phototherapy and photochemotherapy, 200, 201
Plasmapheresis, 197
Platelet activating factor (PAF), 14
Polymorphonuclear neutrophils, 15
Pseudo angioedema, 135
Psychological therapies, 201

R

Rituximab, 196

S

Saccharomyces cerevisiae, 94
Sarcocystis, 91
Schnitzler syndrome, 136
Serum sickness-like reaction (SSLR), 208
Sinusitis, 89
Skindex, 49
Solar urticaria, 13, 116–118
Spontaneous angioedema, 27
Spontaneous MC-AE, 138
Staphylococcus aureus, 90
Streptococcus spp. infection, 90
Strongyloides stercoralis, 91
Sulphasalazine, 179, 180
Superficial wheals, 10
Symptomatic dermographism (SD), 110, 111

T

Tacrolimus, 196
TempTest®, 113, 118
Tezepelumab, 238
Thiopurine methyl transferase (TPMT), 189
Toxocara canis infection, 90
Toxocara canis seropositivity, 91
Tranexamic acid, 180, 181
Trichophyton antigens, 93

U

Unified scoring systems, 29
Union of medical specialists (UEMS), 228
Urticaria
    cellular and molecular basis, 2–3
    chronic "idiopathic" urticaria, 3, 4
    history of, 2
    treatment, 5
Urticaria activity score (UAS), 73
Urticaria activity score 7 (UAS7), 31, 229
Urticaria control trest (UCT), 35, 47, 172
Urticaria factitia, *see* Symptomatic dermographism (SD)
Urticaria pigmentosa (UP), 29, 214
Urticaria vasculitis, 11, 214

V

Vibratory angioedema (VA), 119
Vitamin D deficiency, 197

Index

W
Warfarin, 195
Wheals
   annular wheals, 27
   characteristics, 28
   histamine-induced wheals, 31
   spontaneous wheals, 28
   superficial wheals, 27

X
Xolair pregnancy registry, 219

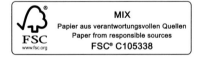

Printed by Books on Demand, Germany